DR RICHARD H
and
DR JANE FOLEY

Self-health

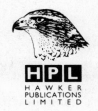

HPL
HAWKER
PUBLICATIONS
LIMITED

Hawker Publications Limited
13 Park House,
140 Battersea Park Road,
London SW11 4NB

Copyright © Dr Richard Hawkins and
Dr Jane Foley 1992

The Author asserts the moral right to
be identified as the author of this work

A CIP catalogue record for this book
is available from the British Library

ISBN 0-9514649-8-1

Printed by Redwood Press, Melksham, Wiltshire

Set in Melior

All rights reserved. No part of this publication may be
reproduced, stored in a retrieval system, or transmitted,
in any form, or by any means, electronic, mechanical,
photocopying, recording or otherwise, without the prior
permission of the publishers.

This book is sold subject to the condition that it shall not,
by way of trade or otherwise, be lent, re-sold, hired out or
otherwise circulated without the publisher's prior consent
in any form of binding or cover other than that in which it
is published and without a similar condition including this
condition being imposed on the subsequent purchaser.

Contents

Dedicated with the greatest affection to Rory, Lois and Kit.

Preface

The human body and mind are amazing. They can recover and heal themselves from injuries and diseases which would have immediately put computers or robots on to the scrapheap!

However, they do need help. So the purpose of this book is to provide practical information on how you can look after yourself and reduce your chances of developing illnesses. It also provides down-to-earth advice on coping with conditions as different as anaemia, food poisoning or jet lag, and on when you should seek professional help.

As doctors we have certainly found that our training and daily experience helped with the writing of this book. But we know that health cannot be isolated from the rest of life, so we have also written it as members of a community, as husband and wife, as parents, as people who have experienced emotions ranging from loneliness and tiredness to love and happiness and recognize how important these feelings are to total well-being.

We have a positive message: that each of us can make a real contribution to our own and other people's health and happiness. We hope *Self-health* can play a part in helping you make that contribution.

We would like to thank the very many people, including friends, relatives and patients, who have helped with this book.

R. L. H.
J. A. F.
London 1992

Dr Jane Foley has had wide medical experience. She is now a consultant in London, specializing in treating people with arthritis and rehabilitating those who have serious illnesses or injuries. These are often long-term conditions so she has developed special skills in discussing medical problems with patients.

Dr Richard Hawkins is a surgeon in London. He has a special interest in writing about medical matters for the public, including editing the patients' magazine *Good Health*.

Dr Foley and Dr Hawkins are married to each other and have three children – an experience which they believe teaches them as much as their medical experience!

1 Healthy Eating

BY DR RICHARD HAWKINS

Eating is fun. It should also help you to look good, feel great and enjoy a fit and healthy life. To give yourself the best chance of enjoying the benefits of a healthy diet it is worth knowing about the composition of food, which is made up of different proportions of carbohydrates (including fibre), fat, protein, vitamins and minerals. Then you can decide for yourself how to eat the balanced diet that is the secret of healthy eating.

CARBOHYDRATE

The sugar and starch in food is known as carbohydrate. Some people think of carbohydrate as just a constituent of prepared foods such as cakes, biscuits, sweets and jam. But sugar and starch are found in many fresh foods too. For example, there are natural sugars in milk and fruit, and starch is present in cereals, potatoes, rice, flour, pulses and some root vegetables. In this form it is known as complex carbohydrate. It is important to choose carbohydrate foods that contain a range of nutrients, and complex carbohydrates do just that. Fruit and starchy foods, especially wholemeal varieties, are highly nutritious, containing vitamins, minerals and fibre as well as carbohydrate.

At one time, carbohydrate-rich foods were regarded as the baddies in our diet, and slimmers were advised to cut out starchy foods as well as sweet ones. Now we know that most of our daily energy intake should be in the form of starchy carbohydrate foods.

Both starches and sugars are digested in the body and converted to the simplest forms of sugar, such as glucose, before being absorbed into the bloodstream and carried to the body's cells to provide energy. This energy is needed for growth, body maintenance and all our daily activities, so a balanced diet should include plenty of carbohydrate foods each day. However, certain types should be restricted. Sweets, syrups, many cakes and biscuits, and other sugary foods are high in calories and low in nutritional value. What's more, they are not very filling, and this makes it easy to consume too many calories which can lead to overweight. The same applies to sugary and alcoholic drinks. Drinking alcohol is an easy way to take in too many calories.

There is no harm in the odd sweet treat, but do try to cut down on bought cakes and biscuits and reduce the sugar you add to drinks and use in cooking. Try using fruit, with its extra nutrients, instead of sugar to sweeten cakes and puddings.

Fibre content of every day foods

	Serving size	Fibre content grams		Serving size	Fibre content grams
BREAD			Wheat biscuits	38g	3.7
Wholemeal	25g	1.5	Kellogg's Fruit 'N Fibre	30g	2.1
Brown	25g	0.9			
White	25g	0.4	**BISCUITS & PASTRY**		
			Crispbread – rye	25g	2.9
FLOUR			Digestive	12g	0.3
Wholemeal	25g	2.3	Gingernuts	12g	0.2
Brown flour	25g	1.6	Oatcakes	25g	1.5
White flour	25g	0.8	Shortbread	25g	0.5
Oatmeal – raw	25g	1.7	Short pastry	50g	1.1
Rice – brown	25g	0.5			
			ROOT VEGETABLES		
NUTS			Carrots	75g	1.9
Almonds	25g	1.9	Beetroot	75g	1.9
Brazils	25g	1.1	Swedes	75g	2.6
Chestnuts	25g	1.1	Potatoes – jacket	100g	1.4
Hazelnuts	25g	1.6	Potatoes – new	100g	1.1
Coconut	25g	1.8	Potatoes (peeled & boiled)	100g	1.2
Peanuts	25g	1.6			
Peanut butter	25g	1.4			
Walnuts	25g	0.9	**LEAF VEGETABLES**		
			Spinach	100g	1.6
BREAKFAST CEREALS			Broccoli tops	100g	3.0
Kellogg's All-bran	40g	9.6	Spring greens	100g	3.6
Muesli	30g	1.8			

FIBRE

Fibre refers to a special group of carbohydrates which aren't really nutrients as they are not absorbed by the gut. They are found in plant foods and there are two kinds: insoluble and soluble.

Insoluble fibre is found in wholewheat flour, bread, pasta and rice, wholegrain breakfast cereals and fibrous fruit and vegetables. It absorbs water which adds bulk to food, making it pass easily through the bowel. This helps prevent constipation and may also

Fibre content of every day foods

	Serving size	Fibre content grams		Serving size	Fibre content grams
Sprouts	100g	4.8	Avocado pear	125g	5.5
Cabbage	100g	2.1	Banana	150g	1.7
Cabbage – raw	50g	1.6	Blackberries	100g	3.1
Cauliflower	100g	1.6	Cherries	75g	0.9
Celery – raw	100g	1.3	Dates – dried	7g	0.3
Leeks	100g	2.3	Figs – dried	14g	1.1
Lettuce – raw	25g	0.3	Black grapes	50g	0.3
			Grapefruit	125g	1.6
OTHER VEGETABLES			Melon	150g	0.8
Peas – frozen	75g	3.9	Orange	100g	2.1
Peas – canned	75g	3.0	Peach	100g	1.5
Peas – fresh	75g	2.2	Pear	100g	2.2
Broad beans	75g	4.1	Raisins	25g	0.5
Butter beans	75g	5.2	Raspberries	75g	1.9
Baked beans	75g	2.6	Strawberries	75g	1.1
Runner beans	100g	2.3	Sultanas	25g	0.6
French beans	100g	3.1	Pineapple	150g	1.8
Lentils – split	50g	1.0			
Corn-on-the-cob	75g	2.0	**FRUIT (COOKED, WITH SUGAR)**		
Sweetcorn – can	75g	1.1	Blackcurrants	100g	2.8
Tomatoes – raw	50g	0.6	Gooseberries	100g	1.9
Onions	150g	2.7	Plums	100g	1.6
			Prunes	75g	2.0
FRUIT (RAW)			Rhubarb	100g	1.4
Eating apples	75g	1.4			

protect against other bowel disorders.

Soluble fibre is found in dried beans, lentils and peas (pulses), most fruit and vegetables and some grains, including oats, barley and rye. One of its useful effects is that it can delay the absorption of some nutrients, such as glucose, making it helpful for diabetics. It may also reduce the amount of cholesterol in the blood.

Fibre plays an important part in the efficient working of your body. It does this by absorbing water as it passes from the stomach through the intestines, forming the soft bulk that stimulates the muscles of the lower bowel to expel waste from the body easily and quickly.

Without fibre the faeces become small and hard and do not have enough bulk to stimulate regular movement of the muscles of the bowel. So it is recommended that you eat between 18 and 30 g of fibre a day to make sure you are regular and avoid the unpleasant effects of constipation. Surveys show that most people only eat about 12 g of fibre a day, so you may need to increase your fibre intake by a third or more. Aim to get this extra fibre from a selection of food rather than just high-fibre breakfast cereals (see table below). You should also make sure that you drink plenty of fluids to help the fibre do its work.

Like any other part of the diet, too much fibre can be harmful. It can reduce the absorption of some essential minerals such as iron, calcium and zinc. And too much fibrous food can fill up young children before they have taken in the energy-rich food they need to grow and be healthy.

PROTEIN

Bodybuilding proteins are found in every cell of the body. Some are needed for making, growing and repairing body tissues, while others are needed for making enzymes and hormones which control vital processes like fighting infection and healing wounds.

Proteins are made up of twenty amino acids which combine together in various ways to make all the different proteins our bodies need. The body can make many of these amino acids itself, but there are eight 'essential amino acids' which can be provided only by the food you eat.

Milk and dairy products, eggs, meat, poultry and fish contain 'complete protein', i.e. they contain all the essential amino acids.

Apart from soya, though, all plants that contain protein – such as nuts, beans, peas and grains – lack sufficient quantities of at least one essential amino acid. This means vegetarians should make sure they get all the essential amino acids they need by combining different types of proteins. Examples of this include baked beans on toast, cereal and milk, or rice and dahl.

FAT

Many of us need to eat less fat but a balanced diet should contain some fat. It is needed as an energy source (weight for weight it gives twice as much energy as protein and carbohydrate do). It is vital for the health of all the body's cells and for making some hormones. It protects the body's vital organs, acting as a shock-absorber, and helps control the body's temperature. It is also needed to help absorb vitamins A, D, E and K from food.

Fat comes in many different forms. Some, like butter and lard, are solid; others, like cooking oil, are liquid. The fat on meat and some other foods is visible, but as much as two-thirds of the fat we eat may be 'hidden' in foods such as biscuits and eggs. It is these hidden fats which you must avoid if you are to cut down the amount of fat you eat.

Fat is made of substances called fatty acids which, according to their chemical make-up, are either saturated or unsaturated.

Saturated fats (including cholesterol) are thought to be the most harmful to your health because they coat the lining of your arteries and may eventually block them completely. If this happens to vital arteries in the heart it causes a heart attack. As a general rule, saturates are found in fats which are solid at room temperature, and in animal products like meat and dairy foods. White meat and oily fish contain fewer saturated fats.

Soft margarine may contain fewer saturates than butter but harder margarines are made by changing unsaturated fats into saturated ones so they usually have a similar saturated fat content to butter. In this sense they are no more healthy than butter. Coconut and palm oil contain high levels of saturates.

The other fatty acids, the unsaturates, include polyunsaturates and monounsaturates. Health educators used to believe that polyunsaturates were the most healthy but recent research has suggested that a diet including monounsaturates is best. There

Some foods containing a high concentration of polyunsaturates

Liver	Some soft margarines	Soya bean oil
Herring	Corn oil	Sunflower oil
Tuna	Safflower oil	

Some foods containing a high concentration of monounsaturates

Beef	Eggs	Olive oil
Chicken	Some margarines	
Pork	Ground nut oil	

The amounts (grams) of different types of fat in some typical food portions

Food	Total Fat Content	Saturates	Mono-unsaturates	Poly-unsaturates
Stewed steak (casseroled), 168g	18.5	7.8	8.8	0.7
Roast chicken (with skin), 168g	23.5	7.8	10.5	3.5
Pork chop (grilled, lean, fat and bone), 168g	31.5	12.5	14.1	2.5
1 Mackerel (fresh), 150g	24.5	5.9	9.4	6.1
Milk 190 ml, (1 glass)				
(whole)	7.6	4.9	1.9	0.2
(semi-skimmed)	3.1	2.0	0.8	0.2
(skimmed)	0.2	0.1	trace	trace
1 Egg (boiled), 50g	5.5	1.7	2.2	0.6
Cheese (Cheddar), 28g	9.6	6.2	2.2	0.2
(Cottage), 112g	4.4	2.8	1.1	0.1
Yogurt (low fat), 1 carton, 150g	1.5	0.9	0.5	trace
Sunflower oil (1 tablespoon), 15g	15.0	2.0	4.8	8.0
2 Biscuits (chocolate digestive),	10.1	5.0	3.7	0.7
Peanuts (roasted), 1 small packet, 56g	27.4	5.2	13.2	7.8
Sausage roll (flaky pastry) 112g	40.5	16.0	17.6	4.5
Butter, 10g	8.1	5.2	1.9	0.2
Margarine (hard), 10g	8.1	3.0	3.5	1.4
(polyunsaturated), 10g	8.1	1.9	1.6	4.2

has also been a lot of interest in research into Eskimos, which suggests that the omega-3 fatty acids found in oily fish (e.g. mackerel, herring, tuna, salmon, trout) may prevent heart disease by stopping the coronary arteries from becoming clogged with fat, and making the blood less sticky. It is suggested that one or two meals of fatty fish are needed each week to have a beneficial effect. This may also help prevent another heart attack if you have had one already.

VITAMINS

Everyone needs vitamins daily in small amounts. Since the most natural source is food, a mixed diet including lean meat and fish, or pulses, some dairy produce, fresh fruit and vegetables and mainly unprocessed foods should provide enough for most people.

Vitamins are good for us but it does not follow that the more we eat the better. In fact, fat-soluble vitamins can accumulate in the body and be dangerous if taken in excess. Too many water-soluble vitamins will simply be lost in the urine. So before you buy supplements, check with your doctor.

WHICH FOODS?

Fast foods, convenience foods and confectionary are best avoided, because vitamins and minerals are lost during processing. These foods also tend to be high in fat and sugar.

Here is a list of the best food sources of vitamins and their various functions.

Vitamin A

A fat-soluble vitamin found in dairy produce such as milk, cheese and butter. Margarine is fortified with vitamin A. Oily fish – mackerel, herring, salmon and trout – are good sources, as is liver.

The body can convert carotene, the deep yellow substance that colours oranges, apricots (fresh and dried), carrots and other yellow or dark-green vegetables into vitamin A.

Vitamin A can be stored in the liver so deficiency is unlikely. Excessive amounts can be dangerous.

Function: Needed for seeing in dim light, for healthy mucus-excreting tissues such as the lungs, intestines and urinary linings. It also helps the body to resist infection and is good for the skin.

Vitamin B complex

There are several different B vitamins which act together and tend to be found in the same foods. They are water-soluble and the body cannot store them, so regular intake is essential. Taking supplements of one B vitamin in isolation can upset the balance, so if you do need extra B vitamins a Vitamin B Complex preparation is probably best. But again, check with your doctor.

VITAMIN B₁, THIAMIN

Thiamin is found in milk, meat and offal (e.g. liver, kidney), eggs, vegetables, fruit, wholegrain cereals and fortified breakfast cereals, wholemeal bread and wheatgerm. Some breakfast cereals and white flour are fortified with thiamin, and yeast extract is a good source.

Function: Needed for releasing energy from carbohydrate foods. Unrefined carbohydrates are rich in thiamin, but white flour products are not and sugars and alcohol contain none. Thiamin also contributes to healthy nerves and muscles. It is destroyed by overcooking.

VITAMIN B₂, RIBOFLAVIN

Milk is an excellent source of riboflavin but the riboflavin is destroyed by light, so take the milk bottle off the doorstep early, or buy it in cartons. Riboflavin is also found in cheese, meat, eggs and other foods which contain thiamin.

Function: Like thiamin, riboflavin is essential for converting carbohydrates into energy. It is a bright yellow substance and is used as a 'natural' food colouring with the E numbers 101 and 101a.

VITAMIN B₆, PYRIDOXINE

The main sources are potatoes and other vegetables, meat and milk.

Function: Needed by the body to make protein and haemoglobin, the oxygen-carrying part of the blood. Deficiencies are rare but women who are pregnant or on the Pill may need extra. Very high intakes are dangerous.

VITAMIN B₁₂, CYANOCOBALAMIN

Vitamin B_{12}, is found in meat (especially liver), white fish, dairy products and yeast. A deficiency can cause anaemia. The liver can store B_{12} for a few years, after which vegetarians and vegans may become deficient.
Function: Works with folic acid to make bone marrow, which in turn makes blood. Also needed for building healthy nerves and skin and using protein.

FOLIC ACID

The best sources are offal and raw, green, leafy vegetables, yeast, wheatgerm, soya flour, pulses, wholemeal bread and eggs. Cooking partially destroys it or changes it so that the body cannot use it so well – on average, fruit and vegetables lose about forty to fifty per cent of their folic acid during cooking.
Function: Needed with vitamin B_{12} to make blood. Both are also needed for body cells to divide rapidly. Pregnant women may need more folic acid for the developing fetus. If you are on the Pill or taking anti-epileptic drugs you may also need more.

NIACIN

Also called nicotinic acid and nicotinamide. Best sources are meat, cheese and fish, wholegrain products, peanuts.
Function: Same as thiamin.

PANTOTHENIC ACID

Best sources are yeast, liver, wholemeal bread, brown rice and other whole grains, peas and beans, eggs, pulses and nuts.
Function: Needed to release energy from fat and for tissue growth.

BIOTIN

Biotin is found in offal and egg yolk, nuts, oats and wheatgerm.

Function: Like pantothenic acid, this is essential for the metabolism of fat. Very little is needed and it is probably made by 'friendly' bacteria that live in the gut.

CHOLINE AND INOSITOL

These are found in eggs and offal, yeast, wheatgerm, oats and nuts.

Function: Essential for a healthy liver and to help prevent a build-up of fats in the body.

Vitamin C, Ascorbic Acid

The best-known sources of vitamin C are citrus fruits, blackcurrants and rosehips, but we obtain most from potatoes (not instant, unless fortified) and fruit juice. Frozen fruit or vegetables may contain more vitamin C than fresh because they are frozen very soon after harvesting, whereas fresh vegetables take time to reach the shops and the vitamin is lost during storage. Fruit juices and some foods are fortified with vitamin C.

Function: Vitamin C helps the body resist infection and keeps cells, blood vessels, gums and teeth healthy. It is also needed for healing wounds. It helps the body absorb iron from vegetables, so it is important for vegetarians. A lack of vitamin C leads to scurvy. It is also used as a food additive, E300.

Vitamin D

This fat-soluble vitamin is found in the same foods as vitamin A. The best sources are oily fish, which includes canned fish such as sardines. Breakfast cereals may be fortified with vitamin D, and so is margarine. It occurs naturally in butter. Vitamin D is known as the 'sunshine vitamin', because it can be manufactured in the skin by sunlight.

Infants who do not get enough may develop rickets. Pregnant and breast-feeding women, and babies and children up to five years old, may need supplements. A vegan diet may also be deficient in this vitamin.

Function: Helps the body absorb calcium and phosphorus to build healthy bones and teeth. Deficiency in the elderly can lead to osteoporosis (mineral loss from the bones), resulting in brittle bones. Too much vitamin D can lead to bony deposits and kidney damage.

Vitamin E, Tocopherol

Another fat-soluble vitamin found in vegetable oils, whole grains, wholemeal bread and wheatgerm, egg yolks, green vegetables and nuts. There is very little in animal fats, meat and fruit.

Function: Known to be essential for health, although the exact function is not fully understood. It is needed for fertility and muscle function in animals – possibly in humans too. It is an antioxidant, so it stops fats being oxidized which makes them rancid. Eating more foods rich in polyunsaturated fats that are readily oxidized, such as some soft margarines, may increase our need for vitamin E. It is used as an antioxidant food additive, E306 (natural) and E307-9 (synthetic).

Who needs vitamin supplements

- **Babies and children under five** may be prescribed vitamins A and D. Young Asian children in particular may need extra because some traditional diets do not supply enough and because their darker skin, which is often well covered by traditional clothing, is unable to make vitamin D in weak British sunlight.

- **Pregnant and nursing women** may need more vitamins. Nausea and sickness during pregnancy may make it difficult to eat nourishing foods, and women at risk of spina bifida births may need extra B vitamins.

- **The elderly** sometimes find eating difficult, and ageing can make it harder for the body to absorb nutrients. Lack of activity also reduces appetite, which restricts the intake of a wide variety of foods.

- **People on long-term medication** might also have trouble absorbing or using vitamins and their doctor might decide they need extra. For example, women on the Pill may need extra vitamin C.

- **Vegetarians and vegans** (who do not eat animal or dairy produce) may need supplements of vitamin B_{12}, because this comes mainly from animal foods. Any special diet that restricts the variety of foods eaten, such as some slimming diets, can reduce vitamin intake.

Vitamin K

The K is short for 'koagulations' (Danish). The richest sources are green vegetables, cereals, soya beans, liver and vegetable oils, but it is also made in the body by 'friendly' intestinal bacteria.

Function: Needed for normal clotting of the blood.

MINERALS

The body needs about twenty minerals, all with different functions. They come indirectly from the earth via the vegetables and fruit we eat and the meat and milk from animals which have also eaten mineral-rich food.

Use the chart below to check that your diet includes enough of

Some common minerals, where they're found and what they do

CALCIUM
Some good sources: Milk, cheese, yogurt, canned fish, green leafy vegetables, white bread, hard tap water

Functions● Healthy bones and teeth, blood clotting, and healthy muscle and nerves

IRON
Meat (especially cooked liver and kidney), bread, flour and cereal products (such as wholewheat breakfast cereals and wholewheat pasta), potatoes, vegetables, eggs

● Red blood cells, oxygen transfer, enzymes, drug metabolism

MAGNESIUM
Milk, bread, cereal products, other vegetables

● Bones, muscles, enzymes and many energy processes including repair and maintenance of body cells

PHOSPHORUS
Milk, dairy products, bread, cereal products, meat and meat products (such as sausages and beefburgers)

● Found in all cells, energy storage, growth and reproduction

the mineral-containing foods, since a shortage of any of the minerals can affect your health.

Eating a balanced diet with plenty of different foods should ensure you get enough of the minerals you need throughout life.

Calcium

Calcium is a most important mineral. It is needed for healthy muscles and nerves and for blood clotting. Getting enough calcium in the diet every day is also essential for building and keeping strong bones and teeth.

Building strong bones in early life is particularly important because it means you will have a good store of calcium ready for the time in later life when you start losing bone calcium. Without this store of calcium the bones may become brittle and break

POTASSIUM

Vegetables, meat, milk, fruit and fruit juices

- Found in all cells, controls the balance of fluids in the body, many metabolic processes including healthy nerves

SODIUM AND CHLORIDE (salt)

Table and cooking salt, cereal products, meat products

- Water and fluid balance in the body, many metabolic processes including healthy nerves

FLUORINE

Water, tea

- Necessary for healthy teeth and bones

IODINE

Fish, milk, meat, eggs

- Necessary for the thyroid hormones which regulate many body processes

ZINC

Meat and meat products, milk and dairy products, bread, cereal products

- Necessary for many enzymes and for many metabolic processes such as growth, bone, sexual maturity and fertility

easily (known as osteoporosis) or in extreme cases the spine may shrink and become rounded. Women are particularly at risk of osteoporosis (see p. 335) when they reach the menopause, because the protective calcium-holding effect of female hormones is lost.

The best way to build strong bones is to eat plenty of calcium-rich foods while bones are still growing (up to the mid twenties) and take plenty of exercise throughout life. Calcium is found in only a few foods (see table below). One of the richest sources is milk; in fact milk and its products provide more than half the calcium in the average diet.

Pregnant and nursing mothers should eat extra calcium (see table below) so that they provide plenty for their babies without reducing their own stores.

Calcium content of some typical foods

Food	Calcium Content (mg)
⅓ pint whole milk	234
⅓ pint semi-skimmed milk	244
⅓ pint skimmed milk	254
5oz (140g) yogurt	252
1oz (28g) Cheddar cheese	206
4oz (112g) dairy ice-cream	157
2oz (56g) sardines	258
2 slices (60g) white bread	60
4oz (112g) broccoli	85
4oz (112g) spring cabbage	34
4oz (112g) baked beans	50
2oz (56g) peanuts	34
2oz (56g) dried apricots	52

UK recommended daily amount (RDA) of calcium

Group	UK RDA
Infants (0–1 years)	600 mg
Children (1–8 years)	600 mg
Adolescents (9–14 years)	700 mg
Young adults (15–17 years)	600 mg
Adult men (over 18 years)	500 mg
Adult women (over 18 years)	500 mg
Pregnant women	1200 mg
Breast-feeding mothers	1200 mg

Iron

Iron plays an important role in maintaining health. It is an essential part of haemoglobin, the red pigment of the blood, which carries oxygen from the lungs to all parts of the body. If you are short of iron, you will be short of haemoglobin (i.e.

anaemic) and notice symptoms such as shortness of breath, tiredness, and pale skin.

An active man should eat 10 mg iron a day. Women need more because the blood lost in their periods needs replacing. Women aged eighteen to fifty-four need 12–18 mg a day. Your body can store iron, so the rate of absorption of iron from food is decided by the level of stores – the more iron the slower the absorption and vice versa.

You will need more iron at times of rapid growth, for example, during adolescence, especially if you are starting your periods, and during pregnancy. Toddlers who are reluctant to take solids or formula milk may also be at risk. A newborn baby of normal birthweight is born with adequate stores of iron for a year's growth, but after a year the iron must be provided by the diet. Small or premature babies may need supplements earlier. Breast milk has some iron but not enough to replenish stores.

The best sources of iron are liver, kidney, dried apricots and figs, peanuts, green, leafy vegetables such as cabbage, Brussels sprouts, cauliflower, celery, cucumber, courgettes, green peppers, cereals such as cornflakes and Weetabix, wholewheat bread and oily fish such as mackerel, pilchard, sardine and tuna. Spinach is a good but not exceptional source of iron; the myth about it arose because the German scientist who did the original research made a mistake, making it appear to have ten times more iron than it has, and Popeye did the rest.

Magnesium

Magnesium is the second most common mineral after potassium in the cells of the body. It is important for bones, muscles, enzymes and many energy processes including repair and main-tenance of body cells. The average daily intake should be 400–800 mg but since it is found in so many different foods deficiency is rarely a problem. Magnesium deficiency has been linked with conditions such as raised blood pressure, osteoporosis and pre-menstrual tension but the scientific evidence is still thin.

A balanced diet will provide you with the magnesium you need. Good sources include nuts, whole grains, milk, bread, cereal products, green vegetables (the greener the vegetable the more magnesium it has), potatoes and tap water in hard-water areas.

People most at risk from magnesium deficiency are those who

drink a lot of alcohol or suffer from long-term diarrhoea. In such people supplementation is probably wise. The cheapest form is magnesium oxide, 100 mg provides about 60 mg of elemental magnesium.

Phosphorus

Phosphorus is a mineral found in every cell in the body. Like calcium it is mainly used for making bones and teeth, but it is also necessary for energy production, storage and release.

Phosphorus is widely available in foods such as milk and milk products, meat, fish, vegetables, cereals and nuts, so deficiency is almost non-existent in the Western world. Some doctors prescribe it with calcium and hormone replacement therapy to post-menopausal women to prevent and treat osteoporosis, but its value in this role is unproven.

Potassium

Potassium is a mineral which every cell in the body needs. It is especially necessary for the correct working of the heart, the muscles and nerves, and for keeping the levels of glucose in the blood normal.

Potassium is found in high concentrations in fresh vegetables, pulses and fruits. It is impossible to eat so much potassium (in the UK the average intake is 2,000–4,000 mg daily) that you put yourself in danger, but if you have illnesses such as kidney disease, severe dehydration or adrenal glands disease the levels of potassium in your blood may rise dangerously. You will need careful medical supervision for these conditions.

Equally, potassium is so widespread that almost all diets (and especially vegetarian diets) include enough potassium. Only if you have problems with your gut (for example due to longstanding diarrhoea), or if you take special types of 'water' (diuretic) tablets do you need to worry about becoming deficient. Ask your doctor if you are concerned about this.

Salt

Salt is the only mineral that many people eat too much of. Though the body needs salt, too much can worsen conditions such as high blood pressure and heart disease. The best way to cut down on salt is to add as little as possible to food when cooking and to avoid highly processed foods.

Iodine

Iodine is an essential mineral. It is needed for production of thyroid hormones, which are vital for controlling the body's metabolism. An intake of 100–1,000 mcg of iodine is regarded as safe, with a recommended minimum of 100 mcg per day for adults and 150 mcg per day for children, adolescents and pregnant and breast-feeding women.

The best sources of iodine are dairy products (e.g. milk, eggs and cheese), meat (e.g. pork), fish (e.g. haddock, halibut, sardines and tuna) and vegetables (e.g. lettuce, spinach and green peppers).

Deficiency is rare in Western countries, but worldwide two million people are said to suffer from iodine deficiency. The main reason is lack of iodine in the soil. Such people can be treated by adding iodine to water or iodized salt to food.

Eating too much iodine is rare. There is one well-known case of some Japanese fishermen who ate a high-seaweed diet containing 10,000–200,000 mcg of iodine a day and all developed goitres (swelling of the thyroid gland). Some experts, though, believe that we are gradually eating more and more iodine since it is now used in the dairy industry, dough conditioners, and colouring dyes for example, and that such additives should be better controlled by the government.

Zinc

Zinc is essential for many chemical reactions in the body including enzyme reactions, tissue growth and repair, wound healing, fertility, the immune system and normal sight, smell and taste. A healthy adult needs about 15 mg a day.

A balanced diet should provide more than enough zinc for ordinary use. More is needed during pregnancy, after major surgery, burns or severe stress. The best sources of zinc are oysters (if you can afford them!), lamb chops, steak, nuts, ginger root, whole wheat (including bread), peas, potatoes and milk.

Estimating your zinc status is difficult, so do not be led astray by wild claims from 'specialists' and laboratories. Levels estimated in blood, urine and hair are inaccurate. Only the analysis of sweat is accurate and this requires specialist equipment.

CALORIES

To lead an active, enjoyable life you need energy, which is measured in calories. This energy is actually provided by the carbohydrate, protein and fat in your food and drink. Starchy carbohydrate should supply most of your daily energy needs.

Energy is essential for all the body's functions and is also burned up by our muscles during exercise. However, it is important to choose energy foods that are rich in a variety of nutrients. Foods that provide only calories, such as many sweet foods, should not be our main source of energy.

How much energy do you need?

The following are recommended daily amounts of energy (kilo-calories) needed for people of different ages.

AGE	BOYS Energy (k. cal)	GIRLS Energy (k. cal)
1 year	1200	1100
2	1400	1300
3 to 4	1560	1500
5 to 6	1740	1680
7 to 8	1980	1900
9 to 11	2280	2050
12 to 14	2640	2150
15 to 17	2880	2150

Recommended Daily Amount of Energy (DHSS, 1979)

Note: These guidelines are based on 'average' body weight and for adults of smaller build may be too high.

MEN	Energy (k. cal)
18 to 24	
Sedentary	2510
Moderately active	2900
Very active	3350
35 to 64	
Sedentary	2400
Moderately active	2750
Very active	3350
65 to 74 (Sedentary)	2400
75 and over (Sedentary)	2150
WOMEN	
18 to 54	
Most occupations	2150
Very active	2500
55 to 74	1900
75 and over	1680
Pregnant	2400
Breast-feeding	2750

Typical energy content of food

Now you have an idea of the quantity of energy (kilocalories) you need each day, this chart shows how much energy typical portions of various foods contain.

Food	Energy (k. cal)	Food	Energy (k. cal)
BREAD, CEREALS AND POTATOES		Peanuts (1 small packet, 50g)	285
Bread, wholemeal (2 slices, 60g)	109	Baked beans (small tin, 200g)	128
Cornflakes (1 serving, 28g)	103		
Rice, polished, boiled (1 portion, 150g)	186	**FRUIT**	
Spaghetti, boiled (1 portion, 225g)	263	Apple (1 medium sized, 150g)	53
Potatoes, new boiled (1 portion, 170g)	129	Banana (1 medium sized, 175g	82
Potatoes, old chipped (1 portion, 150g)	380	Cherries (1 portion, 75g)	31
		Orange (1 medium sized, 180g)	47
MILK AND DAIRY PRODUCTS		Strawberries (1 portion, 113g)	29
Cheese, cheddar (1 portion, 56g)	231		
Cheese, cottage (1 small carton, 113g)	108	**VEGETABLES (WITHOUT SAUCE OR DRESSING)**	
Cream, single (2 tablespoons, 30g)	60	Beans, runner, boiled (1 portion, 112g)	21
Milk, fresh, whole (1 glass, 190ml)	129	Brussels sprouts, boiled (1 portion, 112g)	20
Milk, semi-skimmed (1 glass, 190ml)	91	Cabbage, spring, boiled (1 portion, 112g)	8
Milk, fresh, skimmed (1 glass, 190ml)	65	Carrots, young, boiled (1 portion, 112g)	22
Yogurt, low fat (1 small carton, 150g)	78	Lettuce, raw (1 portion, 56g)	6
		Peas, fresh boiled (1 portion, 112g)	58
FATS AND OILS			
Butter (1 portion, 10g)	73	**SUGAR AND PRESERVES**	
Margarine, all kinds (1 portion, 10g)	73	Chocolate, milk (1 bar, 50g)	265
Vegetable oil (1 tablespoon, 15g)	135	Ice-cream (2 small scoops, 50g)	83
		Jam (2 heaped teaspoons, 15g)	40
MEAT, FISH, EGGS, NUTS AND PULSES		Sugar, white (2 teaspoons, 10g)	39
Pork, roast leg, lean and fat (2 slices, 85g)	243		
		ALCOHOLIC DRINKS	
Chicken, roast (with skin, 85g)	183	Dry white wine (1 glass, 113ml)	75
Ham, boiled, lean and fat (2 slices, 56g)	67	Beer, draught bitter (½ pint)	91
Lamb, leg, roast (2 slices, 85g)	226		
Cod, steamed (1 portion, 113g)	94		
Plaice, fried in batter (1 portion, 130g)	363		
Eggs, fresh, whole (1 boiled)	74		

Source: The Composition of Foods by R. D. McCance and E. M. Widdowson (Medical Research Council and HMSO)

Each of us varies in our calorie requirements depending on our age, sex, size, metabolic rate and activities. If we eat more calories than we need for energy they are stored as fat. So, to keep your weight steady you must take in no more calories than you use up. The energy table below gives an approximate guide to how many calories you need.

Children under five need lots of energy and nutrients in relation to their size because they are very active and their bodies are growing fast. But, being small, it can be difficult for young children to eat enough food to supply their needs. So they must have foods which are concentrated in both energy and nutrients such as whole milk (silver top).

A BALANCED, HEALTHY DIET

Now that you know more about the nutritional value of food you should be able to select a healthy diet. But don't deny yourself your favourite foods all the time, just because they may be less healthy. Eating is about enjoyment, too, and the benefits of delicious food, eaten perhaps with friends or family, cannot be ignored. One tip is that if you eat a selection of foods from each of the following groups every day you will be eating an excellent diet.

Food Groups	Eat this number of servings each day
Meat, fish, poultry, game, eggs, nuts, beans, peas, lentils	2
Milk, cheese, yogurt	3
Bread, rice, cereals, potatoes, pasta	4
Fresh fruit, vegetables, salads	4
Fats, oils	Small amount

Some people have decided to take their healthy eating a step further. They have become worried by the effect of artificial fertilizers, chemical sprays and pesticides and have made a conscious decision to select only food that has been grown in organic conditions. Most supermarkets now stock organic food, though it still tends to be more expensive. Healthfood stores usually stock organic food. If you cannot find organically grown fruit and vegetables in your area you can reduce the amount of chemicals you absorb by washing and scrubbing the food before eating or cooking.

You might like also to consider growing your own food without chemicals or fertilizers, either in your own garden or in an allotment. The soil can be improved by compost, leaf mould or peat, and insects can be kept away by harmless compounds like derris dust.

An increasing number of people are reducing the amount of meat in their diet or cutting out meat and fish completely (vegetarians). Although meat is a rich source of protein and iron it is perfectly possible to get plenty of both provided you eat a good selection of dairy products, cereals, pulses and nuts. And because vegetarians usually eat a diet rich in vitamin C they tend to absorb iron more efficiently than those who do not.

Eating enough of all the vitamins should not be a problem for vegetarians because vitamins are so plentiful in dairy products and fruit and vegetables. The only vitamins which they might become short of are vitamin B_{12} and vitamin D. Although the body can make its own vitamin D from sunlight it may be worth taking supplements, especially if you live in a temperate climate and work indoors. Make sure the supplement contains D_2 and not D_3 which may come from an animal source.

Vegans eat neither meat, fish, eggs, nor dairy products. They need to be more careful about selecting a wide range of food and may need supplements. Vitamin B_{12} for example is not found in plants. Shortage of calcium can also be a problem for vegans, especially for young children who need it to grow strong bones. Soya bean milk can be bought to which calcium has been added up to the levels of cow's milk.

USEFUL BOOKS

Feeding Your Family by Dr Miriam Stoppard, Penguin Books Ltd
Shopping for Health by Janette Marshall, Penguin Books Ltd
Food Facts by Carol Ann Rinzler, Bloomsbury Publishing
The Family Nutrition Workbook by Patrick Holford, Thorsons
   Publishing Group Ltd
The Dictionary of Nutritional Health by Adrienne Mayes,
   Thorsons Publishing Group Ltd

Vegetarian High-Fibre Cooking by Janette Marshall, Thorsons Publishing Group Ltd

Don't Forget Fibre in Your Diet by Dr Dennis Burkitt, Martin Dunitz

High-Calorie Fibre Diet by Dr James Anderson, Martin Dunitz

High-Fibre Cook Book by Pamela Westland, Martin Dunitz

Cooking for Kids the Healthy Way by Joanna Pay, Martin Dunitz

Good Housekeeping. Healthy Eating by Susanna Tee, Ebury Press

Good Housekeeping. Eating for a Healthy Heart by the Coronary Prevention Group, Ebury Press

The Sunday Times Guide to Enlightened Eating by Lis Leigh, Century Hutchinson Ltd

Nutritional Medicine by Stephen Davies and Alan Stewart, Pan

2 Understanding Weight Loss

BY DR RICHARD HAWKINS

Imagine how differently a ballet dancer and a Japanese wrestler think of being overweight. To one as little as 1 kg can make a crucial difference, to the other a 1 kg change would be so insignificant as not to be noticed. So, there are all sorts of definitions of being overweight. But as a general rule, if you are more than twenty per cent over the desirable weight for your height you are overweight. In the UK this means about eight million people are overweight.

Being overweight does not necessarily condemn you to a miserable life. There are fat people who have lived to a ripe old age without problems. But there is no doubt it does make you more likely to suffer a whole range of health problems. Overweight people have an increased risk of heart disease and high blood pressure, diabetes, arthritis and gallstones. Operations are more difficult and carry a greater risk so surgeons may insist on weight loss before surgery. Overweight people are also more likely to experience depression and problems in relationships, both at home and at work. Weight can even influence your chance of a job or promotion.

The more overweight you are, the more likely it is that your health will be affected. How long you can expect to live is reduced in direct proportion to how overweight you are. The good news, however, is that most weight problems can be solved by a sensible, low-fat, high-fibre calorie-controlled diet. And the health problems described above may improve or disappear once the excess weight has been lost.

What makes people overweight?

Food gives us energy, which is measured in calories. Each day you should eat enough (but no more!) calories to give you the energy you need to carry out your daily activities. For women this is usually about 2,200 calories a day, men need more like

2,750 calories a day, although figures vary widely between individuals.

If you regularly take in more calories than your body burns up, the extra energy will be stored as fat.

How can weight be reduced?

The only certain way to reduce weight is to eat fewer calories than your body uses. This means your body will be forced to draw upon its fat stores for energy and as this fat is burned, excess weight is gradually lost.

Eating less is the simplest way of reducing your daily calorie intake – but in doing so you must make sure you still get all the nourishment you need, especially vitamins and minerals. The answer is to eat a variety of foods daily so you get a balanced diet.

What is making you overweight?

Try keeping an eating diary for a week, like the one below. Note down everything you eat – when, how much, and why you ate it.

8 A.M.	cereal and milk	hungry
11 A.M.	bag of crisps	tense
12 A.M.	chicken and chips	hungry
2 P.M.	cup of tea	bored
	3 chocolate biscuits	
4 P.M.	cup of tea, slice of cake	bored
7 P.M.	fish and chips	being sociable

This can help you identify problems. Perhaps you eat too much at mealtimes – so cook smaller amounts to avoid the temptation of second helpings. You may overeat in the evenings through boredom or bad habits, such as nibbling while watching television. Or you may simply eat too much of a fattening food like chips, crisps or chocolate.

Tackle your specific problem and you may find this is all you need to do.

Starting to diet

Once you have decided to lose weight, it's a good idea to have a word with your GP. He or she will check that there are no medical reasons why you should not start a weight-loss diet, can help advise on the most appropriate method of weight loss, and may wish to see you regularly to see how you are getting on. You can feel confident your GP will be pleased you are making the effort to lose weight yourself and will give you useful support.

Make a firm decision to persevere. Here are some helpful ideas:

- Aim for a realistic target, such as getting back into your old jeans or going swimming with the children. Make it something you really want.

- Give yourself small rewards at regular stages. How about treating yourself to a night at the cinema, a new haircut, a new item of clothing, or joining a health club?

- If you have photographs of a younger, slimmer you, keep them out to remind yourself of your target.

- Learn to say 'no' to food you do not really need. The more often you refuse a second helping, the easier it gets!

- Get into the habit of leaving a little of your meal on the plate. Remember that eating more than you need is as wasteful of good food as throwing it away. Of course, you can always save money by making tasty meals from leftovers the next day!

How to eat fewer calories yet stay well nourished

The simplest way to lose weight is to reduce your calorie intake to about 1,200 calories a day. You will still be able to enjoy a good variety of foods. Here are some tips:

- Eat less of the concentrated energy foods like fats, sugars and alcohol.

- Switch to low-fat dairy products such as skimmed milk, low-fat yogurt and low-fat cheese.

- Avoid using fats unnecessarily when you cook – grill or steam rather than fry; bake or braise rather than roast.

- Beware of fats in meat: choose low-fat meats like turkey and chicken, and remove the skin. If eating lamb or beef use only lean cuts, remove the fat you can see, and pour off the juices that come from the meat while cooking. Eat more fish: it's delicious baked, steamed or grilled.

- Choose fruit for your desserts, because it is low in calories and supplies plenty of vitamins. Sugary sweets, puddings and fizzy drinks (except low-calorie ones) are packed with calories and have little nutritional value – avoid them except for the occasional treat.

- Eat more fibre. Wholemeal bread, brown rice, wholewheat pasta, wholegrain and bran-enriched breakfast cereals, pulses, and fresh vegetables contain bulky fibre. These foods are good for your digestion, and have fewer calories ounce for ounce than more refined foods. The bulk also makes you feel full which helps you eat less.

- Choose foods that come in ready portions, such as a slice of bread, a pot of low-fat yogurt, or a chicken leg (without skin). This will help you to work out the calorie content of your meals, and avoid the temptation of leftovers and second helpings.

- When shopping, look at the information on packs and choose the low-fat, low-sugar, high-fibre alternatives. And never go shopping when you are hungry. You might be tempted to buy more than you need!

How quickly will I lose weight?

Cutting down to around 1,200 calories a day for women, 1,500 calories a day for men can result in a gradual loss of around 0.5 kg per week. Women in middle age may require a lower-calorie diet, i.e. around 800 calories a day, because of their lower metabolism. For those who are significantly overweight and who have failed to lose weight on a conventional diet, a very low-calorie diet may be considered. You should discuss with your doctor which diet would be most suitable for you.

Whatever diet you follow, the weight you lose in the first week will contain a high proportion of water, and this weight will be regained at the end of the diet. Aim at a steady weight loss of 0.5–1 kg per week. Weigh yourself regularly – say, once a week – as encouragement, always first thing in the morning. If you are not doing as well as you had hoped, keep a food diary, and carefully weigh the food you are eating – your portions may be more generous than you had thought.

Remember, there are no short cuts to losing weight – you must eat less and choose your foods carefully, so you eat healthy food that is low in calories yet filling. Be suspicious of products which claim to help you safely lose weight without changing your diet, because this is impossible.

Will exercise help?

Regular exercise – about half an hour two or three times a week – helps your circulation and muscle tone, and makes you feel more alert and confident. This amount of exercise will not help you lose a significant amount of weight but it takes you away from the temptation of food at home or at work, and a regular commitment to exercise helps to maintain your new trim figure after a diet.

Commercial weight-loss diets

Slimming Clubs. There will almost certainly be a club in your area. The benefits of joining a reputable slimming club are that you will receive nutritionally sound diet programmes, and have regular contact with other slimmers – a good reason for you to stick to your diet.

Meal-replacement diets. Your local chemist can supply various brands of fortified slimming biscuits, drinks or mueslis. These are designed to replace one or two meals a day with a low-calorie, nutritious food. Make sure your main meal of the day consists of nutritious food containing only 400–500 calories.

Very low calorie diets (VLCDs). VLCDs claim to provide complete nutrition in under 600 calories a day, and come in flavoured formula drinks and soups and sometimes meal-replacement bars. They are usually supplied by chemists and by local diet counsellors who make sure the diet is suitable for you.

The benefits of VLCDs are fast weight loss, an easy-to-follow programme, with a reduction in hunger. Most programmes include personal supervision from your diet counsellor who will support and motivate you. To use these types of diet you should check with your doctor that you are in good health because they can be dangerous. It must be emphasized that they are only needed if you are very overweight and other more conventional types of diet have failed.

How to maintain your ideal weight

Once you have reached your target weight, try not to go back to your old eating habits – they will soon bring back your weight problem. Here are some hints to help you stay slim:

- Weigh yourself once a week. Don't let your weight rise more than 2 kg above your ideal weight without doing something about it. It is not difficult to lose 2 kg, but once you've let a stone creep back on you've got a battle on your hands.

- Learn to be more figure-conscious. A full-length mirror is useful here. Observe your figure and enjoy what you see – and the compliments too!

- Make permanent changes to your eating habits. Follow the advice on page 25 where possible – low-calorie cooking not only keeps you slim, but it's good for your health as well.

- Take regular exercise to remain fit and lean. This will increase your metabolism and help to burn up the calories.

- Don't feel guilty if you overindulge one day, just cut back the next day. That way you can enjoy special occasions yet still feel in control of your weight.

USEFUL BOOKS

A Second Helping by Sue Kreitzman, Bantam Books
Healthy Eating by Anna Bradley, Hodder and Stoughton
T-Factor Diet by Martin Katahn, Bantam Press
The BBC Diet by Barry Lynch, BBC Books
Complete Nutrition by Michael Sharon, Prion
The F-Plan by Audrey Eyton, Penguin Books
The ABC Diet and Body Plan by Oliver Gillie and Susana Raby, Hutchinson

3 Exercise

BY EDWINA CONNER

So much has been said in the press, in magazines, on TV and radio about the role of exercise that it's easy to see the whole subject as a bit of a bore. We *know* we should be running, swimming, cycling, walking and so on. We *know* it's good for us. What more is there to be said on the matter?

It is certainly true that much media attention has been given to the importance of exercise in recent years, and that experts are now more or less agreed that regular bouts of sustained activity are good for us, and, when taken in conjunction with a sensible diet and lifestyle, do help protect the heart and other vital organs from disease.

Long-term benefits of exercise

- Improves the circulation and muscle function, so you have more stamina

- Helps lower blood pressure

- Helps protect against heart disease

- Reduces the tendency of the blood to coagulate or clot

- Helps you lose fat

- Helps control blood sugar levels in diabetics

- Helps reduce stress and tension

- Helps relieve feelings of aggression and anger

- Helps you sleep better

- Wards off depression

- Accelerates the flow of blood to the bones – particularly important for post-menopausal women at risk of osteoporosis (see below)

Everyone who exercises regularly reports that they feel better both just after they have exercised and also in the long term. It is interesting that exercise is now being used by some psychiatrists to help people with mild or moderate depression and to treat tension and anxiety. Nevertheless, despite the attention given to exercise, and government spending on health education, the fact remains that most people still do not take enough. A recent report, 'Women's Health Today' put out by the Office of Health Economics, noted that although women were perfectly aware of the benefits of exercise, and of the health risks associated with a lack of it, only a small percentage actually exercises regularly – though that percentage is increasing slightly. Only a small proportion of men and teenagers take exercise too.

Many people associate 'taking exercise' with a major training programme, involving several days or evenings a week. Needless to say, very few people can suddenly adjust their lifestyle to cope with this amount of disruption to their routine. Finding an extra hour in the day is difficult enough. If you start off trying to fit in an exercise programme that is unrealistic you will not be able to stick to it and before you know where you are you'll be back

---

When taking up exercise:

- Check with your doctor that you are fit

- Choose a form of exercise you know you can keep up

- If it helps, arrange to exercise with a friend or relative

- Make sure you have the right equipment: if you are jogging, good shoes that support your feet properly are essential; if swimming, goggles to protect your eyes from chlorinated water

- Start slowly and build up gradually to at least three half-hour sessions a week

- Vary your exercise routines to avoid straining the same muscles

- Never exercise if you have a viral infection, if you feel at all unwell or are running a temperature

- Do not exercise until at least two hours after a heavy meal or after drinking alcohol

- If you miss a week or two of exercise through illness, remember to return to your routine gently. Don't try and pick up at the point you left off

to slumping in front of the TV in the evenings. The secret is not to completely change your life so as to organize it around your exercise, but to tailor your exercise sessions to fit into your life.

Too old for exercise?

Exercise is not just for the young. A teenager may be able to swim faster than her fit father, but her father may well be able to knock spots off her friend's dad in the pool. So if you are over forty and want to take up a sport, do it with a friend your own age rather than compete with a younger person. That way you'll avoid injury and strain and still make progress.

Is exercise risky?

Occasionally people who are very fit die during or after vigorous exercise. The most famous example is Jim Fixx, an American fitness expert who was at least partly responsible for getting thousands of his fellow Americans to take up jogging. At the post-mortem examination it was discovered that he in fact had coronary heart disease and that it was likely he had sustained several heart attacks in the past.

The vast majority of cases of sudden death during exercise are due to underlying heart disease. It is therefore as well, particularly for men over forty, to have a thorough medical check-up before embarking on a vigorous exercise programme. Women are becoming more susceptible to heart disease too, so it's probably wise for everyone to be cautious. Moreover, if you have any of the following symptoms while you exercise, you should seek medical advice:

- Crushing chest pain which may spread into the arms and be accompanied by pins and needles in the fingers

- Pain in the teeth, jaw or throat

- Dizziness, nausea or discomfort in the stomach and a high degree of breathlessness

- Fatigue and exhaustion after exercise

- Burning sensation or feeling of tightness in the chest, throat or jaw

The other risk that has received publicity is that of becoming addicted to exercise, so that it becomes a compulsion you cannot give up. This is thought to be due to substances called endorphins, which are found naturally in the body and act in a similar way to drugs such as morphine. Endorphins are thought to be responsible for the 'runner's high', experienced by certain long-distance runners and those who exercise strenuously and regularly. Some people describe it as a euphoric sensation, a feeling of elation, or even an altered state of consciousness.

The role of endorphins is complex, but it is possible that some people become addicted to them, and if they are forced to give up exercise they suffer withdrawal symptoms such as irritability, insomnia and depression. This is, however, very rare.

The main dangers of this are not so much physical as mental and social, and seem particularly to affect men who take up exercising, particularly running, over the age of forty. Marriages, work, families can all be relegated to second place, with unfortunate consequences for everyone concerned. It is as well to guard against compulsive exercising and, if you have other responsibilities in your life, to keep your exercise programme to a sensible timescale.

Injuries

Some sports are more likely to cause injuries than others. Again, running seems to be the main culprit, with damaged feet, ankles, tendons and knees among the most common injuries.

If you are taking up running:

- Make sure you buy proper running shoes, not just ordinary sneakers.

- Do not run on concrete if you can help it. Grass or turf is a much safer bet.

- Before starting your run, do some bending and stretching exercises to warm up your muscles and reduce the chances of injury. They do not take long to do but can make all the difference.

- If you are prone to ankle or joint problems, consider taking up swimming rather than running, as swimming cushions the joints.

WHICH TYPE OF EXERCISE?

The main aim of exercise is to increase stamina, strength and flexibility. Stamina is best increased by aerobic exercise. The word 'aerobic' simply means 'with air' and there's nothing mysterious about it. The air we breathe feeds our muscles, heart, lungs and blood all the time. Aerobic exercise is the kind that uses large groups of muscles in continuous activity (e.g. swimming, walking, running) and involves our breathing in more air. If the exercise is continued for at least ten minutes and carried out regularly it improves the capacity of our system. That in turn means we feel fitter.

Strength and flexibility are improved by aerobic exercise but are also helped by exercises for specific muscles – stomach, legs, ankles, pelvic floor, arms – and by the kind of movement taught in body-conditioning and keep-fit classes.

Ideally you should combine regular aerobic exercise with daily exercises for strength and flexibility.

Which aerobic exercise?

SWIMMING

This is a safe and effective form of exercise – particularly if you are unfit and stiff – and good for all age groups.

Start off by doing one or more lengths until you are comfortably out of breath. Take a short recovery break between each length. Then if you can, try two or more lengths without a break in between. Gradually increase the number of lengths and decrease the rests.

When you have cut out the rests altogether, try and speed up. You will soon find you have had enough after about twelve to fifteen lengths. When you feel ready, go on and do more lengths if you wish, but enjoy yourself – don't let it become a chore.

Vary your strokes – breaststroke, front crawl, backstroke, legs only – to keep your interest up.

AIM TO BUILD UP TO THIRTY MINUTES' CONTINUOUS SWIMMING, THREE TIMES A WEEK.

WALKING

Whenever possible try to walk rather than use motorized transport. If you don't own a pair of comfortable walking shoes, invest in some, preferably the kind with padding to help put a spring into your step.

Start by walking for about fifteen minutes. Gradually walk further in that time, so you are increasing your speed. Then if you feel you want to, walk for longer until you end up walking briskly for thirty to forty minutes.

AIM TO BUILD UP TO ONE HOUR'S BRISK WALKING, THREE TIMES A WEEK.

JOGGING

Make sure you have good running shoes and are dressed for the weather.

Start off by jogging for one minute and walking for one minute alternately. Ten minutes will do to start with. Gradually increase the jogging time and decreasing your walking time. You'll soon be able to jog for ten minutes.

You can then think about increasing the amount of time – again by walking and jogging alternately to start with – and then perhaps increase your speed.

Keep up your interest by jogging with a friend, entering a fun run or joining a running club.

AIM TO BUILD UP TO JOGGING FOR THIRTY MINUTES, THREE TIMES A WEEK.

CYCLING

Unless you live in a reasonably flat area without too much traffic about, or too much wind, and can cycle to work, for example, a bicycle is unlikely to be the best choice for regular exercise. However, if you are already a cyclist and conditions in your area are good, then it is an excellent way to build up stamina and strength.

AIM TO BUILD UP TO THIRTY MINUTES' BRISK CYCLING, THREE TIMES A WEEK.

STAIR-CLIMBING

If you can't get to a swimming pool and you hate running and walking, you could try stair-climbing. This is an excellent form of aerobic exercise that you can do in the warmth and comfort of your own home without any special clothing or shoes – all you need is a flight of stairs!

Start by walking up and down one flight of stairs until you are comfortably out of breath. Have a short recovery break and try again. Count how many times you go up and down and how long it takes you. Soon you will be able to climb the stairs more times in fewer minutes and with fewer breaks.

Then add another flight to your programme, or go up and down the same flight once or twice more in the same space of time. Five minutes of this will leave you very tired to start with: even the very fit will find twenty minutes enough.

AIM TO BUILD UP TO TWENTY MINUTES' FAST STAIR-CLIMBING THREE OR FOUR TIMES A WEEK.

EXERCISE CLASSES

Classes can be an excellent way to get fit and to improve your strength and flexibility. If you join an exercise class of any kind do be sure:

- that the teacher is qualified

- that the exercise studio floor is resilient and preferably properly sprung. Do not exercise for any length of time, if at all, on concrete

- that the class suits your own level of fitness

- that you understand *why* you are doing a particular exercise and how it should be done correctly

EXERCISES TO DO AT HOME

If you don't want to go to a class, follow a home exercise programme – every day if you can, but at least three times a week.

Work, stress and exercise

If you are tied to the office during the day, going out to expense-account lunches, and bringing home work in the evenings, you are likely to suffer from stress, not to mention a bulging abdomen and flagging muscles. Unless you take exercise, of course.

Middle-aged men with responsible, sedentary, tiring jobs are at risk from heart disease and other illnesses related to stress and lack of exercise, such as constipation, diabetes, high blood pressure and haemorrhoids (piles).

Some offices and factories now organize exercise classes for their employees, and even if yours doesn't there may be a swimming pool, squash court or park nearby where you can get out for an hour at lunchtime. It really is worth the effort.

Other stresses, such as divorce, bereavement, or children leaving home, can also make you susceptible to illness. Regular exercise cannot solve your problems but it can give you the energy to deal with them.

EXERCISE AFTER A HEART ATTACK

It is natural that someone who has suffered a heart attack should be nervous of taking up or resuming an exercise programme. It is certainly important to consult a doctor about the kind and amount of exercise, but some form of activity is very therapeutic, both physically and mentally. Make sure you get expert advice from your GP.

A LIFETIME OF EXERCISE

Children and exercise

Young children spend plenty of time running about and getting exercise. As they grow older though, and have to spend more time at a desk doing schoolwork, many children, apart from those who are obviously talented at sports and get into their school teams, become more sedentary and less interested in sport. This fact has seriously worried the British Medical Association. Teenagers are growing up overweight and unfit, hardly able to get themselves once around the netball court without getting puffed out. Then, once they're at home, homework and TV take up their evenings. Once this pattern of inactivity sets in it could persist for life.

The answer is to encourage children to take up physical activity out of school hours. Perhaps the family could go swimming together, or go out every weekend for a good long walk or cycle ride. A morning jog around the park would help too. If there is a dog in the family, it could provide an extra incentive for the children to get out and about.

Dancing classes (tap, jazz ballet, ballet, modern), keep fit, judo, kung-fu, badminton, tennis and karate are all available for children, are very enjoyable and very good exercise.

Exercise in pregnancy

Many women use pregnancy as an excuse to become overweight. After years of dieting and sporadic efforts at attending local keep-fit classes, they start to overindulge – eating for two and forgetting all about exercise.

It is best to start a sensible exercise programme *before* you get pregnant, so that you are fit and have a manageable routine.

Of course, it is important to look after yourself during pregnancy and an exhausting game of squash the day before the baby is due would not be sensible, but, as long as there are no complications which mean bedrest or a hospital stay, it is perfectly possible to take the right kind of exercise almost up to the last minute. That way your back, stomach and leg muscles will be in good working order and that will help you during labour. It will also mean that you will get your figure back more quickly after your baby is born.

Swimming, where the muscles and skeleton are well supported but the whole body is exercised gently, is an excellent choice. There are plenty of fashionable, cover-up-type swimming costumes on the market, should your usual costume become too tight.

The other perfectly safe exercise is walking. Try to take a good hour's brisk walk every day, or at least three times a week. You could perhaps alternate this with thirty minutes' swimming.

Dancing, either at a class or socially, is good for you too, and helps to keep your body flexible. So let your hair down when you get the chance.

It is equally important to take plenty of relaxation during pregnancy, so do put your feet up for at least fifteen minutes each day. If you are working, take time out during your lunch break to relax, or give yourself quarter of an hour immediately after work when no one is allowed to disturb you.

Postnatal exercises

You should be able to take up regular exercise after your doctor has pronounced you fit at your six-week postnatal examination. Fitting this in with looking after your baby may not be easy, but perhaps you can take it in turns with a friend to look after each other's children for an hour three times a week, or get out in the evenings. Not only will this help you get back into shape after your baby is born, it will also ward off any possible tendency to become depressed, and give you more energy to cope with the rigours of child-rearing.

Exercise, the menopause and osteoporosis

Young people should take plenty of exercise while their bones are still developing; this is the best way to ensure a strong and healthy skeleton which will help keep osteoporosis at bay later on. Osteoporosis is a condition affecting many people – particularly women after the menopause – when the bones become thinner and more likely to fracture. This happens for various reasons related to ageing, too little calcium in the diet, a decrease in the female sex hormone oestrogen, and lack of exercise.

If you are already going through the menopause or are over it, it is not too late to start taking regular exercise and to consider extra calcium in the diet, as well as a course of hormone replacement therapy (HRT) if your doctor recommends it. Such precautions could mean that you will avoid a painful wrist or hip fracture later in life.

Many local authorities run special exercise classes for the 'over fifties' or 'over sixties'. These are specially geared for older people who may need to take special care of their backs and joints. Enquire at your local reference library.

*   *   *

The arguments for taking up exercise are very strong. You will feel better, look better, sleep better and are very likely to live longer and have fewer aches, pains and serious illnesses.

Try not to put it off – get started as soon as you can, and encourage the rest of the family to join you!

USEFUL BOOKS

Why Exercise? by David Ashton and Bruce Davies, Blackwell
Food For Sport by Karen Inge and Peter Brukner, The Kingswood Press
Fitness and the Urban Walker by Eric Taylor, Blandford
Health and Fitness for Over-40s by B. Watson, Stanley Paul
Physical Fitness, Royal Canadian Air Force Exercises, Penguin
F/40 – Fitness on Forty Minutes a Week by Malcolm Carruthers and Alistair Murray, Futura
Age and Vitality by Irene Gore, Age Concern
Exercise without Exercises by Christopher Pardoe, Merlin Books

4 Enjoyable Sex Life

BY ANTONIA ROWLANDSON

YOUNG TEENAGERS

However much a young person has been told about sex and relationships, there is always a great deal that can only be learned through practical experience. Initial explorations of sexuality can be both extremely exciting *and* fraught with misery and uncertainty. But with the right approach, first sexual experiences can be very enjoyable.

Some basic knowledge about sexual functioning is obviously a good idea before you start relationships. Unfortunately everyone assumes that in this enlightened age all teenagers have more than enough sex education. But there are still many who don't seem to get enough of the right information. Sex-related problems – including unwanted pregnancies – are still common in the teenage years. Some parents tend to assume that their children get all the information they need from their school and friends, and so spend very little time discussing sex and related issues with their children.

Don't believe everything your friends tell you or that you read in magazines, but try to get accurate information and advice from books written by specialists or from organizations such as The Family Planning Association.

The more information you have, the easier it will be for you to form your own opinions about sex and relationships. Having clear-cut ideas about these things is particularly important these days when there are so few rules and social expectations to guide you.

THE FIRST TIME

Some women looking back at their first sexual experiences don't remember them as being very enjoyable. Some had sex just because they thought all their friends were already involved in sexual relationships. They didn't find their partners particularly attractive or special so weren't very aroused and found the experience painful and uncomfortable. They also felt guilty or were worried about getting pregnant. Boys may boast about their first experiences but often they feel that the first attempts are all over quickly and don't quite live up to their expectations.

First sexual encounters are much more likely to be enjoyable if they are with someone to whom you are strongly attracted and also that you know and like reasonably well – someone you can trust, talk to and relax with. You can't learn everything about sex from a book – it's not like maths or cookery where if you know the right formula or recipe you have a good chance of success – but if your first experiences are with someone with whom you can discuss the physical and emotional aspects of sex, and with whom you can laugh about its more amusing aspects, you will learn to enjoy it much more quickly, and hopefully with much less distress.

One practical aspect of sex which isn't always discussed, perhaps because of reluctance to draw attention to differences between boys and girls, is that arousal is much less straight-forward in girls than in boys. Boys become sexually aroused very easily – most teenage boys will have experienced the embarrass-ment of erections at inappropriate times. But for girls arousal is a longer process and often more dependent on emotions. During arousal the vagina becomes lubricated and the sex organs swell and move their positions slightly. A woman will probably find sex uncomfortable if these changes have not taken place, so it is important that her partner takes time to arouse her, both emotionally and physically, before attempting to have sex.

It is possible to have a physical relationship with someone without having full penetrative sex. Hugging, kissing and touch-ing each other's genitals, perhaps until orgasm is reached, can often be just as satisfying.

However, some people have a strong urge to have full sexual experiences at an early age and to have many different partners. If you feel like this, it is worth considering why this might be in your case. Perhaps you don't have much confidence or self-esteem and are tempted to have sex with someone just to get their approval or affection, or maybe you have been led to think that this is the way to behave by books, films and advertising.

Everyone has to make their own decision about when they begin to have sex and with how many partners, but it is worth remembering that a lot of partners doesn't necessarily mean a good sex life. In fact a succession of less-than-satisfactory relationships may even eventually put you off sex. Also the more sexual partners you have, the more likely you are to pick up sexually transmitted infections, particularly if you don't use condoms all the time.

However, even if you wait to have sex with someone with whom you have a special relationship and it doesn't seem to be all that enjoyable, don't be disappointed. Like most things, sex gets better with time and practice. Masturbation before you have sexual relationships with others is a good way of finding out what excites you most, and you can then use this knowledge to guide your partner to touch or stroke you in the right places. Learning to explore a new partner's body and finding out what gives him or her pleasure is also an important part of enjoyment in sex – giving pleasure is often just as much fun, and as arousing, as receiving it.

And never go further than you want to, or do things that you don't want to do. Partners who don't respect your feelings are probably not worth bothering about.

Contraception

Make sure you get some advice on contraception before you start having any sort of sexual contact. You should *never* have unprotected sex – unwanted pregnancy, or simply worrying about it, will not add to your sexual enjoyment. Go to your local family planning clinic for advice, and read **Contraception** in the A-Z section of this book.

LATE TEENS AND EARLY TWENTIES

Many people don't start having proper sexual relationships until their late teens or their twenties. When you start makes absolutely no difference. Everyone is unique and will have different desires, attitudes and opportunities, and you're not going to be 'better' at sex or enjoy it more because you started at an early age. When you start, what you do and with whom is up to you alone – you are unlikely to enjoy a sexual relationship if you're having sex just because you think you ought to.

One-night stands may be quite common in this age group, particularly for those who are living away from home for the first time, perhaps living in a flat with friends or at university. The desire to have new experiences and to experiment can be very strong but although some people find one-night stands very enjoyable at the time, they can also be rather unsatisfactory in the cold light of the morning. Furthermore, the more sexual partners you have, the greater the risk of disease.

An enjoyable sex life and happy sexual relationships depend to a large extent on what sort of person you are and how you approach those relationships. A selfish person who has little concern for the feelings of other people may get some physical pleasure from sex but a satisfying sexual and emotional relationship will be more difficult to sustain.

Some measure of confidence and self-esteem is also vital if you are going to enjoy sex. If you don't think much of yourself, then other people won't respect you either. You may end up having sex with partners who aren't necessarily right for you just to get attention and some sort of affection. Do try to be yourself — pretending to be someone that you aren't will probably lead to misery, as you will tend to attract the wrong kind of partners who are unlikely to make you happy.

Happiness in sex also involves keeping your attitudes to sex and sexual situations under control. Don't go further than you want to just to keep up with your friends, and don't let sex dominate your life. Non-sexual friendships and relationships with your family can be much more lasting and supportive than sexual relationships, so invest time in these and in keeping up a wide range of interests outside study and work.

HOMOSEXUALITY

Homosexuality describes the preference, in men or women, for sexual and emotional relationships with those of the same sex. Homosexual men generally refer to themselves as 'gay', homosexual women as 'lesbian'. Around five per cent of the male population are exclusively homosexual in adult life. A much higher proportion have had sexual relations with another man at least once. These figures are lower for women. Homosexuality is no longer regarded as a disorder, although in certain countries it remains illegal for religious or other reasons. It is a part of human society, and is in no way associated with psychological or physical abnormalities. The apparently homosexual adolescent can be sure of emotional and sexual fulfilment in adult life, although the pressure within society to conform may mean that a full acceptance of his or her sexuality may take a little longer than for a heterosexual. Many people experience sex with both male and female partners before establishing their sexual preference. For some, physical relations with both sexes continue into adulthood. These people are known as bisexual.

Most homosexuals will establish long-term loving relationships with an adult partner. Homosexuals are not a threat to children, and homosexuality cannot be 'acquired' through chance encounters or childhood experimentation. In fact, the 'causes' of a homosexual preference are unknown, and for most homosexuals are not relevant. Homosexual is how they are and how they wish to be.

Because of the nature of the physical relationship between men, which may, more often than between men and women, involve oral and anal sex, certain sexually transmitted diseases are more common among promiscuous homosexuals than among heterosexuals. These include hepatitis and AIDS. Homosexual women are not at increased risk of these diseases.

Sexually active homosexual men will usually be aware of the risks associated with promiscuity, and should take the same precautions as anyone else to prevent themselves becoming infected or giving an infection to their partners (see **Sex, Safe**).

ENJOYING SEX IN A PERMANENT RELATIONSHIP OR MARRIAGE

Once you have found someone who is a good friend and lover and with whom you want to spend a lot of time, or even the rest of your life, you may find your sexual enjoyment increases considerably. At last many of the insecurities and lack of trust which can interfere with sexual relationships are resolved and you can both relax and enjoy yourselves. But unfortunately some couples find that this satisfaction can, in a few years, turn to boredom and lack of interest, so that sexual activity gradually decreases. The demands of work and the arrival of children can also limit opportunities for sex and cause exhaustion, contributing further to the decline in sexual activity. To awaken your interest in sex, try to have sex in a different place, perhaps in the shower, or at a different time – last thing at night is often the time when people are most exhausted and arousal can be difficult. If you have children, try to arrange a weekend away from them now and then to give you a chance to catch up on your sex life – and your sleep!

There are many good books that suggest in a tasteful and lighthearted style new ways of making love and of stimulating your partner. Reading one of these or a sexy novel together, discussing possible new sexual activities or sexual fantasies can often help rekindle the fire of the early days of your relationship. But never do anything unless both of you are entirely happy about it.

SEX IN LATER YEARS

Young people are always amazed to think that their parents enjoy active sex lives, but some couples continue to have sex well past the age of retirement, though perhaps with less exertion and frequency than in their youth. Sexual activity may be temporarily restricted by illness, for example, but a loving couple who have always enjoyed sex should be able to pick up their sexual activity again when everything is back to normal. One of the secrets of a healthy sex life in later years is to sustain sexual activity. Once a couple gets out of the habit of it, it can be quite difficult to start again. Also a healthy lifestyle with plenty of exercise, a good diet, and not too much drinking or smoking helps to keep the sex organs functioning well so that sex can still be enjoyed. Close physical contact of any kind, whether it involves full sex or not, can be extremely beneficial for the mental and physical well-being of elderly people.

One reason many couples stop enjoying sex and eventually give it up is that they don't seek professional help when the woman goes through the menopause. Many women sail through the menopause, when the ovaries cease producing oestrogen and periods stop, without any problems, but others suffer from depression, irritability, hot flushes, dry vagina and thinning of the vaginal walls, and repeated urinary infections – none of which is conducive to an enjoyable sex life.

It is well worth going to your doctor to talk about these problems, as there is much that can be done to help. A lubricant such as KY jelly, which you can buy from the chemist, may be all that you need. But it is also possible that you could benefit from hormone replacement therapy, in which your doctor prescribes a course of low-dose, natural hormones to make up for the decreased production by the ovaries. Many women find that this treatment relieves many of the problems associated with the menopause, and at the same time helps them to enjoy sex.

Other disabilities and illnesses in old age, and the gradual decline in sexual function, may also be obstacles to enjoyable sex. But if you want to go on enjoying sex the key is to be flexible. Change your lovemaking positions and explore new ways of giving each other pleasure – to accommodate the discomfort of a bad back, for example. And don't forget that mutual trust and support and the ability to communicate with each other in a sympathetic way are the basis of a good sexual relationship – at any age.

USEFUL BOOKS

First Love First Sex by Kaye Wellings, Thorsons (recommended by the Family Planning Association)

Sexual Happiness For Men and *Sexual Happiness for Women* both by Maurice Yaffé and Elizabeth Fenwick, Dorling Kindersley

Living, Loving and Ageing by Wendy Greengross and Sally Greengross, Age Concern

Contraception. Your Questions Answered by John Guilleband, Pitman

The Joy of Sex by Alex Comfort, Quartet

5 Safety in the Home

BY HAZEL COAD

Every year about 5,500 people die and about three million need medical treatment after an accident in the home. For all the security that the home symbolizes and the safety it should offer, almost as many people die in domestic accidents as on the road. A third of all injuries needing hospital treatment happen in the home.

The late sixties and throughout the seventies saw a downward trend in the number of fatal accidents at home, but since 1982 these figures have levelled off. Unfortunately in the case of non-fatal accidents there has been an overall increase in reported incidents. Statistics clearly show two vulnerable groups: children, particularly from birth to four years old, and elderly people. Children have the highest rate of accidents at home, while elderly people run the greatest risk of an accident proving fatal.

Making the home a safer place for young or old is often a matter of common sense. It need involve little or no cost but may necessitate rethinking the way we carry out ordinary, everyday activities that have become second nature.

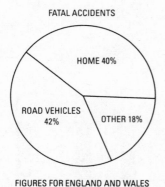

FATAL ACCIDENTS

HOME 40%

ROAD VEHICLES 42%

OTHER 18%

FIGURES FOR ENGLAND AND WALES

SOURCE: OPCS MORTALITY STATISTICS 1984

ACCIDENTS TREATED IN HOSPITAL

ROAD VEHICLES 9%

HOME 34%

OTHER 57%

ESTIMATES FOR ENGLAND AND WALES

SOURCE: HASS LOCATION OF ACCIDENT SURVEYS FOR 1984 SAMPLE HOSPITALS

HOME ACCIDENT RATES BY AGE AND SEX
(GREAT BRITAIN 1984)

RATE OF FATAL HOME ACCIDENTS PER MILLION
POPULATION PER YEAR

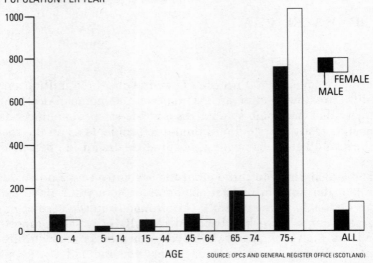

AGE   SOURCE: OPCS AND GENERAL REGISTER OFFICE (SCOTLAND)

RATE OF HOME ACCIDENTS RECEIVING MEDICAL TREATMENT
PER THOUSAND PER YEAR

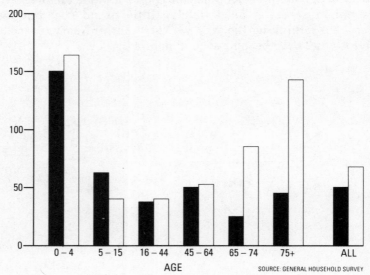

AGE   SOURCE: GENERAL HOUSEHOLD SURVEY

SAFETY FOR YOUNG CHILDREN

The birth of a new baby is a time of adjustment for parents, but for siblings it can be a time of intense rivalry. Jealous of the newcomer, an older child may cause an 'accident' to happen.

Cot death is still an ill-understood phenomenon. Some medical opinion suggests that such deaths are due to a sudden infectious or allergic reaction; other paediatricians are debating whether there is a link between whooping cough vaccine and cot deaths. Nevertheless, there are some basic guidelines for the safety of the sleeping child:

- Children under one year old should not have a pillow.

- Avoid open-textured bedclothes in which little fingers may get caught, very fluffy fabrics, the fibres of which a child may inhale, and tight-fitting top sheets or blankets.

- Don't let a pet sleep with a young child as this may cause suffocation.

- Don't allow your child to sleep with you if you have been drinking or taking medication. Either of these may make you sleep more heavily than usual and you may not awake if the child is in distress.

From a very early age (as soon as hand/eye co-ordination has been established at around three months) children instinctively put things in their mouth. But their sense of taste, which differentiates pleasant from unpleasant and good from bad, is almost non-existent until the age of around three years, as is their awareness of danger. From these early months, and especially when a child starts to crawl at around six months, close supervision is essential. This isn't always possible, so it is worth investing in a play pen and a stair gate. Both should conform to British Standard specifications. It is easy to identify those items that have British Standard approval by the familiar 'kite' mark, and a four-digit number preceded by the letters 'BS'.

Toys, too, should be BS approved. Horror stories of toy animals whose eyes can easily be pulled out, and the use of toxic paint, have highlighted the desirability of buying reputable goods, albeit slightly more expensive, which conform to a national standard. Toys should be appropriate to the age of the child: what is perfectly safe in the hands of a seven-year-old – for example a construction kit – could prove lethal to a baby. So watch yours if he or she is playing with older children.

Some foods are hazardous to young children. Nuts, for example, are small and easily inhaled, often salty and, if lodged in the respiratory tract, can be a source of irritation and infection. Because they are hard they don't break up during coughing and don't dissolve.

Statistics from the Home Accident Deaths Database (HADD) set up by the Department of Trade and Industry's Consumer Safety Unit show that suffocation and choking are second only to house fires as the main cause of fatal accidents in children between birth and four years old. Too often parents will go out and leave a young child sleeping unattended, or in the care of a teenage babysitter. It sounds unbelievable but it happens, and there can be little wonder that, if a fire does break out, the babysitter cannot cope with the emergency and young lives are lost. No one under the age of sixteen can legally be held responsible for the care of others.

In the league table of causes of fatal accidents to young children, falls come third. But falls are the most common cause of non-fatal accidents requiring medical attention in the under-four age group. Around 2,000 children every year are injured by falls on the stairs, while nearly 3,500 are injured in falls on the same level or between two levels. Falls on the same level occur mainly in the kitchen, living/dining areas, and outside in gardens and yards. Possible explanations for these figures are the presence of hard flooring in the kitchen, furniture in dining areas on which a child may sustain injury, and unyielding, rough surfaces outside which can cause fractures and abrasions.

Falls between two levels occur mostly in the bedroom, possibly from beds and bunk beds, and in the living/dining areas, perhaps from chairs and high chairs. A stair safety gate should be removed as soon as a child starts to try to climb over it; for the safety of young and old, rugs and carpets should be well secured, worn lino replaced, and slippery floor surfaces avoided. Climbing is part of a child's exploration of the immediate environment and is inevitable, so make sure that furniture and shelves cannot be tipped over or pulled down.

By far the highest incidence of accidental poisoning is among the very young: approaching 2,000 cases in the under-fours, and around 130 in the five to fourteen age groups. Keep all household cleaning fluids and decorating materials in locked cupboards, and avoid storing these substances in, for example, old lemonade bottles.

A child may suffer lasting damage from burns and scalds, and kitchens are a particular danger zone. Ideally, children should be kept out of the kitchen when cooking is in progress. If this is not possible, make sure that saucepan handles are turned away from the front edge of the cooker. Electricity power points should be shuttered (safety covers are available from mother and baby shops), and flexes and cables must be kept out of reach.

Though it seems to be stating the obvious to suggest that prams and pushchairs should be stable, this point is often forgotten when a heavy shopping bag is hung at one end. A shopping tray under the pram is much safer. Other factors to consider when investing in this major item for a child are: does the pram/pushchair comply with British Standards? Is there a harness for the child? Do the brakes operate on both sets of wheels and not just one?

Every area of the house and garden should be considered from the angle of your child's safety: door locks inside and out, and especially on the garage or garden shed, should be raised so that the child doesn't lock him or herself in. Consider replacing plate glass with safety glass. Run cold water in the bath before hot water, and never leave a child alone while bathing. Decorative balcony rails, or those with any horizontal bars, are easy to climb – and easy to fall from.

SAFETY FOR ELDERLY PEOPLE

Safety features to consider for elderly people start from a recognition of the effects of declining health and faculties. A child may meet with an accident while exploring the new and unfamiliar with critical senses that have not yet developed. Most accidents to the elderly occur while doing the familiar – tasks that have been carried out countless times before and which are now second nature. But failing to take account of loss of agility, poor sight, hearing impairment or the presence of some physical disability may make even the most innocent of activities potentially dangerous.

The Consumer Safety Unit's Home Accidents Surveillance System (HASS) has compiled statistics that show falls to be the most common cause of non-fatal accidents in the over-sixty-fives, with a significant increase in incidents when over seventy-five, particularly among women. And falls are also the most common cause of death in people over sixty-five years of age, and there are almost three times as many deaths from falls in the over-seventy-fives.

Loneliness, depression, and poor diet are some of the other factors that affect an old person's ability to recover from a fall. All too often he or she will succumb to a secondary problem, such as a blood clot or chest infection, and this may prove fatal.

To make the home a safer place for an old person, it is first necessary to recognize that there is a problem. To some, this may signify the end of their independence but in fact, accepting that there is a problem and dealing with it early on is more likely to lead to a happy, safe existence in the home of their choice.

The house should be well lit, and the lighting should be even to avoid confusing shadows. Light switches must be placed within easy reach, and a bedside light, night light, or even a torch, will reduce the danger from trips to the bathroom during the night.

The homes of elderly people are often cluttered with furniture and bags and boxes containing the memories of several decades. While it would be heartless to suggest disposing of this, plenty of manoeuvring space is important, especially if the old person needs to use a walking stick or walking frame for stability.

Rugs, mats and carpets, including stair carpets, should be nailed down; loose mats are just asking to be tripped over. Worn lino or floor tiles need to be replaced, and non-slip floorings in the bathroom and kitchen are advisable.

An extra banister rail will make getting up and down stairs safer. If the time comes when even this extra aid is insufficient, consideration should be given to moving the bed to a downstairs room. If access to a toilet is then difficult, local community nursing services may be able to supply a commode for use in the new 'bedroom'. Alternatively, the social services department can offer financial help with installing a stair lift.

Small grab handles, sited at strategic points around the house, may prove helpful when getting up from an easy chair, for example, or negotiating steps at the front of the house or to the back garden. Getting out of comfortable lounge chairs frequently presents problems to the old and infirm. The seat height of all chairs in the house should be around 43 cm. Most dining chairs fit this specification and some easy chairs can be raised to this height on blocks, but a high seat or high-backed chair purpose built for the elderly may prove a sound investment.

Baths are dangerous places because of the combination of hard and slippery surfaces. A small seat in the bath and a rail on the wall will facilitate getting in and out. A rubber mat or non-slip adhesive strips on the floor of the bath will help prevent feet from slipping.

A rail on the wall beside the toilet, possibly in combination with a high seat extension, will make it safer to use. Old people should be persuaded not to rely on the handbasin, towel rail, or toilet-paper holder for support.

Advice on all aspects of safety equipment is available from disabled living centres or from social services departments.

As mobility becomes more difficult, food intake, and the nutrition gained from food, decreases. The winter months close in, and the cost of heating the house appears formidable. All elderly people run the risk of hypothermia. Early warning signs are drowsiness, confusion, slurred speech, and a drop in body temperature from 37° C to 35° C or less. It is preferable to heat one room well rather than a number of them inadequately, and autumn may be the time to consider using one room as a bedsitter. Several layers of clothing are recommended and, as a high proportion of body heat is lost through the head, it is wise to wear a warm hat.

Oil and paraffin heaters are not recommended for use by the elderly. An electric fan heater, or oil-fired electric radiator, is considered the safest type of portable heater. The Gas Board will carry out a free safety check of all appliances for senior citizens.

That old faithful of heating appliances, the hot-water bottle, should be replaced as soon as signs of perishing appear. A hot-water bottle should never be used with an electric blanket. Don't let an elderly person keep medication at the bedside. Waking up during the night, he or she may forget that a dose was taken earlier and take another, resulting in an overdose. Dosage specifications should be observed at all times, though for medicines that are bought over the counter some elderly people may find the adult dose excessive.

Old people living alone may feel reassured that help can be summoned in an emergency if supplied with a personal alarm. This could be a body-worn device, like the simple anti-mugging alarm, or a more sophisticated radio alarm which can have a range of up to 100 metres. An alternative is a system of pull cords or push buttons situated around the home, which the elderly person can activate in time of distress and which will trigger an alarm or flashing 'help' sign in a front window or door.

Outside, pathways should be kept free of debris and material such as leaves, which can become very slippery in the rain. The dustbin should be easily accessible and kept in a well-lit area. It is recommended that greenhouse glass and cloches should be replaced with plastic, and that plate glass around the house be replaced with safety glass.

HASS has made an interesting analysis of the occurrence of non-fatal accidents in the home: more accidents happen in May and July than in any other months, with February and November the safest months. During the week, most accidents occur on Sundays, with Thursday the safest day, closely followed by Wednesday and Friday. But be careful between four o'clock in the afternoon and eight in the evening, as this is the time when by far the most accidents happen. So, if you want to minimize your chances of an accident at home, after taking heed of all the advice in this chapter, do whatever you have to do between midnight and seven in the morning, on a Thursday in February.

USEFUL BOOKS

Play it Safe, Health Education Authority, London
Safety in the Home, Health Education Authority, London
First Steps to Safety, Royal Society for the Prevention of Accidents, Canon House, The Priory, Queensway, Birmingham B4 6BS

6 Stress and Mental Health

BY DR JOAN GOMEZ

One person's emotional meat and drink is another's intolerable stress. An IRA bomb attack injuring a bus-load of soldiers in London meant stimulus, with a chance to use his skills to the full, for the chief surgeon: he worked all night without strain. But that bombing caused persistent nightmares and other anxiety symptoms to some unharmed bystanders, while the soldiers' relatives suffered acute distress. Unlike the surgeon these others felt helpless. The essence of stress is the individual's sense of his or her incapacity to respond effectively to a situation.

Stress may arise from a single event such as divorce or a traffic accident, or from a series of experiences, especially if they follow on within a matter of months. What might seem trivial in normal circumstances may become the last straw after months of stressful incidents. Having to move house, followed by the death of a pet dog may plunge someone into severe depression if she has built her life round the animal since the recent loss of her husband.

Stress comes in several styles: physical, emotional, or more often, a combination of the two. It can occur as separate events, single or repetitive, or a long-term state of tension. It can crop up at work or at home.

Stress can cause physical, psychosomatic (in which an emotional state underlies a physical condition) and psycho-emotional symptoms. The latter are always present. Women are generally better at recognizing and expressing it, whereas men tend to (and are expected to) deny distress, depression or anxiety. Their pent-up feelings are forced into physical effects, from indigestion to a coronary attack.

One of the problems of the modern world is the lack of an appropriate active response to stress. Neither fight nor flight is possible when, strapped in the car seat, a driver sees approaching danger in the shape of a top-heavy truck, or his girlfriend sitting beside him says that she has found another man. Something has to give – what and how depends on the victim's make-up and reaction-type, and how he or she perceives the situation: transiently unpleasant or devastating.

By far the most common stress symptoms are vague, often unrecognized, and attract little sympathy. There may be an out-of-sorts feeling, difficulty concentrating, mental and physical tiredness, and a short temper. Normal tact disappears, making relationships uncomfortable. Competence and confidence decline, at first imperceptibly. Drinking, smoking, overeating or gambling may increase but only make matters worse.

This type of stress reaction merges into one kind of depressive illness. Symptoms are poor, unrefreshing sleep, restlessness, and failure to find any satisfaction in usually pleasurable pursuits, including work. There is a tendency to put off decision-making and to avoid decisive action, a loss of sociability and, most importantly, of self-esteem.

As depression becomes worse, the self seems worthless, the outside world meaningless, the future hopeless. The sufferer wakes early and longs for the day to end. Food has no taste, sex no joy and the whole of the past life seems to have been wasted. Work, or indeed any activity, becomes impossible. In this mood there is a big risk of the sufferer resigning from a good job or turning down a worthwhile proposition: a reaction that will be regretted later. If life no longer seems worth living suicidal ideas can slide into the mind. Successful suicide or non-fatal self-harm both arise when the subject is suffering stress beyond his or her tolerance level and can see no other escape.

Some people may respond to overstress differently by developing an anxiety state. Acute anxiety may be caused by a personal attack such as mugging; or discovering that a close companion has the AIDS virus; or because an important examination is due soon and failure is a terrifying possibility. Acute anxiety symptoms include palpitations, trembling, vomiting, or very rapid breathing. In the summer examination season of 1987 two physically healthy young students died suddenly – from examination anxiety.

Fortunately anxiety is usually far less intense. Acute anxiety was a rare response to battle stress in places such as Vietnam, or Beirut, but less severe symptoms are common: difficulty in getting to sleep, upsetting dreams, endless worrying, apprehension about something relevant or something apparently pointless. Fear amounting to panic may become associated with, for example, travel, lifts or social situations. Menstrual periods and digestion may be disturbed in stress-related anxiety.

Chronic tension is closely related to anxiety. It tends to develop in perfectionists who are exposed to long-lasting stress, such as an unhappy marriage, an invalid relative to care for, a job with too much or too little responsibility, or financial problems. Tension shows in miserable and unpredictable moods, tears in some, and quarrelsomeness in others. It may also cause many physical symptoms: migraine and other headaches, backache and muscle pains, including over the heart area, painful periods and other abdominal disturbances, high blood pressure, heart attack, peptic ulcer, or asthma.

Some fraught and tense people will turn increasingly to distractive habits such as alcohol, tobacco, tranquillizers, food or drugs. Others when stressed and tense unconsciously attempt to reduce their discomfort by obsessional rituals of counting, checking and repeating even their most trivial actions. Living slows to a snail's pace and nothing is accomplished.

In contrast to the cautious, obsessional personality is the reckless action man or woman who boils over under pressure into angry, antisocial behaviour and violence. People enduring the difficult stresses of unemployment in the inner cities are statistically more likely to kill or commit suicide. Less dramatic but similar responses are shoplifting, drug abuse, promiscuity, delinquency and minor street crime – usually in an adolescent who has few inner resources as yet and inadequate steadying external support.

People suffering from schizophrenia may suffer an acute relapse after upsetting life events or long-term social stress, particularly if they are trying to cope without tranquillizing medication.

Everyone has limits and will break down if subjected to too much stress, but some are more prone to breakdowns than others. Vulnerability factors can be divided into those that are unalterable and those that can be adjusted or improved. Among the former are such factors as a genetic disposition to one of the two major psychiatric illnesses, schizophrenia and manic depression (fortunately these are comparatively rare), and a life-experience that includes the loss of a parent in childhood. If the parent has died the child grows up to be more vulnerable to depression; if the loss is a consequence of divorce or desertion the child is more likely to become neurotic or to react with antisocial behaviour when put under strain. Unhappiness, abuse or milder personal insecurity in childhood leaves the adult less confident to cope in later life, as does missing schooling, from whatever cause. An introverted, conscientious and conscience-laden personality, with a limited capacity for laughter, makes a person more likely to succumb to stress.

Men differ from women in that they report fewer symptoms of minor emotional disorder, but on the other hand they do not stand up to the stress of bereavement as well as women, nor to serious illness in themselves. Married men are cushioned from the worst effects of stress more than single men, and more than homosexuals in a steady partnership. A mother with three or more children aged under fifteen is vulnerable to stress, but their father is not. Having no job outside the home is another risk factor for women, particularly in big cities. Adolescence and the post-retirement years are particularly vulnerable periods for everyone, plus the years around menopause for women, when self-confidence is low and children leave home.

SPECIAL SITUATIONS OF STRESS

Disasters

The Bradford football stadium fire of 1985, the Zeebrugge ferry sinking in March 1987, and later that year the Hungerford massacre by a gunman gone mad occurred respectively in a happy sports crowd, to soldiers and holidaymakers returning home, and in a peaceful English village in summer. The incongruity, sudden-ness and scale of catastrophes such as these makes the effects more severe for the people involved: worse, for instance than loss or disability resulting from a domestic accident, or bereavement through disease. There is less normality to hold on to, and there is an urgent need of support, someone with whom to weep and to talk it all out: preferably someone near and dear, but someone for certain.

Supportive human involvement should be given for at least a year. At some time during the first two months the victim is likely to feel he or she has got over it, only to relapse more severely later, when public and neighbourly sympathy has subsided. Persistent anxiety and nightmares are especially likely to be troublesome. Two years after the Aberfan disaster in 1966, in which a school was destroyed and many children killed, the villagers still suffered two or three times more physical and psychiatric illness than previously. At that time the importance of talking, even when sufferers were reluctant, was not realized.

Burglary, mugging and rape

These are equally sudden, unexpected disasters from outside, but intensely personal. Added to anxiety and depression, the common responses to stress, are humiliation, anger and – unexpectedly – guilt. All of these emotions damage the victim if they are kept bottled up: they must be expressed verbally and in tears, over and over again, until they have lost their sting. This usually takes at least three months. In the case of rape the woman feels so defiled and ashamed that it is difficult for her to tell her family and partner about it: it is vital that she does so or her ability to have affectionate relationships will be permanently impaired.

Stresses concerned with work and family

Most stresses are more run-of-the-mill, affecting both people in work and those unemployed.

BURNOUT

Burnout is the stress disorder *par excellence* of the person at work. It affects workers such as casualty officers, police officers, teachers and troubleshooters, who work directly with people and perceive themselves as responsible. At the other extreme, boredom can cause burnout in a job that is repetitive and carries little acknowledged responsibility or value.

Emotional exhaustion shows itself in continual tiredness, edginess, proneness to accidents, awkwardness with colleagues, and a sense of low achievement. The burnt-out is in urgent need of treatment. To provide reward and satisfaction to the worker a job needs plenty of variety both in content and routine. Overstressed workers need verbal as well as monetary reward, and interested supervision to underscore the importance of the job, as well as opportunities for discussion with colleagues.

If no change in working conditions seems likely the stressed worker must improve his or her out-of-work life to provide sufficient stimulus.

UNEMPLOYMENT

Whether it is caused by so-called early retirement, redundancy, real retirement or from being surplus to requirements from day one of leaving school or college, unemployment is a blow to one's self-esteem. It hits like a bereavement: first comes a shock to the system after years of little freedom; then a sense of holiday – time to pull a weed, paint a door – which lasts about three weeks. After that the stress sets in: money becomes a source of worry; family tensions increase – particularly if the partner's career is flourishing; energy, interest and drive diminish; depression creeps over everything.

The first important step to recovery is to impose a structure on the day, for example not getting up late. The second is to value work as work, whether paid or unpaid. The third is to refresh existing outside contacts and to explore new ones. A new life plan needs drawing up, with new horizons and achievable objectives.

WOMEN

For women even more than men emotional conflicts and disappointments are a major stress. A wife whose only adult contact of importance is her husband is dangerously dependent on him for interest, sympathy and entertainment as well as affection, and he may feel oppressed by the situation. Women who have some paid employment have a more positive sense of self and fewer psychological disorders.

Communication problems are at the root of much marital and family tension. Both partners tend to assume that the other one must know how he or she feels and thinks. Very often the assumption is false, and such mistakes can be lessened by asking specifically, and in good time.

ADOLESCENTS

Adolescents need space – from their families – and support without critical comment. Even implied criticism can be so stressful for a timid seventeen-year-old that she may develop anorexia nervosa.

The keynotes for adolescents to help them survive inevitable stress are to keep in good repair a confiding relationship with at least one person, and to maintain good relationships with the extended family, colleagues, friends and neighbours. It is also important to keep in good physical health, taking medication if advised, moderate any potentially bad habits and nourish a sense of fun, while maintaining a healthy balance between study and social activities.

Tips for reducing stress at home

- Improve what you eat so that you can benefit from a healthy, balanced diet.

- Take regular exercise – at least half an hour three times a week. Frequent moderate exercise is better for you than occasional violent exercise.

- Make time for yourself every day – even as little as twenty minutes can make all the difference.

- Involve your partner and family in any problems you may have and encourage them to involve you. Tensions inevitably build up in any family but they are better released than bottled up. However, think carefully about an appropriate time for this release – late at night when everyone is tired may not be the best time to mention your partner's most irritating habit.

- Make sure you have interests outside the home. Research shows that those who are too dependent on the home for their every need are more prone to the ill-effects of stress.

- Try to get the sleep you need. This may vary from four to ten hours a night for different people but, as every sleep-deprived parent of young children will tell you, a good night's sleep makes stressful events the next day less difficult to cope with.

- To reduce your stress level try relaxation exercises. There are many different types but they are all intended to relax the muscles of the body. Here is one technique:

1. Choose a regular and quiet time of the day when you know

you can have twenty minutes undisturbed. Disconnect the phone or put it on the answering machine.

2. Make sure the room is warm (but not hot) and quiet. Most relaxation teachers do not recommend background music.

3. Loosen any tight clothing then choose a comfortable position. Any position will do provided it can be held with minimum effort. One is the 'coachman position' in which you sit in a chair with the head and body leaning forwards and the forearms resting on the thighs. Another is the 'lotus position' which yoga teachers recommend.

4. Make an effort to clear your mind of any worrying thoughts.

5. Breathe deeply and regularly – about fourteen breaths a minute for two minutes – and imagine you are feeling happy, drowsy and warm. Think of your favourite place.

6. Gradually start to relax all the muscles of your body. Begin at one end, for example the toes, and then systematically work to the other end. Think of each group of muscles in isolation. Some people find it helps to tense the muscles first to identify them before relaxation. Spend about ten minutes relaxing in this way and a further ten minutes gradually coming back to normal. You will find yourself greatly refreshed for the rest of the day.

- Meditation is useful for some people. It is beyond the scope of this book to describe the techniques in detail but they vary from formal techniques like transcendental meditation to your own techniques which you know work for you.

Tips for reducing stress at work

- Consider changing jobs to reduce the time spent travelling to and from work. A recent survey showed that over half the white-collar workers in London found travelling and working in London stressful.

- Reduce the level of noise. Noise over eighty decibels is a common source of irritation and mental and physical stress. Internal noise (e.g. from machines) can be reduced by carpeting, subdividing large offices or workshops, and ensuring noisy machines are fitted with 'noise guards' and located away from people.

  External noise can be reduced by locating workplaces away

from heavy traffic areas or airports and by such measures as double-glazing.

- Work areas should be at a comfortable temperature. For desk work 20–21°C is an ideal temperature. Humidity levels should be between forty and fifty per cent.

- Attention should be paid to the colour of the workplace decorations. Too much red causes restlessness, loss of concentration and over-stimulation. Too much blue causes lethargy and loss of vitality. Yellows and oranges are popular with workers.

- Take holidays to give you a chance to step back and think about your life and priorities from a distance. They will refresh you and make you less prone to the ill-effects of stress. If you have a boring job take an active, exciting holiday; if your job is very busy and stimulating take a peaceful holiday. If you work in the city go to the countryside or sea. In these ways you will achieve a balance in your life which reduces stress.

- Set yourself attainable career goals and when you have achieved them learn to recognize and enjoy the fact that you have achieved them. Too many people always imagine the grass is greener elsewhere and never allow themselves the pleasure of enjoying their successes.

- If work is very stressful do not be ashamed to 'let off steam' to your partner or close friend. Studies show that people who keep a stiff upper lip at all times do worse than others who 'let go' at an appropriate time. Others find that what psychologists call a 'displacement activity' helps: they run or play squash or go to aerobics classes to burn up some of the adrenaline produced by stresses at work.

USEFUL BOOKS

Executive Stress by Donald Norfolk, Arrow
The Human Zoo by Desmond Morris, Jonathan Cape
Stress Without Distress by Hans Selye, Hodder and Stoughton
Overcoming Depression by Andrew Stanway, Hamlyn
Anxiety, Nervousness and Depression by F. R. C. Casson, Family Doctor Publications

The Mind Gymnasium by Denis Postle, Macmillan
Stress Management. A Comprehensive Guide to Wellness by
 Edward Charlesworth and Ronald Nathan, Souvenir Press
Women and Tranquillizers by Celia Haddon, Sheldon Press

7 Screening and Preventive Medicine

BY DR MICHAEL SPIRA

To enjoy good health you need to do two things: one, live a healthy lifestyle, and two, take advantage of every aspect of preventive medicine that is available. It is this second feature that this chapter is concerned with.

Most people imagine the role of doctors is to cure illness, to make people well again. But this is a little like keeping the bath water topped up by leaving the taps running rather than using a plug to prevent water running out of the bath. Far better to prevent water loss with a plug than to have to keep replacing it from the tap. The tap is the traditional curing role of doctors whereas the plug is the more effective preventive role. Preventing coronary heart disease, for example, saves far more lives than treating the disease.

There are two main elements of preventive medicine. The first is screening, which means looking for early signs of disease with the intention of taking steps to prevent the disease becoming severe or to minimize its effects. The second is preventing disease from occurring, the most important area being immunization against infectious conditions.

The process of screening and immunization goes on throughout life from before birth into old age.

BEFORE BIRTH

Screening and preventive medicine are aimed at two people – the mother (antenatal care) and the unborn child (prenatal screening).

Antenatal Care

There are several components of antenatal visits, which usually take place monthly in early pregnancy and increase to weekly towards the end of pregnancy. These include:

- Physical examinations by the doctor or midwife to check the health of the mother and the baby and to see that the pregnancy is progressing satisfactorily.

- A blood test at the start of the pregnancy to test for anaemia, blood group, syphilis, rhesus and rubella antibodies. Blood is taken at fifteen to twenty weeks to test for a substance called alphafetoprotein, high levels of which point to fetal abnormalities (see Prenatal Screening below). Further blood tests at twenty-eight and thirty-six weeks check again for anaemia and for rhesus antibodies (if the mother is rhesus negative).

- Urine tests to detect urinary infection, pre-eclampsia and diabetes.

- Ultrasound scan to measure the growth of the fetus, to ensure that the placenta (afterbirth) is not in a position where it might cause problems during labour, and to check for obvious abnormalities in the baby.

- Amniocentesis and chorionic villus sampling (see below).

Prenatal Screening

There is one important difference between prenatal screening and all other types of screening. Instead of looking for conditions for which treatment is available prenatal screening detects disorders for which the only 'treatment' is termination of pregnancy.

The main test is called amniocentesis. This consists of the withdrawal of a small amount of fluid from the sac surrounding the baby in the womb in order to detect abnormalities of the fetus. It is carried out at sixteen to eighteen weeks when there is sufficient fluid present but it is not too late for the pregnancy to be terminated if necessary.

Several conditions are screened for. Lack of development of the brain, known as anencephaly, occurs about once in 500 pregnancies, and the affected baby would either be stillborn or would die within a few days of birth. Severe forms of spina bifida, a condition in which the bones of part of the lower spine are not properly formed, leaving part of the spinal cord exposed, may be detected too, although in about eighty per cent of cases a simple and cheap test on the mother's blood will detect an abnormally high amount of a substance called alphafetoprotein.

Because amniocentesis involves a small risk of miscarriage, the test is carried out only if the mother has already had a baby affected by a congenital abnormality such as Down's syndrome or if she is over the age of forty (when the possibility of a Down's syndrome baby is greater than average) or if she is over thirty-five and has had several miscarriages or unexplained stillbirths.

Another group of conditions screened for are those in which females carry the genes (the carriers of genetic information) but only males are affected. If a woman has previously given birth to a baby with one of these sex-linked disorders, such as haemophilia or Duchenne's muscular dystrophy, or if there is a family history of such a disorder, amniocentesis will show if the baby is a male and therefore whether it *might* be affected, so that the parents may then wish to consider termination of pregnancy.

One problem with amniocentesis is that results are often not available until three weeks after the test is done, so that if termination is necessary it may not be performed until around the twentieth week of pregnancy. For this reason chorionic villus sampling (CVS) is becoming more widely available.

The developing embryo has two membranes, of which the outer one is called the chorion. Outgrowths, known as chorionic villi, invade the wall of the mother's womb and serve as a means of transferring nutrients from the mother's blood to the embryo. Later in the pregnancy part of the chorion is formed into the placenta.

It is now possible to look for congenital abnormalities by drawing off cells from chorionic villi through the cervix during the first three months of pregnancy. At the time of writing the risk of inducing abortion is not known, but if CVS proves reliable, early termination, if necessary, would be possible.

GENETIC COUNSELLING

Conditions that arise as a result of inheritance are called genetic disorders. They are much more common than is generally realized and occur in about one in twenty live births. Furthermore, long-term (chronic) disease in which inheritance plays some part occurs in about ten per cent of the adult population. Examples of such genetic conditions are haemophilia, sickle cell anaemia,

Huntington's chorea, muscular dystrophy, cleft lip, cleft palate, cystic fibrosis and Down's syndrome.

It is understandable that people with possible genetic disorders or with relatives who have genetic disorders want to know about the risks to themselves and their children. In addition first cousins who intend to have children together should know that there is a risk of genetic disorders.

Genetic counselling advises prospective parents. Often such advice is available from a GP, paediatrician or obstetrician, but in some cases advice is needed from a specialist trained to recognize rare genetic disorders.

Cancer

Fortunately very few cancers seem to be inherited. However, familial polyposis of the colon, a condition in which polyps develop in the large bowel, is so clearly inherited that careful screening and sigmoidoscope examination of the bowels of all relatives at risk is important. Other examples of malignant or potentially malignant inherited conditions are neurofibromatosis and retinoblastoma, an eye tumour. Breast cancer occurs most often in daughters of affected women and self-examination of the breasts is particularly important for such women.

CHILDHOOD SCREENING

The aims of screening and preventive medicine in childhood are:

- To prevent illness, mainly by immunization (see table).

- To detect and to correct defects, such as congenital heart disease and hypothyroidism, so that children may lead normal lives.

- To detect defects such as spina bifida, where treatment and training can avoid many problems so that children may lead as normal lives as possible.

Newborn babies

All newborn babies are screened for two conditions – phenylketonuria and hypothyroidism, the tests being carried out on a tiny specimen of blood obtained from pricking the baby's heel. Phenylketonuria is an inherited disorder resulting in the deficiency of a particular liver enzyme or chemical, which leads to mental retardation and fits. The harmful effects of the disease, once diagnosed, can be prevented by a diet low in an amino acid called phenylalanine. This involves substituting proprietary foods, known as casein hydrolysates, and amino acid mixtures for normal high-protein foods such as milk. Low-protein natural foods such as fruits and vegetables are allowed.

Congenital hypothyroidism, or underactive thyroid gland, is an important cause of mental retardation. The sooner the condition is diagnosed and the earlier treatment is started the fewer the effects of the illness.

Newborn babies are also examined for physical abnormalities such as spina bifida, Down's syndrome, congenital dislocation of the hip, congenital heart disease, and undescended testicles.

Children

During their pre-school years children are examined at child health clinics, run either by local health authorities or GPs. At six weeks old and then again some time between two and three years of age the GP and health visitor check on the general development of the child, as well as looking for specific problems such as mental and physical handicap, defects of vision and hearing, and behaviour disorders. If speech is poor at three years this aspect of a child's development will be kept under review so that speech therapy may be sought later if there is no improvement. The six-week check-up is also a suitable time for parents to discuss immunization plans with their doctor.

As the child grows older the parents may suspect problems with hearing or vision. For example, the child may always insist on the television being turned up very loud. Or at school the child may complain that he or she cannot see the blackboard unless sitting at the front of the class.

Further examinations take place during the school years and include, in the early teenage years, a simple physical test to detect scoliosis, a potentially painful and disabling twisting of the upper spine. Between the ages of eleven and thirteen all girls should be immunized against rubella.

Childhood immunization

	Diphtheria	Whooping cough	Tetanus	Polio	Measles	BCG	Rubella	Mumps
3 months	●	●	●	●				
4½ years	●	●	●	●				
8½–11 months	●	●	●	●				
15 months					●		●	●
4½ years	●		●	●				
11–13 years						●[1]	●[2]	
15–19 years			●	●				

[1] For children who have a negative turberculin test
[2] For girls only if missed earlier

THE HUMAN MOT

Although the human body is a wonder of biological engineering things can and do go wrong with it long before the end of its natural lifespan. Sadly, some illnesses are not detectable sufficiently early to be curable; this applies especially to certain kinds of cancer. But the good news is that there are many other diseases that can be detected at an early enough stage to prevent serious problems developing. For example, cancer of the cervix is easy both to detect and to cure. High blood pressure, too, is simple to detect, and if it is controlled by weight reduction, medication, or both, its harmful effects may be prevented or at least minimized.

A more comprehensive MOT might include a blood test, chest X-ray, electrocardiograph (known as an ECG) to test the heart, lung-function tests, and vision and hearing assessments. Some GPs will carry out this sort of screening but otherwise you might have to go to a private clinic.

The blood test is not in fact just one test but a dozen or more separate tests carried out on a single blood sample. Conditions looked for include various forms of anaemia, kidney disorders, liver problems such as alcohol damage, high cholesterol, and diabetes.

The ECG is a useful, though not infallible, screening test for coronary heart disease, which is the single commonest cause of middle-age death in the Western world.

Lung-function tests often provide reliable, objective evidence of the damaging effects on the lungs of smoking, and the results may encourage smokers to give up the nicotine habit.

The wide range of tests offered may be complemented by a consultation with a doctor, which includes a detailed medical history and physical examination. This is also an opportunity for the doctor to record the family history for risk factors, especially those associated with coronary heart disease. Smoking, over-weight and alcohol consumption may be noted, and appropriate advice given.

Perhaps the most useful benefit of such a comprehensive health assessment is the reassurance and boosting of confidence that stems from a set of normal results. But even the most comprehensive MOT is no substitute for a healthy lifestyle − avoiding tobacco, excess stress, and alcohol, eating a well-balanced diet, and taking a reasonable amount of exercise.

BREAST EXAMINATION

Discovering a lump in the breast can be a frightening experience. But rather than panic consider the facts:

- Often a lump is felt only before a period and disappears a few days after the start of the period. Do not worry about such a lump, which is completely harmless.

- Most breast lumps which do not disappear are *not* cancer. A lump is most likely to be either a cyst or a collection of fibrous tissue or gristle called a fibroadenoma. But because of the possibility of cancer you should always consult your doctor. Even a doctor may not be absolutely certain about it and you *may* have to have fluid removed from the lump via a needle, or part of the lump may need to be removed for examination. This is known as a biopsy. If you are advised to have these tests it is because it is better to be 100 per cent certain rather than only ninety-five per cent.

  Examining your breasts once a month takes only a few

moments and enables you to get to know what is normal for you. The best time is the last day of each period or, if you are no longer having periods, the same date of each calendar month, for example the first day of each month.

The changes you are looking for are:

1. Any change in the size of either breast.
2. Any change in either nipple, especially recent turning in of a nipple or discharge or bleeding from a nipple. Always inspect the inside of your bra for any signs of discharge of blood.
3. Any dimple or puckering of the skin of the breasts.

In order to look for any changes strip to the waist. Then examine your breasts and nipples in the following positions:

1. Stand or sit up straight in front of a mirror and look carefully at your breasts.
2. Raise your arms above your head and turn from side to side.
3. Lower and raise your arms again and check that each nipple moves the same distance.
4. *Gently* squeeze each nipple to check for any discharge or bleeding.
5. Lean forward and examine each breast and nipple in turn.
6. Lie down on your bed or carry out the next part of the examination whilst you are in the bath. With your left hand under your head use the flat of the fingers of your right hand, the fingers kept straight and close together, to examine your left breast. Start at the armpit and move across the breast above the nipple to the centre of your chest pressing in *gently* to feel for lumps. Then do the same again but lower down across the line of the nipple, and then again below the line of the nipple. Finally feel for lumps in the dip above your collarbone and in the armpit.
7. Examine your right breast in exactly the same way using your left hand.

Breast Screening Units

There are now many units offering screening for women, including breast screening, the recommended interval between visits being about three years. The procedure includes a clinical exam-

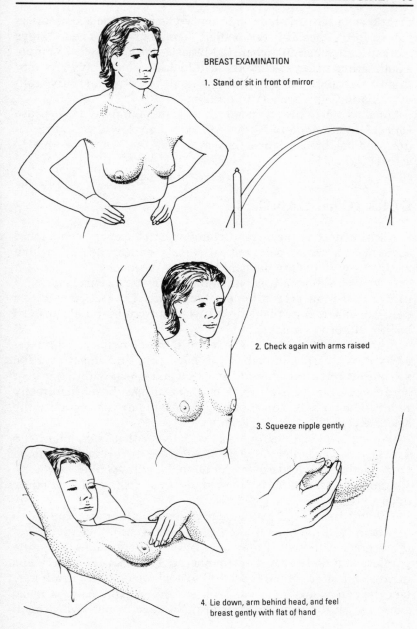

BREAST EXAMINATION

1. Stand or sit in front of mirror

2. Check again with arms raised

3. Squeeze nipple gently

4. Lie down, arm behind head, and feel breast gently with flat of hand

ination as described above and, for women over the age of thirty-five or forty, special X-rays called mammography. These X-rays are especially helpful when the breasts are large (when simple examination using the hands is difficult). The X-rays are very useful but are not infallible, which is why monthly self-examination remains very important.

Some women are worried that mammography may cause cancer. In fact modern X-rays use extremely low doses of radiation and no breast cancer has ever been shown to be due to screening.

CERVICAL CANCER

Cervical cancer is the second commonest cancer in women and accounts for three per cent of female cancer deaths, which compares with twenty per cent from breast cancer.

However, although it is one of the commonest cancers cervical cancer is also the easiest to detect and cure. The test, known as a cervical smear, is available to all women from their GPs or local health authority clinics.

Every sexually active woman should have a cervical smear test every three years, although if you have your first smear over the age of thirty-five you should have a second smear within one year because of the possibility that a smear has been incorrectly reported as normal. You should continue to have smears until the age of seventy.

Women who are highly sexually active − that is, women who first have sexual intercourse before the age of seventeen, women with many sexual partners, or women with genital herpes − should have smear tests more often than five-yearly, possibly once a year.

The test involves a gentle vaginal examination and the taking of a sample of the cells in the neck of the womb (the cervix) and the vagina. Although it may be a little uncomfortable it is quite painless and takes only a few moments. The cells are placed on a microscope slide which is sent off to a laboratory. The result may take several weeks to come back to your doctor. Always make sure you get the result of your test. No news is not always good news.

If the test shows that cancer might develop you will probably be asked to have a further test, known as a cone biopsy, in which a very small area of tissue is removed from the cervix. This may necessitate your staying in hospital for a day or so. The test does not affect your sex life or your ability to have children.

TESTICULAR SELF-EXAMINATION

Testicular cancer, though uncommon, can be detected early and therefore cured. Self-examination once a month, shortly after a warm bath or shower, is the key to finding this condition which typically affects men aged fifteen to forty.

1. Support the testicles in the palm of the hand. You may notice that one testicle is larger than the other. This is not unusual and, unless the increase in size is recent, does not indicate that anything is wrong. But if one testicle feels *heavier* than the other, early cancer *may* be present.
2. Using both hands gently roll each testicle between the thumb and fingers. On the top and back of each testicle you will find an irregular, sausage-like structure. This is a normal organ called the epididymis, whose function is to store sperm.
3. Feel each testicle for any lumps, irregularities or change in firmness.

If you find any abnormalities or if you feel a dragging or heaviness in the scrotum you should see your doctor at once. The probability is that you do *not* have cancer, but if cancer is present it is curable *if it is treated early.*

OTHER FORMS OF CANCER

People often ask how effective screening is at detecting cancer. At present the most important way of screening for cancer is keeping a watchful eye for any important changes in your body. Regular self-examination of the breasts and testicles will reveal the presence of a lump that was not there before. The appearance of a new lump anywhere on the body, or blood loss from a bodily orifice, or an alteration in your bowels or bladder, should alert you to the *possibility* that all may not be quite right. In all probability the cause will be quite benign, but medical advice should be sought just to be sure.

With the exception of breast and cervical cancer there are as yet few actual tests for cancer. One of the problems is that cancer is not a single disease but is as varied as the number of different organs there are in the body. Nevertheless, scientists hope that eventually there will be a simple test, perhaps a blood test, that will show immediately if a cancer is just starting to develop anywhere in the body. The smear test for cervical cancer is the best example. Examination of the large bowel by a doctor using an inspection tube, such as a sigmoidoscope or a colonoscope, is offered to all patients over forty years old attending some screening centres, especially in the USA. Tests on stools to detect early bowel cancer can be performed by laboratories, and there are now kits available from chemists, which enable patients to carry out tests on their own stools.

OLD AGE

People are now living longer than ever before. Although this is good news it does mean that many more people must expect to experience the health problems of old age such as deafness, failing vision, breathing problems, arthritis, wear and tear of the spine, foot defects, Parkinson's disease, faints and 'funny turns'.

The severity of many of these problems may often be prevented by a healthy lifestyle throughout life and by screening. Glaucoma is an example. This condition of abnormally high pressure within the eyeballs is a major cause of blindness. This is due mainly to the fact that it may be present quite unnoticed for several years by which time irreversible eye damage has already occurred. Unfortunately it is not yet a condition that is easily detected except by specialists. However, glaucoma often runs in families, and so if anyone in your family has glaucoma you should have your eyes checked by an optician periodically from the age of about forty.

Some people may look upon screening and preventive medicine as hypochondria. But you service your car, manufacturers look after their plant and machinery, so is it not prudent to do at least as much for your body? After all, machines are replaceable – your body is not. It is only sensible to look after it.

USEFUL BOOKS

The Sunday Times New Book of Body Maintenance by Oliver Gillie, Celia Haddon and Derrik Mercer, Peerage Books

An Introduction to Preventive Medicine by John Simpson, William Heinemann

Prevention and Health; Everybody's Business, HMSO

Prevention is Better . . . by Andrew Stanway, Century

SELF-HEALTH
AN A–Z

A

ACNE

Acne is a skin condition that causes spots mainly over the face, neck, shoulders, back and sometimes chest and buttocks. It is so common amongst teenagers (seventy per cent suffer from it) that it is almost regarded as an inevitable part of growing up.

Normally the skin is lubricated by grease/sebum from the sebaceous glands. With acne, however, the glands may become blocked by dead skin cells or grease, something that often happens during puberty when hormones stimulate the glands to produce more grease. The result is a blackhead or, if the blockage is deeper, a whitehead. Sometimes the whole area of skin may become infected with bacteria, leading to inflamed, tender, red spots.

Acne cannot be entirely prevented but there are things you can do to help yourself.

Self-health

- See your doctor as soon as blackheads and whiteheads start to appear. It may be that early treatment will prevent the condition getting worse.

- Do not cover your face with greasy make-up (e.g. foundation cream) because it might block the glands further and make the acne worse. Instead use stick make-up or a concealer stick to hide the spots.

- Get as much sun as you can, because ultra-violet light is good for acne sufferers. Hot weather, though, may cause the condition to worsen, probably due to a combination of perspiration, high humidity and suntan lotions.

- Avoid working in a greasy atmosphere, such as kitchens or

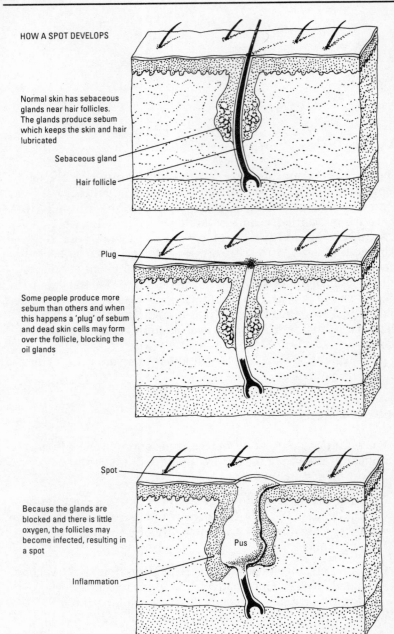

HOW A SPOT DEVELOPS

Normal skin has sebaceous
glands near hair follicles.
The glands produce sebum
which keeps the skin and hair
lubricated

Sebaceous gland

Hair follicle

Plug

Some people produce more
sebum than others and when
this happens a 'plug' of sebum
and dead skin cells may form
over the follicle, blocking the
oil glands

Spot

Because the glands are
blocked and there is little
oxygen, the follicles may
become infected, resulting in
a spot

Pus

Inflammation

fast-food restaurants. People who work with chlorinated hydrocarbons used in varnishes, paints, pesticides and some roofing materials may develop a kind of acne called chloracne.

- Most experts agree that diet has little effect on acne. But it is worth experimenting to see whether cutting out chocolate, sweets, coffee, tea or cola improves your skin.

- Although exercise is good for you, it does not prevent or help cure acne.

- Nor does hygiene have any effect. Excessive dirtiness does not cause acne and excessive washing will not cure it. When washing your face do so gently and dry it with a rough towel. Lank, greasy hair hanging over the face does not cause acne.

- Some researchers believe stress may bring on acne because it affects the hormones that control the production of grease in the skin. This may also explain why taking the contraceptive pill – which contains hormones – can sometimes make acne worse.

- In its earliest stages, before any signs of inflammation or redness have developed in and around the blackheads, the only treatment is lotions, gels or creams containing various types of antiseptics. Some are available over the counter at chemists; others need to be prescribed by your doctor. Antiseptic washes, although advertised a great deal, are unlikely to help much. The evidence is that the most effective skin treatment is benzoyl peroxide. This is available from chemists under many brand names and is very helpful in most cases, though it may irritate the skin a little or cause excessive dryness, particularly on very fair skins. It is best to start with a weak version to avoid any risk of skin soreness, and slowly build up to a stronger version which improves the skin but does not cause it to become too dry.

  Benzoyl peroxide has been used for many years in the UK and is very safe. Few people show signs of allergy. You may have to use it for several months to clear the blackheads and to stop them returning, and there is no danger in this.

- The only other effective skin treatments are antibiotics, usually in lotion form, and vitamin A. Few doctors like to use antibiotic lotions because they may cause skin allergy or the bacteria may build up a resistance so that the antibiotic no longer works. Anyway, they have not been shown to be any more effective than benzoyl peroxide. Vitamin A (known as tretinoin) applied to the skin can sometimes be helpful but can also make the skin quite sore.

- If your acne becomes worse and you have a lot of tender spots, then skin treatment alone will not be enough. Your doctor will prescribe one of several pills. Oxytetracycline is the most common. It has been used for many years and found to be very safe. It needs to be taken on an empty stomach half an hour before meals with a glass of water only, to ensure that it is fully absorbed. This may be difficult if you have a busy schedule, but it usually works well. A modern version of oxytetracycline is minocycline. This is expensive, but it is easily absorbed no matter what you have eaten or drunk, so it is a more practical treatment. Another acne drug is erythromycin, but this can cause stomach upsets.

  Whichever antibiotic you are prescribed, you will probably have to take it for at least six months. This may seem a long time, but acne responds very slowly, and treatment must be continued until it is well under control and all signs of inflammation have disappeared. You will probably be prescribed lotions or cream at the same time, and asked to use these even after stopping the antibiotic tablets.

- A combination of skin treatment and antibiotic tablets should control your acne. If it does not respond to this, there are other treatments available on prescription. The most effective drug of all, called isotretinoin, is available only through a hospital doctor.

ACUPUNCTURE

Acupuncture (or needle puncture) was definitely in use in China two thousand years ago, and may well have been up to five thousand years ago. In the West it has been regularly used for about 180 years, since Dr Berlioz first described it at the Paris Medical School in 1810.

The Chinese believe that good health depends on the free flow of the energy fluid Ch'i along special channels throughout the body. In sickness these channels become blocked but can be released by placing shallow needles very precisely along them to restore free flow. The placing of the needles need not necessarily be close to the diseased organ but could be in distant areas such as the ear lobe, hand or foot.

The theory behind acupuncture is not well understood except that many Western doctors (e.g. Melzack in 1977) have noticed that the acupuncture points match their 'trigger points' for pain very well. In some conditions, particularly painful ones, acupuncture works well and it is gradually being accepted by the medical establishment. In fact a recent survey of young British GPs showed that up to three-quarters would consider using acupuncture for treating certain conditions.

A practitioner will make a diagnosis by noting your symptoms, palpating the affected parts of your body and feeling your pulse. He or she will then stick very fine needles into the appropriate points. There are over 350 of these points but usually only ten to fifteen are used at any one time and most practitioners regularly use only forty to fifty in their entire practice. Depending on the diagnosis and the practitioner's own preference the needles may be left in for just a few minutes or up to half an hour. Do not worry that these needles will be painful; generally you only notice a tiny pinprick.

Self-health

- The Chinese have used acupuncture as a form of preventive medicine for thousands of years; the patients have regular treatment to ensure good health and pay the doctor only when well. Payments stop immediately if illness develops. However, this form of preventive medicine is not practised in the West.

- The question most people in the West ask is which conditions should they consider most appropriate for treatment by acupuncture. The answer is that it is best for painful musculoskeletal conditions such as arthritis (both osteo and rheumatoid), backache and tennis elbow. It is also good for neurological conditions such as trigeminal neuralgia and migraine. In skilled hands it may be useful for conditions such as asthma, colitis, depression, anxiety, and peptic ulcers. It can also help people stop smoking (twenty per cent were still not smoking six months after treatment, a recent survey showed), and possibly lose weight, though research is awaited to confirm this. It has little or no role for serious illnesses like cancer or heart disease.

- Acupuncture is available from three types of practitioner:
  1. Non-medically qualified acupuncturists who work outside the NHS and charge private fees.
  2. Medically qualified practitioners who may or may not charge fees depending on their status. Names can be obtained from the British Acupuncture Association (see p.463).
  3. Recently some physiotherapists have begun to practise acupuncture.

- Acupuncture has many advantages (not least lack of side effects) but also some disadvantages. The most serious is that you might catch hepatitis or AIDS from previously contaminated needles. It is also time-consuming and can be expensive. If the treatment has not worked after three or four sessions you should seriously think about stopping it.

ADDITIVES

An additive is a substance that is added to food to preserve it or improve it in some way (e.g. its flavour, colour or texture). For example an anti-spattering agent may be added to oil so that, when hot, it does not spurt out of the frying pan when food is immersed in it.

Self-health

- There has been much concern recently about food additives, particularly after the labelling system was simplified by the addition of E numbers so that consumers could check what they were eating (see table on p. 87). Some of this concern is justified, but equally there is no reason to get obsessive about additives, since many have a useful function, particularly in preserving food. It is sensible to eat as few as you can while enjoying a healthy diet but there is no evidence to suggest you should not eat any at all.

- There are about 3,500 additives used in the UK so it might seem daunting to keep track of them all, but it is possible to learn enough about them to decide which ones are useful and which are designed just to 'improve' the taste or colour of the food.

- E numbers 212–217 should be avoided by asthmatics, because they may make the condition worse, and by people who are allergic to aspirin because they may have a similar effect. Nor should they be given to babies or young children.

- The following additives are not allowed in baby and infant food: E310–E312, E320, E321, E420–E422, E621–E623, E627, E631, E635.

- Hyperactivity in children (see separate entry) has been linked with additives. Tartrazine (E102) is probably the worst offender but hyperactive children should also avoid the following additives: E104, E107, E110, E120, E122–E124, E127, E128, E131–E133, E150, E151, E154, E155, E180, E210–E220, E250, E251, E311, E312, E320, E321, E621–E623, E627, E631, E635.

- If despite your efforts, you are still worried about your diet, or your child's diet, see your doctor.

The major E-number groups

E100–E180	Permitted food colourings
E200–E297	Preservatives
E300–E321	Permitted antioxidants
E322–E495	Emulsifiers, stabilizers, thickeners
E500–E529	Acids, bases and others
E530–E578	Anti-caking agents
E620–E637	Flavour enhancers and sweeteners
E900–E907	Glazing agents and others
E920–E927	Bleaching agents and others
E1400–E1442	Starches

AIDS

Acquired Immune Deficiency Syndrome (AIDS) is so called because it is a disease in which the body's defence (immune) systems have been so destroyed by the human immunodeficiency virus (HIV) that they are no longer able to fight infections. Patients therefore die of chest infections and cancers that the body would otherwise have eliminated.

The virus passes from one person to another, most commonly by sexual intercourse. The World Health Organization estimates that so far between five and ten million people worldwide have been infected. If the lower estimate is accepted, about two and a half million are in Africa (mostly Central and East Africa), two million in the USA, half a million in Europe and the remainder worldwide. In the UK the Department of Health estimates that at least 20,000 people are infected. Dr Harold Jaffe, an AIDS expert, has predicted that AIDS could become the second biggest cause (after heart disease) of premature death in the USA, with more deaths from it in a single year than from the entire Vietnam war.

In Britain, Europe and the USA most cases of AIDS involve homosexual or bisexual men. However, increases among intravenous drug users and their sexual partners and babies are being noticed, while the homosexual epidemic may have plateaued out.

In Africa most people acquire AIDS heterosexually. Why there should be a difference between Africa and the rest of the world is not yet fully understood. However, the number of people getting AIDS heterosexually is slowly increasing everywhere and now makes up about four per cent of the total USA cases for example.

Self-health

- Prevention is crucial, because there is as yet no cure for AIDS. It is now thought that everyone who has been infected by the virus will eventually develop AIDS, whether in a matter of months or after many years without symptoms.

- AIDS cannot be caught from sitting next to someone with it, or from sharing their cups or plates. Nor is it possible to get the disease from lavatories or bed linen. Despite a lot of speculation it is probably not possible to catch it from saliva or teardrops.

- It is not possible to get AIDS from donating blood for transfusions (providing, of course, sterile equipment is used). So there is no reason, in developed countries, to stop donating blood because you fear AIDS.

- In the early and mid 1980s, however, there were tragic cases of haemophiliacs (see **Haemophilia**) being infected after transfusions of blood from donors who were unaware they had the virus. In developed countries such as Britain and the USA this is no longer possible because of strict controls on blood, but in other parts of the world where controls are less strict it may still be possible to get AIDS from infected blood transfusions.

- The simplest safeguard against getting AIDS is not to make love with anyone who falls into the high-risk group (male homosexuals, bisexuals, and drug addicts who use contaminated needles to inject drugs into their veins). Male homosexuals are most at risk possibly because the anal tissues are more delicate than those of the vagina, allowing the virus to get into the bloodstream.

- If you want to make love with someone who you suspect or know is in the high-risk group, it is important you practise 'safe sex' techniques (see **Sex, Safe**).

- If you want to make love to someone whose sexual history you don't know well, it is essential to use a condom. Remember, every time you make love to someone you are making love to everyone that person has had sex with in the past. And it only takes one infected person, on one occasion, for you all to become infected too.

- If you are HIV-positive (i.e. you are infected with the HIV virus) but have not yet developed the symptoms of AIDS, you must get specialized medical advice about how to live. There is no reason why you should not lead a 'normal' life, and even have sexual relations provided you use 'safe sex' techniques. Some HIV-positive people seek partners who are also HIV-positive so that they can share their worries and anxieties and are not in danger of infecting each other.

- If you have full-blown AIDS you will need specialized medical and spiritual care. You may find great comfort and practical support from self-help groups (see p. 464).

Screening

- At the time this book goes to print there is great confusion about the role of screening. Some experts believe everyone at risk should be screened (regardless of whether they consent or not) and told if they are HIV-positive; others believe everyone at risk should be screened but those positive should not be told (because of the trauma this would involve for them); still others believe a sample of the whole population should be screened so accurate estimates of how many people are affected can be made.

    Our belief is that people at risk should have the AIDS test and that anyone found positive should be told in as sympathetic and supportive a way as possible because, if they are not, they represent a terrible danger to all their sexual contacts.

- One difficulty with voluntary screening is that some life insurance companies automatically regard as high risk anyone, regardless of reason, who has had an AIDS test. Since they may refuse you life insurance (or charge a high premium) for this reason alone, you should consider this problem before having the test.

ALCOHOLISM

The World Health Organization defines alcoholics as 'those excessive drinkers whose dependence on alcohol has attained such a degree that it shows a noticeable mental disturbance or an interference with their bodily or mental health, their personal relations and their smooth social and economic functioning, or who show the early signs of such development'. In England and Wales alone there are about 750,000 people with a serious drinking problem.

Everyone has different abilities to tolerate alcohol. Women are more at risk of alcoholism than men because their bodies contain less water to dilute the alcohol and their livers are less efficient at processing it.

Safe limits are difficult to set but a Scotsman, Dr Francis Austie, first recommended 'Austie's limit' in 1864 and this has recently been endorsed by the Government. It states that safe drinking should not exceed half a bottle of wine a day, or two pints of strong beer or three and a half tots of well-diluted spirits. Recent research suggests that these levels may be lower for women.

Self-health

- Prevention is very important because treatment often does not work. It has been estimated that fifty per cent of dried-out alcoholics start drinking again.

- Prevention is aimed at three levels. First it is important to educate youngsters about the dangers of alcohol. Some experts believe that Jewish, Italian and French people set the safest pattern of drinking by introducing children to alcohol as a normal social activity within the context of the family.

  Second, it is important to make heavy drinkers aware that they run the risk of becoming alcoholic, and to show them how to avoid it.

  Finally alcoholics should be helped to stop drinking so they do not destroy their own and their families' lives and die prematurely.

- There are many steps you can take to make sure you do not drink dangerously:

  1. Try not to drink alone.
  2. Eat plenty of bulky food (such as bread and cheese) before you drink.
  3. Set yourself limits for social occasions, such as weddings, and stick to them. Sip drinks slowly to make them last longer, and take part in activities that will take your mind off alcohol.
  4. Do not serve yourself and guests generous tots. Always measure spirits, and only half fill wine glasses. Help a guest who is drinking too much by serving food and not thrusting drinks on him or her.

5. Alternate alcoholic with non-alcoholic drinks. Have the courage to refuse a drink if you do not want one. If necessary you can always order a drink that looks alcoholic but is not, e.g. tonic water and lime or low-alcohol beer.
6. Reward yourself by buying something special with the money you have saved by not drinking as much.

- Eat a healthy diet containing plenty of fibre and vitamin-rich food because this will help your liver to break down the alcohol. Some treatment centres in the United States take alcoholics off sugar, cigarettes and coffee and put them on a diet of fresh fruit and vegetables, grains and vitamin B and C supplements.

- Many alcoholics are unhappy people with deep personal problems who use alcohol as an escape. Experts believe that alcoholics will stop drinking only when these inner problems are sorted out, perhaps by psychotherapy.

ALLERGIC RHINITIS

Allergic rhinitis is a condition in which your nose runs and may feel stuffy, you sneeze a lot and your eyes may be red, itchy and watery. Occasionally it can cause loss of sense of smell. It is due to an allergy to a specific substance. Grass pollen is the most common, causing hayfever (see separate entry). Other causes include the mites that infest house dust (see **Mites**), spores from fungi, hair, skin or feathers from a pet, strong smells or fumes, smoke, cold air or a dry atmosphere.

Self-health

- Allergies run in families, so if your family suffers from allergies (e.g. asthma or eczema) and you have the symptoms listed above you should try to discover whether you too are allergic to something.

- Discovering what causes your allergy can be difficult. Sometimes it is a question of trial and error, doing some basic detective work. In the past doctors used to try skin testing for allergies but nowadays it is recognized that they can be misleading.

- Having pinpointed your allergy the best medicine is prevention – avoiding the cause as best you can. This may mean clearing the house of mites (see **Asthma**), giving your pets away to a good home, or wearing a surgical mask in appropriate places.

- Often, though, no specific cause is found, or even if it is, you continue to have symptoms. To alleviate these symptoms you can buy medicines from the chemist without a prescription.

  1. Antihistamine tablets can both prevent and treat attacks. The problem is that, to be effective, they have to be taken regularly and they often cause drowsiness (which makes driving or working with machinery dangerous) and an unpleasantly dry mouth, throat and nose.
  2. For quick relief of symptoms you can try decongestant nose drops or spray. These often work well when you first use them but they sometimes become less useful with time and over-use may actually make the condition worse. So, if your symptoms are getting worse do not assume you should use more and more decongestants; you may have to stop them altogether.

- If your symptoms persist despite your efforts, see your doctor. He or she may be able to find the cause or, if not, to prescribe some medicine that will help without causing side effects. In the past a course of desensitizing injections used to be recommended but they are much less popular with doctors nowadays because there are risks and they are often not very effective.

ALLERGY, FOOD

The word allergy comes from two Greek words meaning altered reaction. The affected person suffers physical symptoms (e.g. rash, headache, wheezing, migraine) when exposed to substances to which he or she is sensitive. The most common sources of these allergies are inhaled allergens (see **Asthma**, **Hayfever** and **Allergic Rhinitis**), chemicals and food. Some people are allergic to more than one substance – and from different categories – so identifying the source of an allergy can sometimes be difficult.

Opinions on how common food allergy is vary widely. Some experts believe that up to twenty per cent of children are allergic to some foods at some time or another. Others believe food allergy is rare and much overdiagnosed.

What is certain is that food allergies are more common in children than adults, that they run in families, and that if you are already allergic to one substance you are quite likely to be allergic to others. If you are such a person this may sound rather depressing news as you sneeze and wheeze your way through summer or come out in a rash at the mere thought of shellfish, but the good news is that research has shown that such 'allergic' people are much less likely to get cancer.

Symptoms of food allergy include feeling unwell, tiredness or hyperactivity (see **Hyperactivity, Children**), colic, bloating of the stomach, diarrhoea, nappy rash, other rashes, wheezing, shortness of breath, fluctuating mood changes, palpitations, and unexplained swelling of the hands and ankles, and may include serious conditions such as asthma, migraine, poor growth and epilepsy. Fluctuating weight and food cravings or binges are also common with food allergy.

Self-health

- There is nothing a family can do to prevent its tendency to allergies. The main thing is to recognize that allergy may be a cause of unexplained symptoms and to take sensible avoiding action.

- Some experts believe that giving your baby solid foods (especially protein foods such as cow's milk, egg whites, fish and cereals) before their young digestive systems can cope with them may bring on food allergies. You should therefore avoid solid foods until your baby is about five to six months old and nine to twelve months old for cow's milk.

- Breast-feeding exclusively for the first five to six months of your baby's life seems to help prevent allergies. Breast-fed babies can still develop allergies, though, so do not exclude this possibility. It may be that if a mother drinks a lot of cow's milk when breast-feeding, tiny particles get through into her milk and provoke an allergic reaction in her baby.

- Artificial colourings and flavourings found in many foods may cause allergy (see **Hyperactivity, Children**). Try to eat fresh, additive-free food as often as you can. Check labels if you are suspicious that a food may contain an unwanted additive. Remember, too, hidden allergens such as chemicals on fresh fruit (which should preferably be peeled, and certainly always washed if bought in shops whose likely suppliers are commercial growers).

- Food allergies usually occur in children, and once an allergy has developed it can usually be prevented only by eliminating the offending food from the diet. Discovering this food can be difficult.

  1. First, try to think back to when symptoms began, e.g. introducing cereals or starting school. This may give you a clue to the cause.
  2. If you have no clues, put your child on an elimination diet rather than eliminating one food at a time and watching for any change. It is probably wisest to involve your family doctor at this stage.
  3. The principle of an elimination diet is that you start with a very simple diet which eliminates the common food allergens (see below). This diet allows fresh meat, fresh vegetables and fruit, and mineral water. After seven days your child should start to feel better and have fewer symptoms (if not, the cause is unlikely to be a food allergy so you will have to think again). Then gradually introduce other foods one by one, checking whether the symptoms start again. If they do, you can identify the offending food. But remember, there may be more than one.

- All sorts of food allergies exist but here are some specific examples:

  1. Egg allergy causes the tongue to swell immediately, often accompanied by a rash, nausea, a bloated stomach, or diarrhoea. The short time between eating the egg and the onset of symptoms usually makes diagnosis easy.
  2. Shellfish may cause swelling, vomiting, severe headaches and joint pains.
  3. More than ten cups of coffee or tea a day can cause bad headaches or migraine, palpitations and a hand tremor.

4. Some people (usually children) have a shortage of the enzyme lactose needed to break down milk in the gut. The deficiency causes diarrhoea, stomach pain and bloating, which disappears when milk products are cut out of the diet or special products containing the enzyme are taken with the milk.
5. Infants commonly suffer milk allergy. As well as intestinal problems, this may also cause 'flu-like symptoms, wheezing, eczema, asthma and occasionally arthritis.

- Experimenting with diet can be dangerous. It is important that your child (and you) always receives a nutritious, balanced diet containing all the vitamins and minerals and that your family doctor is consulted if you have any doubts about progress.

Common food allergens

Wheat, rye, oats, corn	Chocolate	Yeast
Dairy produce	Coffee	Citrus fruits
Eggs (especially the	Tea	Tomatoes
whites)	Beef	Alcohol
Cane sugar	Pork	Shellfish

ANAEMIA

Anaemia is a shortage of the red (or oxygen-carrying) cells in the blood. It is the commonest blood disease and is usually caused by a deficiency of iron to make the red cells, or the body losing blood faster than it can make it.

Because not enough energy-giving oxygen is being carried to all the body's organs, the person may notice tiredness, or shortness of breath, faintness, headaches, palpitations or a pale face. Not every pale person is anaemic, though – some may just have a thicker skin than the rest of us!

Self-health

- A good diet with plenty of iron is essential. Meat, fish (especially sardines), cereals, potatoes, black pudding, and green, leafy vegetables (but not especially spinach) are all rich in iron.

- Third World and vegetarian diets may cause a problem because much of the iron is bound to phytic acid in the cereals which makes it less easily absorbed from the gut. In the Third World, too, millions of people are infected with worms which cause a steady loss of blood from the intestines.

- Pregnancy and breast-feeding are times when the body needs plenty of extra iron. Although women are better than men at absorbing iron, they may still need to take iron tablets to be sure of getting enough. Sometimes these tablets cause constipation and nausea.

- It may also be necessary to take folate tablets. Folate is a vitamin needed to build all the cells of the body, including the red cells of the blood. Because there is so much building going on during pregnancy and breast-feeding, some women need extra to prevent the body running short.

- You should look for (and talk to your doctor about) any unusual or excessive loss of blood. Some women have very heavy periods which are impossible to treat, but others may be helped. Untreated piles may bleed continuously over the days and years adding up eventually to a large volume – they should be treated early. Stomach and duodenal ulcers may bleed and cause anaemia – you should tell your doctor about severe heartburn and especially if you notice blood in your stools.

ANAL IRRITATION

Anal irritation (also known as pruritus) is common among adult males, although not among men of African origin. It is usually due to the skin around the anus becoming inflamed, perhaps by soiling from faeces or perhaps by infection.

Self-health

- Try not to scratch; it will only make the irritation worse.

- After you have opened your bowels adopt scrupulous hygiene to remove all traces of faeces from the skin round your anus. Washing may be necessary. Some people's anatomy is such that removing all faeces can be difficult, so persevere.

- Take a daily bath or shower; two may sometimes be needed.

- Avoid strong soaps, powders and ointments as a general rule – they themselves may irritate the skin. Some contain anaesthetics combined with steroids, which may encourage secondary infections, e.g. thrush.

- If you practise anal intercourse, be gentle and scrupulously hygienic.

- See your doctor if your own efforts to cure anal irritation fail. Your doctor may wish to investigate you for piles, other skin conditions like eczema or psoriasis, diabetes, threadworms or thrush (see separate entries).

ANOREXIA NERVOSA

Anorexia nervosa is a mental condition in which the person refuses to eat food – or deliberately vomits after eating (see **Bulimia Nervosa**) – because of an overwhelming and unreasonable fear of becoming fat. It affects ten times as many women as men and is most common between the ages of fifteen and thirty-five. It is becoming more common in the Western world. Twelve and a half thousand people in the UK have anorexia severely enough to need medical treatment and there are many more people with less serious forms. On the whole it is middle-class girls who are affected, especially from families who are upwardly and socially mobile (in other words the parents may have come from a lower social class). One survey showed that two-thirds of fathers of affected daughters were professionals. Another showed that a comprehensive school with 2,331 girls under sixteen had no cases whereas an independent school might expect one in 200 girls to suffer from anorexia. The highest incidence is found in dance and modelling schools (up to one in fourteen pupils affected). There is a link, too, with intelligence and academic pressure (up to one in fifty university students are affected).

First the girl (as it usually is) decides she is overweight (a few are overweight, but most are not) and starts to avoid food.

Gradually she becomes thinner until at seventy to eighty per cent of her expected weight she starts to think and act as an anorexic. She may be moody, inward-looking, restless, occasionally euphoric but often depressed. Her periods may stop and she may develop fine hair all over her body. She will become emaciated but will try to hide this by wearing loose-fitting clothes like jerseys and jeans, jackets and scarves. She will become weak, prone to accidents, and puffy round the ankles and eyes. In more serious cases she may force herself to vomit (especially when she has just eaten) and take large quantities of laxatives of all types.

Self-health

- Do not be too alarmed about media reporting of anorexia nervosa which tends to emphasize the dangers. Overall about half those who have suffered are back to a normal weight within five years, although some still admit to an abnormal obsession with food. In the UK there is a one to four per cent death rate. In America death rates as high as eleven per cent have been reported.

- It is probably unrealistic to ask hard-working, ambitious families to take the pressure to succeed off their children. However, there is no doubt this pressure may start the illness in a girl who is otherwise prone to it.

- It is vital that the early signs of illness are recognized and acted upon. It may be possible to gain the anorexic's confidence and persuade her that her body image is disturbed and her lack of self-confidence is unjustified. Most sufferers, though, will need professional help either as outpatients or within hospital. The longer the girl has suffered from anorexia, the longer it will take to recover. Interestingly though, there is no close link between severity of symptoms and failure to respond to treatment quickly.

AROMATHERAPY

Aromatherapy is a system of healing which uses natural oils from flowers, trees, plants and other biological substances to treat a wide variety of illnesses. Practitioners claim that complaints such as acne, eczema, psoriasis, arthritis, rheumatism, poor circulation, and depression may be helped. The system comes from ancient Eastern traditions and most recently has been developed by Marguerite Maury and her homeopathic husband.

Practitioners analyse a blood sample to find out which essential oils you need. The appropriate oils are then massaged through the skin in what most people find is a very pleasant experience.

Aromatherapy is very enjoyable and totally harmless. Its healing value is unproven but few people can fail to benefit in one way or another.

ARTHRITIS

Arthritis means inflammation of a joint. There are two main kinds:

Osteoarthritis is the commonest kind and happens when the soft cartilage covering the bone surfaces of the joint becomes worn away (usually by age), exposing the hard bone. Bone rubbing on bone makes a bad joint so the owner feels pain, stiffness and swelling.

Rheumatoid arthritis is less common, affects all ages and is due to inflammation destroying the joint, its lining, ligaments and muscles.

Self-health

- Although osteoarthritis cannot be prevented, it is possible to slow down destruction of the joints.

  Losing weight is worthwhile because it helps reduce wear and tear on the joints.

  Exercise keeps joints mobile and muscles round them strong. Many joints (like the knee) depend on their muscles for stability. If muscles are weak and slack, joints become unstable and more prone to arthritis. Non-weight-bearing exercises like swimming and cycling are the best. It is always worth warming up gradually before any exercise and making sure you have the right equipment and clothing. Long-distance runners, squash and badminton players, for example, should wear good-quality, shock-absorbing shoes.

- It is not possible to prevent rheumatoid arthritis. It comes out of the blue and may as quickly go. It is this fluctuating course that makes it so difficult to tell whether a treatment is working – and explains why so many 'miracle' cures are recorded.

- It is tempting to hope there is an ingredient in the diet which, if avoided, would prevent the disease. Fat, gluten, sugar, salt and refined foods have all been suggested but never proved. Others think that diets low in minerals, trace elements (e.g. zinc) and vitamins (especially vitamin C) are the cause but again there is no proof. The answer is to eat good, healthy food and consider diet as only a rare cause of arthritis.

- For those with arthritis, early physiotherapy, especially in water, is important to prevent the joints becoming stiff and weak. Drugs and splints may be necessary to prevent limbs becoming deformed. Best of all is a positive attitude to life and a refusal to bow to the illness.

ASTHMA

Asthma is a condition in which a fluctuating narrowing of the air passages of the lungs may cause difficulty with breathing, cough or chest tightness. Children are particularly prone to the *extrinsic* type which comes on after exposure to allergic substances like pollen, pets or certain foods. This type often runs in families also affected by eczema and hayfever. Adults develop *intrinsic* asthma, the cause of which is unknown.

Self-health

- If there is a family history of asthma, eczema or hayfever it is worth trying to breast-feed alone for up to six months because cow's milk early in the diet may play a part in bringing on asthma. Later, eggs and nuts can also cause problems.

- Smoking should be avoided. If there is a smoker in the family, a good air filter helps an asthmatic. Some asthmatics also find sudden draughts of cold air, air pollutants, chemical, paint and petrol fumes, and hair sprays start symptoms.

- It may be necessary to avoid furry pets like cats or dogs if they are causing troublesome attacks. Certainly ban them from bedrooms.

- Some children are allergic to the house-dust mite (see **Mites**). If so, vacuum mattresses thoroughly and enclose them in plastic covers. Synthetic bedclothes and regular damp dusting also help.

- Asthmatics should be encouraged to take plenty of exercise but some find it brings on attacks. Small doses of bronchodilating drugs to expand the narrowed airways before exercise can help.

- Stress should be avoided as much as possible (see chapter on Stress and Mental Health).

- Chest infections must be treated promptly to avoid asthmatic complications but remember that some antibiotics (and aspirin) can themselves cause asthma.

- Certain asthma-causing allergies, particularly to grass pollens, mould spores and house-dust mites, can be prevented by desensitizing injections.

- Some medicines can help prevent attacks of asthma. One of the best known is sodium cromoglycate which prevents the allergic reactions that narrow the airways. Also important are inhaled steroids, which damp down the inflammation of the tubes.

- Other drugs can prevent symptoms becoming serious. These bronchodilators (such as salbutamol and aminophylline) reverse spasm in the tubes.

- Many asthmatics will benefit from using a peak flow meter. This simple instrument (which can be used at home) measures how well or badly the lungs are performing and can give early warning of an asthma attack.

ATHLETE'S FOOT

A fungal infection of the skin which most commonly affects the soles of the foot and between the toes. It is a type of ringworm which flourishes in damp, warm places.

Self-health

- Since the likeliest places to pick up the infection are changing rooms, swimming pools and gyms, wearing rubber or wooden sandals will greatly reduce your chances of infection.

- Keep your feet cool by going barefoot if possible. Sweaty socks and shoes should be changed after activities. Shoes should be roomy and made of natural materials so that feet can 'breathe' easily.

- Dry the feet well after swimming or bathing, particularly between the toes.

- Dust your feet and socks with anti-fungal powder if you know you are in a high-risk place.

B

BACKACHE

We have all probably suffered from backache, however minor, at some time in our lives. In most cases there is no obvious cause and it is probably due to a strained ligament or vertebral joint causing the surrounding muscles to go into painful spasm. Usually the pain gets better over three to four days and may disappear never to return, or not for many years. If it lasts longer, or you notice numbness, weakness or tingling in your legs, or trouble with your bowels or bladder, you should consult your doctor immediately.

A few unfortunate people suffer from long-standing pain which makes their lives a misery. There is likely to be a more definite reason for this type of pain, such as arthritis or osteoporosis, and a cure is less likely.

Self-health

- Poor posture is an easily avoidable cause of backache. The spine is not well designed for sitting – even when sitting correctly the pressure within the spinal discs is twice that when standing (which in turn is twice that when lying). So choose chairs and car seats that support the small of your back and are not soft or bucket-shaped. Avoid slumping down – it might seem more immediately comfortable but it will not be in the long run. Some people find sitting with their knees higher than their hips helpful. On long plane journeys, walk about frequently, and when driving long distances stop the car for a few minutes' walk every two hours or so.

- When walking, try to maintain the natural curves of your back. Keep your head up, your shoulders back, your tummy pulled in and your lower back hollow.

- Wear low-heeled shoes whenever possible (especially for long walks or heavy lifting) because high heels throw the hips forward and put an extra strain on the lower back.

- Athletes and sports players should wear thick-soled shoes that will prevent the shock waves from hard roads or gymnasiums being transmitted directly to the back.

- Lifting incorrectly is a common cause of backache. Never lift a heavy weight on your own when someone else could easily help. Always bend your knees, not your spine; never get into an awkward position (or you may stay there permanently!) and try to lift with a straight spine and the load carried evenly between your hands. And always do everything slowly.

- Avoid carrying heavy shopping in one hand – split it so that you are evenly balanced.

- Garden by going down on one or both knees, getting as close to the weeds or plants as possible. If you bend from the hips with straight legs, both you and the garden will get in a terrible mess while you spend two or three weeks flat on your back.

- Lying is the least stressful position for the back – providing your bed and mattress are firm. Matresses older than ten years usually need replacing, but the problem of sagging bedsprings can be solved by a board placed under the mattress. Try not to sleep with two pillows; you may find a pillow between your knees helpful when lying on your side.

- Keep slim. Being overweight (especially round the tummy) throws extra strain on the lower back, weakens the important back and tummy muscles and makes correct lifting difficult.

- Exercise regularly. Non-weight-bearing exercises like cycling and swimming are best. Always warm up gradually before exercise and warm 'down' afterwards.

- Never work through back pain – even a twinge. You might manage to finish your lifting or sport but you will more than pay for it afterwards.

BAD BREATH

Bad breath is usually caused by decaying teeth, gum disease or dirty dentures. Throat infections may result in an unpleasant smell, as do sinus and lung infections, especially the condition known as bronchiectasis. Smoking gives a characteristic nasty smell, as do certain foods such as garlic, onions, and spices. In some cases no cause is ever found.

Self-health

- Keep your gums and teeth healthy by regular brushing, by cleaning between the teeth using dental floss, by avoiding sugary snacks and by regular visits to your dentist.

- Crisp foods like apples and celery do help but are no substitute for regular cleaning. If you think you have plaque on your teeth you can buy disclosing tablets from the chemist. On chewing, these stain the plaque so you can see where it is and remove it.

- Visit your doctor for treatment if you have persistent infections of the sinuses, nose, throat or lungs.

BALDNESS

Even before Julius Caesar, while courting Cleopatra, combed his remaining hairs round the bald patch on the top of his head, people have tried to prevent, disguise or restore lost hair.

Nine out of ten Britons who experience hair loss have male-type baldness – receding hairline and loss at the crown of the head. This results from the body's male hormones. Some researchers have shown that baldness is associated with higher than normal levels of these hormones, but this is by no means proven. Heredity is also important but it is a fallacy that a son will lose hair like his father, particularly as his mother's side plays an equal role.

Self-health

- If your hair loss seems unexpected, very fast or you feel

unwell, see your doctor immediately because there are one or two conditions (such as anaemia or too much thyroid hormone) which first show themselves with hair loss.

- There are no certain ways to prevent baldness. All sorts of remedies such as brewer's yeast or apple cider have been suggested but none consistently works.

- Treating hair gently will make it healthy and more likely to last. Avoid vigorous brushing.

- Wearing a hat or even a wig will not cause baldness. Hair does not have to 'breathe'.

- A new drug, minoxidil, has been reported to re-grow hair. However, the hair appears wispy and thin. About thirty per cent of men using minoxidil report an improvement.

BEDSORES

Anyone stuck in bed for more than a few days is at risk of developing bedsores, especially if he or she is seriously ill, cannot move easily or has poor circulation. The sores happen most commonly on the heels, buttocks, hips, elbows, knees, shoulders and back of the head. Check these places for the red, tender, inflamed skin which warns that a sore is starting.

Self-health

- The more a person moves, the less likely he or she is to develop bedsores. Even wriggling the toes, stretching the body, bending and straightening the arms and legs can help.

- People who cannot move should be turned at least every two hours. Make sure you always lift or roll them, and *never* drag them because this will damage the skin. Be careful you don't scratch the skin with fingernails or jewellery.

- Make sure that sheets are taut and breakfast crumbs removed. Wet, soiled sheets can hasten bedsores by chafing the skin, so think about preventing incontinence and change sheets quickly when the occasional accident happens. To be healthy, skin must be clean and dry.

- Sheepskins (preferably synthetic, washable) are useful. You can get large ones to cover the whole bed or smaller ones held over vulnerable areas (like the heels) by a bandage, stocking or fastening.

- Bed cradles keep the heavy weight of the bedclothes off the body and so encourage movement. Ask your health visitor or local British Red Cross Society about loan arrangements.

- Occasionally a ripple bed can also be loaned from local health services for a very immobile person. Its 'rippling' changes the pressure the bed exerts on the skin and so helps prevent bedsores.

- If an area of skin does become inflamed keep it clean and dry and keep all weight off it until the redness disappears. If it breaks down to become an ulcer, see your doctor at once.

BEDWETTING

Most children become dry at night between the ages of three and four years. About one in seven children over five years, however, is wet at night and one in 100 may still be wet at night aged fifteen. Boys are more commonly affected than girls.

Self-health

- If your child wets the bed he or she needs your patience and support. Anxiety and anger will only make the condition worse. Never use punishment; always praise dry beds.

- When you go to bed sit your child on the lavatory or potty for a few minutes. Most children go back to sleep at once and remember nothing in the morning.

- Limit drinks before bedtime so the bladder does not get quickly full.

- Use a nightly calendar with stars for dry beds.

- You should see your doctor if your child still regularly bedwets (despite your efforts) over the age of six or seven. Very occasionally congenital abnormalities of the urinary system, diabetes or urinary tract infection may be the cause. You should also consider whether the child is under excessive stress – especially if he or she has been dry and then starts to wet again.

- Electrical gadgets that ring to awaken the child as soon as he or she wets a sensitive pad in the bed are sometimes helpful for the older child. Consult your doctor or health visitor.

BLOOD CLOTS (VEINS)

Occasionally a blood clot (thrombus) may partially or completely block a vein in the leg. If it affects a superficial vein near the skin (thrombophlebitis) it causes pain, redness, itching and a cord-like swelling along the vein. If it affects a deep vein (deep vein thrombosis) swelling of the whole calf or thigh is more common and the main danger is that a piece will fly off into the circulation, and lodge in the lungs, causing an obstruction to the circulation there. A difficulty is that many clots cause no symptoms at all so the person is unaware of the possible dangers.

Self-health

- Try to keep as mobile as possible.

- If you are going to be immobile for any reason (for example after an operation) make sure your legs are up, and keep the circulation active by wriggling your toes and moving your ankles, calves and knees. Elderly and overweight people or those taking oestrogen either in the contraceptive pill or as hormone replacement therapy are particularly at risk.

- Do not constrict your leg with tight bandages or straps as these slow circulation.

- Try to avoid long, sustained pressure on veins – especially during long car or plane journeys.

- If you have varicose veins see your doctor to decide whether treatment is necessary.

- If you have had a clot before be particularly careful and be sure to warn the doctor before an operation or childbirth.

BLOOD PRESSURE

If you have high blood pressure (hypertension) you are about four times more likely to have a stroke and about six times more likely to develop heart failure than those with normal pressure. In addition, you may damage your kidneys, eyes and all the arteries in your body. So it is very important to keep it within the normal range for your age. The fact that you are feeling fine does not mean your blood pressure is normal – many people have no symptoms until irreversible changes have started.

Self-health

- Anyone over thirty-five should have their blood pressure checked about every three years. People with special risk factors such as a family history of high blood pressure or diabetes should consider having it checked earlier and more often.

- For many overweight people, getting back to a suitable weight for their age, sex and height is, itself, enough to bring the blood pressure back into the normal range.

- Stop smoking, because smoking also causes hardening of the arteries and the combination of the two could be disastrous.

- Salt your food less generously. No direct link in all people has been established between salt intake and raised blood pressure but there is no doubt that some people are affected, and as it is impossible to tell whether you are such a person it seems sensible to cut down your salt intake and that of your children. Remember that salt in processed and preserved food probably adds up to much more than salt added when cooking.

- Take plenty of exercise. It helps to keep your weight under control, to reduce 'stress' levels and make you feel good.

- Try to avoid stress and crises. Occasional excitement is probably good for you, but not continuously.

- Blood pressure machines (sphygmomanometers) have recently become available in better chemists. Most are accurate to within five per cent. Do not worry about the occasional high reading – it is general trends that matter. See your doctor or practice nurse if you have any worries.

- If self-help measures fail, your doctor may recommend a drug to keep your blood pressure normal. If this drug makes you feel unwell, tell your doctor (especially if, as a result, you stop taking it!) because there is such a variety of modern drugs that one will be found to suit you.

BOILS

A boil is a pocket of infection in a hair follicle, the tiny pit in the skin from which a hair grows. Cells which form part of the body's defence system gather at the site of the infection and kill the germs causing the pus.

Self-health

- If you have a boil your friends and family are at risk of catching the infection. Make sure you wash your hands carefully before preparing food. Put disinfectant in the bathwater and certainly don't share it or your towel with other family members.

- If you tend to get lots of boils think about whether you are eating a healthy diet (especially fruit) and getting plenty of relaxation because these will help to build up your resistance.

- If you are still getting many boils despite your own efforts, see your doctor. There is usually no obvious cause but one that your doctor may wish to rule out – by a urine test for sugar – is diabetes.

- Just occasionally your doctor may decide that antibiotics might help, either by mouth or spread as a cream. Although in theory this sounds a good idea, the danger is that the germs may become resistant to the medicines, making treatment more difficult.

BOWEL, CANCER

Cancer of the bowel is a growth of the large intestine and rectum. The growth may ulcerate, causing anaemia and bleeding through the anus, or it may block off the intestines, causing constipation and colic. If allowed to progress it may spread to other structures nearby or through the bloodstream to other parts of the body. It is common in Western countries; in Britain it is the third most common type of cancer.

Self-health

• There is good reason to believe that a high-fibre diet will reduce your chances of developing this cancer. Third World countries where a high-fibre diet is eaten have little bowel cancer but it is common in Western countries where a highly refined diet is usual. You should aim to eat about 30 g of fibre each day in the form of cereals, vegetables, pulses, and fruit,

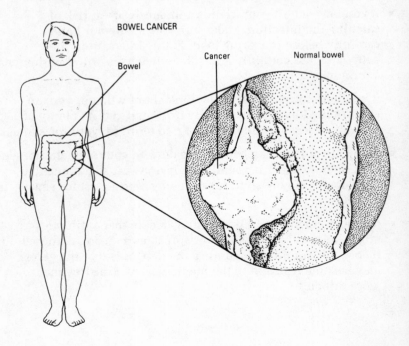

BOWEL CANCER

Bowel

Cancer

Normal bowel

rather than as bran sprinkled on to your food. Fibre probably works by reducing the length of time faeces and cancer-causing agents are in contact with the bowel. It may also work by increasing the bulk of the faeces and so diluting the cancer-forming agents, and by encouraging natural bacteria to grow, displacing and discouraging bacteria that may be involved in producing cancer-forming agents.

- Some researchers think a low-fat diet will reduce your chances of developing cancer of the bowel. They point to the Japanese, who eat little fat and have low rates of bowel cancer, but who develop similar rates to Americans when they emigrate to the USA. They also point out that recently the Japanese have begun to eat more fat and their rate of bowel cancer has started to rise. However, these ideas are by no means proven and there may be many other factors involved.

Screening

- It is most important that bowel cancer is detected early, because if it is there is an eighty per cent chance of a complete cure.

- Some families are prone to this cancer. So tell your doctor if you have one or more close relatives who have died young from bowel cancer. Your doctor may decide to investigate your bowel with X-rays (barium enema X-rays) or a long, bendy telescope (colonoscopy).

- It is possible to buy kits from the chemist that detect blood mixed in with faeces. This can be a valuable test for cancer but be sure to follow the instructions carefully because it is easy to get false results.

BREAST ABSCESS

A breast abscess is an area of infection within the breast. It often happens while mothers are breast-feeding. Germs enter through a cracked nipple and infect the milk ducts and glands. As the germs multiply they cause a painful lump. Sometimes the glands under the armpits are also affected.

Self-health

- Breast abscesses appearing out of the blue *cannot* be prevented. Cracked nipples leading to breast abscesses *can* be prevented. Make sure your baby is on your breast correctly – if necessary, ask your midwife or health visitor to check the position. Do not wash your breasts after every feed as this removes natural oils and makes the skin more likely to get damaged. Change your feeding position often so your baby's gums press on different parts of the breast. Start feeds on alternate sides and keep your nipples dry between feeds, using disposable breastpads or cut-up nappies. Many mothers do not need cream or sprays but they may help if your nipples remain obstinately sore and liable to crack.

BREAST CANCER

Breast cancer is the most common female cancer affecting about one woman in fifteen. A lump, usually painless, grows in the breast. Any part of the breast can be affected but the upper, outer position is the most common. Sometimes the lump creases or puckers the skin lying over it. Sometimes there is a discharge from the nipple, or the nipple itself may be drawn inwards.

Self-health

- If you have a close relative (e.g. mother or sister) who has had this cancer, or if you started your periods early or continued them longer than normal (fifty is the average age for the menopause) or you have had no children, take particular care to examine your breasts regularly as you are slightly more likely to develop this cancer than others.

  At the time of writing, no link between the contraceptive pill and breast cancer is proven.

- Examine your breasts every month (see p. 73), because the earlier the cancer is found, the better your chances of cure.

- Women over fifty are ten to twelve times more likely to develop breast cancer than those in their thirties. The best way to detect the cancer is by a special X-ray known as mammography. The Government has announced plans to provide a breast screening programme including mammography to all women between the ages of fifty and sixty-four. Meanwhile, if you are in this age group find out about screening from your GP, local Health Education Unit or Well Woman Clinic.

BREAST-FEEDING, BLOCKED DUCTS

One of your milk ducts may become blocked due to engorgement (see **Breast-feeding, Engorgement**), rushed or missed feeds, or pressure from clothing. This causes a painful, red area of skin overlying a lump.

Self-health

- It is important to keep the milk flowing to unblock the duct so do not give up breast-feeding. Breast-feed frequently, particularly on the affected side.

- A warm bath, shower or flannel will help milk to flow.

- Gently massage the lump towards the nipple.

- Express as much milk as possible by hand or pump.

- If your symptoms are no better within twenty-four hours, or if you start to feel feverish, you should see your family doctor because you may be developing mastitis (see **Breast-feeding, Mastitis**).

BREAST-FEEDING, CRACKED NIPPLES

Cracked nipples usually occur during the first few days of breast-feeding, especially affecting fair and red-headed women. They start as small, barely visible cracks which hurt when breast-feeding.

Self-health

- Follow all the advice for sore nipples (see **Breast-feeding, Sore**

Nipples), particularly ensuring the baby's mouth is correctly 'latched on' to the breast.

- Feed on demand so your baby is more likely to treat you gently.

- If feeding is too painful, express your milk and feed to your baby from a spoon or bottle. You will probably need to express by hand but some mothers manage with hand or electric pumps.

- Restrict the time your baby spends sucking and do not allow comfort sucking. A finger or dummy will do instead.

- Be cautious once the crack has healed. Still feed from this side second and restrict feeding time for another two to three days.

BREAST-FEEDING, ENGORGEMENT

Milk engorgement usually starts on the second to fifth day after childbirth when the milk 'comes in'. However, it is not all due to lots more milk – increased blood flow and excess fluid in the tissues also contribute. The engorgement usually goes down after two or three days but you can make yourself more comfortable meanwhile.

Self-health

- Feed your baby often.

- Put ice-cold flannels over your breasts after feeding to narrow the blood vessels and reduce the blood flow through them.

- Splash your breast with warm water before feeding to encourage the milk to flow.

- If your nipples do not protrude far enough:
  1. Try finger stroking away from the nipple to reduce the swelling.
  2. Try a latex nipple shield to start feeding but make sure you remove it once your nipple stands out firm.

- If your breasts are still engorged, express some milk either by hand or pump. This relieves the immediate discomfort of breast engorgement but has the disadvantage of encouraging the breast to produce more milk.

• If your own efforts fail to cope with engorgement consult your midwife, breast-feeding counsellor or doctor.

BREAST-FEEDING, MASTITIS

Mastitis is inflammation or infection of a milk duct. It usually happens when a blocked milk duct (see **Breast-feeding, Blocked Ducts**) traps milk, allowing bacteria to multiply in it.

Symptoms include an area of red, painful skin overlying a tender lump. You may also develop a temperature and feel unwell.

Self-health

• It is often difficult to tell when a blocked duct becomes infected. The most obvious sign is the lump becoming tender. As soon as it does you should see your family doctor, who will probably prescribe antibiotics. Antibiotics will not harm your baby although they may cause diarrhoea, which often makes your baby's bottom sore.

• Opinions vary about whether you should continue to feed from the affected breast. Most experts believe you should and that it will help clear the duct.

• You should also rest, preferably in bed and apply hot compresses to encourage milk flow and cold ones after feeding to soothe the breast. Drink plenty to keep your milk flowing and replace fluid lost by sweating.

BREAST-FEEDING, SORE NIPPLES

Breast-feeding is a pleasurable experience for most mothers but sore and cracked nipples can spoil it. Fair or redhaired women tend to suffer most.

Self-health

- Preventing sore nipples:

    1. Mothers used to be encouraged to 'harden' their nipples before birth with such horrors as nailbrushes. But now it is realized that this causes far more harm than good, so there is no need to prepare your nipples before breast-feeding begins.
    2. The best way to prevent sore nipples is to make sure the baby is 'latched on' correctly. You should get a nurse or breast-feeding counsellor to show you how, but here are some tips:

        a. Choose a feeding position that allows you to relax.
        b. Make sure your baby's head is tilted back in order to get your nipple and areola into his or her mouth. When your baby is correctly positioned, the chin will be against your breast but the nostrils will be free.
        c. If your baby's cheeks are puffing in and out he or she is not on properly. Start again by breaking suction with your little finger put into the side of the baby's mouth and re-positioning correctly.
        d. If you can see the top of your baby's ears wriggling while feeding, you know he or she is on the breast properly.
        e. Check that your baby's tongue is under, not over, your nipple if you are having difficulties.

    3. Start feeds on alternate sides. A safety pin on your bra strap will remind you which side to begin.
    4. Change your baby's feeding position often to rotate pressure from your baby's gums onto different parts of the areola.
    5. Don't wash your nipples before and after each feed; once daily is quite enough. Too much washing will make them soggy and easily damaged. After feeding, let your nipples dry naturally (speeded up by a hairdryer if you like). Some mothers find a drop of expressed milk on their nipples helps prevent soreness.
    6. Keep your nipples dry between feeds by exposing them to the air as much as possible or using one-way disposable nappies cut up. Avoid tissues, which quickly become damp and soften your nipples.

- Looking after sore nipples:

   1. Check all the points above.
   2. Try to relax, have a hot bath, listen to some music before feeding.
   3. Get the milk flowing before feeding starts. Thinking about your baby feeding often helps the 'let-down' reflex.
   4. To minimize the trauma to your nipples, feed your baby before he or she is very hungry.
   5. Start feeding on the least painful side first.
   6. Expose your nipples to the air as much as possible.
   7. By all means use a latex nipple shield but this will reduce the amount of milk your baby gets, so you will have to feed longer and more often.
   8. Beware of sprays and creams because your skin may be allergic to them. Camomile ointment (Kamillosan) is a useful and safe one.
   9. Sometimes the soreness may be due to thrush caught from your baby's mouth or bottom (see **Thrush, Mouth and Skin**). Consult your family doctor about treatment.

BREAST-FEEDING, TOO LITTLE MILK

Some mothers find difficulty in getting their milk to flow freely. Others get the milk flowing but find they are not producing enough to satisfy their baby. In such cases the baby may scream a lot or lose weight at a time when you might expect him or her to be gaining weight.

Self-health

- Start breast-feeding as soon as your baby is born. Do not imagine the apparently watery colostrom or 'first milk' is no good. It is precisely what your baby needs at this time.

- Three to five days later your milk will 'come in'. It may happen gradually or within a few hours. Thereafter you should continue to feed on demand. Ten or twelve feeds a day is not unusual in the first few weeks. The more your baby feeds, the more milk you will produce (which explains how mothers can cope with twins).

- You will need about 550 extra calories per day (equivalent to a good lunch) to make the milk for your baby, and it is a good idea to make sure this contains plenty of calcium.

- Rest as much as you can to give your breasts a chance to make the milk.

- Do not get in a panic about breast-feeding and not having enough milk. Worry and anxiety may themselves stop the milk. Other worries (e.g. other children, money or work) can have the same effect.

- Get yourself well organized in advance before starting your breast-feed. Make sure your chair or bed is comfortable; put on your favourite music or television programme; eat your favourite foods; if you have other children, make sure they have plenty of toys to keep them occupied while you breast-feed.

- Use relaxation techniques (see p. 62).

- A warm bath or shower may start the milk flowing. Feeding your baby in the bath often works.

- Make sure your baby is correctly positioned on your breast (see **Breast-feeding, Sore Nipples**) and that he or she drains them both completely at least once a day. This will stimulate them to produce more milk.

- Occasional milk supplements are useful and may help you at difficult times. But try not to use them frequently because this will reduce the stimulation to your breasts to make milk.

- Beware of some medicines (e.g. laxatives, antihistamines and the combined contraceptive pill) that may reduce milk production.

Screening

- It is a good general rule to allow your baby to decide how much milk he or she needs. Nevertheless, you may worry about whether your baby is getting enough. In this case, take your baby to the baby clinic to be weighed, always making sure he or she has the same clothes on.

BREAST, LUMPY

If you ever notice a lump in your breast you should consult your family doctor without delay. On no account wait to see whether it will go away, and certainly do not try the diets recommended in some irresponsible magazines as being able to get rid of lumps. The chances are that the lump is not cancer (see **Breast Cancer**) but you can never be sure until you have received professional advice.

Lumpy, tender breasts are common, especially just before and during periods. No one knows the cause but it is probably hormonal, because the symptoms may be helped by hormonal medicines (e.g. the contraceptive pill) or disappear after the menopause.

Self-health

- Treating lumpy breasts is so important and difficult that it must be left to experienced medical professionals.

- Your role and understanding is, however, vital for the success of prevention and treatment, whatever form it may take.

Screening

- Women with lumpy breasts have a slightly greater chance of breast cancer than other women, so they should practise breast self-examination regularly (see p. 73) and consult their family doctor or Well Woman clinic if they notice any unexplained changes.

BREATHLESSNESS

We need to breathe in order to obtain oxygen from the air, which is vital for the normal functioning of our bodies. Breathing is also necessary to get rid of waste products such as carbon dioxide. The brain controls these functions and increases or slows our rate of breathing to keep us healthy.

Most of us are not aware of breathing. Normally babies and infants breathe twenty-four to forty times a minute, and older children and adults sixteen to twenty-four times a minute. It is only a change in our breathing pattern that brings it to our attention – for example, breathing hard after a race.

So, breathlessness is not necessarily cause for concern. What matters is if the breathlessness is unusual for you – for example if you suddenly find that you can climb only one flight of stairs instead of two, or that going out into fields in the summer makes you wheezy.

In children there are all sorts of causes of sudden breathlessness but the common ones include inhaling something (e.g. a peanut) into one lung, or the beginning of an asthma attack which needs treatment to prevent it getting worse, or a sudden chest infection.

In adults there are many causes too, but common ones include a heart attack (which may not be accompanied by chest pain), heart failure or sudden pneumonia.

Self-health

- For many thousands of years breathing has been recognized as a way of controlling stress and tension. Many yoga, relaxation and stress-control exercises use breathing as a way of achieving mental and physical peace.

- If you live a fit and healthy life you will breathe deeply and regularly and the rate will quickly return to normal after exercise. The opposite happens if you are unhealthy.

- Any sudden breathlessness for no obvious reason should be taken seriously, and medical help sought immediately in an emergency.

- If you (or your child) are becoming increasingly breathless you should see your doctor because there may be a serious cause (e.g. anaemia, see separate entry) which can be treated. Other symptoms such as cough, high temperature, or loss of energy and appetite should persuade you to go to the doctor immediately.

- Giving up smoking and losing weight if you are overweight are two sure ways of limiting your breathlessness.

Breathing Exercises

- Make a habit of taking deep, slow breaths whenever possible in your everyday life.

- Sometimes it helps (especially if you know you are getting tense) to take a few minutes off twice a day to do the following exercises:

  1. Lie down with your lower back pressed firmly flat against the floor.
  2. Place your hands flat on your chest so you can feel its rhythmic movement. Close your eyes.
  3. Take some slow, deep breaths, gradually reducing the number to half the rate at which you normally breathe. Continue at this rate for up to five minutes (but stop if you feel faint or dizzy). Gradually increase the rate of your breathing back to normal. Open your eyes.

- You can do these exercises almost as effectively by sitting somewhere quiet, consciously relaxing all your muscles (especially in your neck) and breathing slowly for a few minutes.

BRONCHITIS

Bronchitis is an inflammation of the larger air passages leading to the lungs. There are two types, acute and chronic.

Acute bronchitis occurs when germs attack the lining of the air passages, causing inflammation. The lining swells, narrowing the passages and making you breathless because it is difficult to shift air in and out of the lungs. The irritation makes you cough. Usually after a few days it clears and you should have no long-term problems.

Chronic bronchitis is more serious because inflammation over a long time may permanently damage the airways so that you are prone to frequent attacks and become short of breath all the time.

Self-health

- Stop smoking. Research has shown that if you smoke up to fourteen cigarettes a day you are seven times more likely to die from chronic bronchitis than non-smokers. If you smoke fourteen to twenty-four cigarettes daily your chances rise to twenty times those of non-smokers.

- Keep away from smoky or dusty places. If the air you breathe at work is polluted consider changing jobs or persuading the management to clean the air up.

- Regular exercise and breathing exercises may help your body to work more efficiently. A good posture, with upright back and shoulders held back, helps your lungs to work well.

- Don't become overweight because this hinders breathing.

- If you are looking after very young or elderly people be wary of bronchitis because it affects them particularly seriously.

BRUISING

When blood seeps from a damaged blood vessel into surrounding tissues it causes bruising. This may be red or bluish to start with, turning yellowish-green.

Self-health

- The most common cause of bruising is accidental injury. In many cases this cannot be prevented, but read the chapter on Safety in the Home for some useful tips. There are some steps you can take to limit bruising.

- If possible, prevent further bleeding from the damaged blood vessel (see **Haemorrhage**).

- Bruising is a sign that bleeding has taken place and this should warn you to check that there isn't a more serious injury, like a fracture (see separate entry).

- Apply an ice-pack (e.g. bag of frozen peas) to the bruised part.

- Raise the bruised part if possible. For example put a leg up on a stool, or put an arm into a sling.

- Do not be alarmed by the vivid colours of the bruise – it does not mean it is getting worse, just older.

- If you start to bruise more easily after starting to take a medicine regularly (e.g. an anti-inflammatory medicine) see your doctor, who will decide whether a change is needed.

Screening

- Some people bruise more easily than others and there is nothing abnormal about this. However, if you bruise much more easily than others or you notice that you have begun to bruise more easily than you used to, you should see your doctor. There are one or two rare diseases such as haemophilia, leukaemia (see separate entries), or thrombocytopenia, especially in children that may cause this problem.

BULIMIA NERVOSA

Bulimia is also known as the binge/purge syndrome. It is a condition in which the person (almost always a woman) eats enormous quantities of food and then, often overcome by self-disgust, rids herself of the food by self-inducing vomiting or laxative abuse. It affects about one to two per cent of women (especially adolescents), which means up to half a million may be affected in the UK and perhaps as many as a million in the USA. Studies also show that up to fifteen per cent of women have an episode of bingeing and purging at some time in their life.

Affected women come from all social classes, are often extrovert, outgoing, sexually experienced and appear confident and normal in weight. Unlike anorexics (see **Anorexia Nervosa**) they acknowledge their problem and usually seek help.

Self-health

- It is impossible to identify in advance who will suffer from bulimia. However, certain women are at risk: those with a tendency to depression, overweight, alcohol or drug dependency; those with unreal obsessions about slimming or keeping an ideal weight, a proneness to carbohydrate craving before their periods and intolerance or hypersensitivity to certain foods.

- Warning signs that might alert a family that a relative has bulimia include:

  1. Repeatedly avoiding meals

2. Always visiting the bathroom after a meal
3. Dramatic fluctuations in body weight
4. Constant discussion about diets and weight
5. Unaccountable disappearance of food from cupboards
6. Increasing depression and isolation

• It is vital that the bulimic is persuaded or persuades herself to seek professional help. The longer the condition continues, the harder it is to recover from it. Occasionally in-patient hospital treatment may be needed. Broadly there are three forms of treatment: psychotherapy, in which you develop a relationship with a therapist who is able to help you to an understanding of your personal problems and your value as a person; group therapy, in which a group does the same thing; or behaviour therapy, in which the therapist pinpoints the triggers (e.g. anger, loneliness, boredom) to the bingeing/ purging and helps you to overcome them.

• Many women with bulimia have further attacks even after they have been well for years. Stress, unhappiness or overwork may be the triggers. So the bulimic or her family always has to be on the alert for warning signs.

BUNION

A bunion is a deformity of the big toe joint which produces a hard swelling on the inside edge of the foot. If the bunion is rubbed by shoes a callus may develop over it, and if it becomes inflamed a painful condition known as bursitis may develop.

Bunions are common in Western countries. About one in 1000 people (three times more women than men) consult their GP about them, but many more people suffer from them. The cause is not fully understood. Many experts believe they are due to badly fitting, lightweight shoes, particularly those with high heels and narrow toes. However, bunions occur in people who have never worn shoes so clearly there are other causes. It seems that bunions run in families so some people are more likely to get them whatever they do.

BUNIONS

Instead of remaining straight (like the other toes)
the big toe twists outwards, causing a bunion

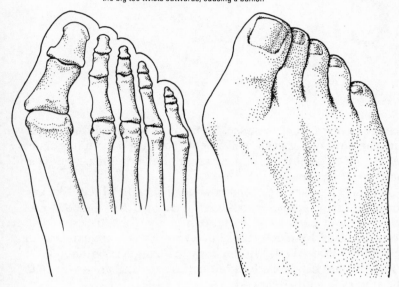

Self-health

- Most experts advise well-fitting, low-heeled shoes, especially
  for children, whose bones are still growing and soft. Shoes
  with a straight inner edge are best.

- Once a bunion has begun to appear it is even more important
  that you should wear comfortable, well-fitting shoes to prevent
  a callus or bursitis developing.

- A bunion shield, available from a chemist, can help if you
  have problems with the bunion.

- Cutting a hole in an old shoe so that the bunion can stick
  through it is useful if the bunion is painful.

- If your own efforts to cope with your bunion are not working,
  consult your family doctor or a chiropodist. Your chances of
  avoiding painful surgery are better if this is done earlier rather
  than later.

C

CANCER

Cancer is not a single disease. There are over 100 different types and the outlook for each is different. To say a person has cancer means little; what matters is where in the body the cancer is and how fast it has spread.

A cancer is made up of many abnormal cells which, like an invading army, spread into neighbouring parts of the body and prevent those parts from working properly. Sometimes collections of these cells break away from the main cancer and spread to different sites in the body, causing further damage. These distant cancers are called metastases and are a sign that the illness is well advanced.

There are no easy answers to the question 'Why do cancers start?' Some people live to a ripe old age despite smoking heavily and eating an unhealthy diet, yet others lead an exemplary life and develop a cancer.

However, scientists are beginning to discover the answers. It seems there are three main influences deciding whether you will get cancer – heredity, the environment, and your immune system (the system that spots and kills cancer cells before they have a chance to grow and become dangerous).

HEREDITY

Some cancers run in families, although the importance of the link varies greatly from cancer to cancer. For example, a high percentage of people with an inherited condition called polyposis coli develop cancer of the bowel. Retinoblastoma, a tumour of the eye, is directly inherited. Close relatives of a person with cancer of the breast run a higher than average risk of developing breast cancer themselves. But there are also many other cancers in which no link has been made.

ENVIRONMENT

The environment in which a person lives is an important influence on whether he or she will develop a cancer. Families who leave one country for another are more likely to develop the cancers common in the new country than those of the country they have left.

There are many different environmental influences, and on p. 130 there are suggestions on how you can avoid some of them. These influences range from a sudden exposure, such as the nuclear radiation caused by the Chernobyl disaster, to the long-term exposure that comes from living with a smoker.

THE IMMUNE SYSTEM

The body is made up of 100 million million cells. These are constantly dividing to make new cells so that organs do not wear out too quickly. With so many cells dividing it is not surprising that a few 'wrong uns' are made. These abnormal cells are immediately spotted by the body's 'policemen' cells (the lymphocytes) and killed before they have a chance to take root and start forming a cancer.

Sometimes, though, the body's defences are not so effective. The abnormal cells slip away, divide and start making a cancer which eventually becomes so strong that the body cannot kill it.

Many AIDS victims, for example, die from cancers which in a healthy body would have been destroyed long before they became life threatening. This is because the AIDS virus damages the body's defence systems, making its 'policing' abilities much less effective.

Researchers have been aware for some time that cancer often strikes when a person has just undergone severe stress, such as divorce, the death of a spouse or being made redundant. Recent research has shown that during this stressful time the body's defence cells, the lymphocytes, are much less effective at killing cancer cells.

Self-health

- There is no certain way of preventing cancer. The best that anyone can do is to reduce the risks as much as possible.

HEREDITY

- At the moment we cannot change our genetic make-up and therefore our susceptibility to cancer, although scientists are working on the problem and there may come a time when the genes responsible for 'hereditary' cancer can be identified and removed. It is important though that everyone takes into account their 'family' illnesses. For example, if your father and grandfather both died of lung cancer, it would be particularly reckless of you to smoke, because the combination of your family genetic make-up and the stimulus of smoking clearly results in cancer. Similarly if a close relative has died of breast cancer it is worth taking extra care with regular self-examination (see p. 75) because your family may have a tendency to breast cancer.

ENVIRONMENT

- **Smoking**.   The greatest single cause of cancer in the world is smoking. In America, for example, one in three cancer deaths is due to smoking. Most people know there is a close link between smoking and lung cancer, but there is also a link with other cancers, including that of the lips, mouth, gullet, bladder and cervix. Clearly a great burden of cancer would be lifted if people were able to stop smoking (see **Smoking**).

- **Too little dietary fibre**.   Nations whose inhabitants eat a high-fibre diet suffer from relatively little cancer of the bowel. Experts believe the reason is that a high-fibre diet makes a bulky stool, which dilutes any cancer-forming substances in the diet thus reducing the effect. Fibre also speeds the passage of the stool through the bowel, giving the cancer-forming substances less time to damage the bowel wall.

- **Sunlight**.   Too much sunlight is closely associated with skin cancer, especially in people with fair skins. Researchers have found that people with an estimated lifetime sun exposure of more than 30,000 hours have a twenty times greater chance of developing skin cancer than similar people exposed to less than 10,000 hours. Recently it has been found that just a few serious sunburns, especially in children, can be almost as harmful as long-term exposure to the sun.

So, the message is clear – protect your skin at all times. Being careless, even only occasionally, could be fatal.

- **Radiation**. Closely associated with sun exposure is the exposure to other types of radiation, including X-rays. If you work with radiation of any kind make sure all the safety precautions are observed.

- **Chemicals**. The risk from environmental chemicals and materials is difficult to assess but estimates suggest they cause one to three per cent of all cancers. The dangerous substances include some chemical dyes (bladder cancer), some compounds of arsenic, chrome and nickel (skin, lung and nose cancer), some wood dusts (nose cancer), some types of tar and soot (skin cancer) and asbestos (lung cancer). Air pollution probably does not cause cancer.

- **Viruses**.   More and more scientists are becoming convinced that viruses are closely linked with some cancers. The closest link is between the Epstein-Barr virus and a childhood cancer of the jaw called Burkitt's lymphoma. Also very important is the link between the herpes virus and cancer of the cervix. In the past, women who have had many sexual partners have been found to be prone to cervical cancer but no one understood why. Now we know that it is because they would have been more likely to pick up the herpes virus from their partners. Reducing the number of sexual partners is the most obvious preventive step, but using a condom or diaphragm ('cap') is also useful. It is important to have regular cervical smear tests in order to detect and treat cervical cells that look dangerous but not yet cancerous.

- **Diet and Alcohol**.   Few foods are closely linked with cancer. Some experts believe that smoking and curing foods produces dangerous hydrocarbons and they therefore recommend avoiding burned, charred or heavily smoked food. Others believe that food preserved by nitrates are dangerous because the body converts these substances into nitrosamines, which cause cancer in animals. No food additive, incidentally, has been directly linked with cancer.

  Alcohol has been loosely associated with cancer of the mouth, throat, gullet and liver but generally it is more likely to cause other diseases than cancer.

Sadly no food has been shown to protect against cancer, although some researchers believe that vitamins A, C and E and the trace metals zinc and selenium can be helpful. Eating a healthy diet is probably the best most of us can do.

Screening

The purpose of screening is to detect cancer at such an early stage that it can be successfully treated. Techniques are rapidly improving. Ten years ago, for example, the only routine way of detecting early breast cancer was by physical examination. Now the X-ray examination, mammography, can detect breast cancers that even the most expert surgeon could not feel. Recently researchers have reported that some time in the near future they will be able to predict who will develop breast cancer by culturing cells taken from breast skin.

USEFUL SCREENING

Breast: Self-examination, mammography
Cervix: Cervical smear
Testis: Self-examination
Mouth and tongue: Dental examination
Large bowel: Testing for blood in the faeces, sigmoidoscopy, colonoscopy (possibly)
Prostate: Examination by the doctor through the back passage
Kidney/Bladder: Testing for blood in the urine
Skin: Check skin regularly to make sure there are no new moles or old moles getting larger or bleeding

Why me?

The question everyone with cancer asks is 'Why me?'. There are now some who answer that it is due to a fault or failure in these unfortunate people's lives, thus adding the burden of guilt to their problems. The truth is that only in a very few cases can we be certain of the cause, and no one should ever be made to feel guilty for having cancer.

See separate entries for individual cancers.

The most common cancers worldwide	Number of new cases each year
Stomach	680,000
Lung	590,000
Breast	540,000
Colon and rectum	510,000
Cervix	460,000
Oesophagus	300,000
Liver	260,000

Cancer survival rates
(Figures from Cancer Research Campaign Factsheets 1987)

Types of cancer	Percentage of new UK cancer cases of this type (1984)		Percentage of patients alive 1 year after registration (England & Wales 1979–80)		Percentage of patients alive 5 years after registration (England & Wales 1979–84)	
	Male	Female	Male	Female	Male	Female
Lung	25	9	20	19	8	8
Skin (excluding melanoma)	11	10	98	99	98	99
Breast	0.2	19	—	85	—	64
Colon	6	7	52	49	37	35
Stomach	6	4	19	20	10	10
Prostate	9	—	71	—	47	—
Rectum	5	4	58	56	37	37
Bladder	6	2	75	63	63	52
Pancreas	3	2	10	10	4	4
Ovary	—	4	—	47	—	27
Cervix	—	4	—	76	—	57
Uterus	—	3	—	82	—	72
Oesophagus	2	2	18	21	8	9
Leukaemia	2	2	44	41	23	23
Other	23	29	—	—	—	—

CARPAL TUNNEL SYNDROME

Carpal tunnel syndrome is a condition in which there is pain and tingling, sometimes numbness, in the thumb, middle and forefingers of one or both hands. It is caused by compression of the median nerve, which runs from the upper arm to the hand, within its bony tunnel at the front of the hand.

It usually affects women and comes on at night or after carrying heavy shopping.

Self-health

- Symptoms often occur during pregnancy because the body has a natural tendency to retain fluid at this time. Try not to become overweight, as this will make the condition worse. Sometimes a wrist splint or hanging the arm over the bed at night will prevent symptoms becoming bad.

- Losing weight, if you are overweight, often causes the symptoms to disappear.

- Occasionally rheumatoid arthritis or an underactive thyroid gland causes this condition. If these are successfully treated, symptoms in the hand may disappear.

CATARACT

A cataract is the formation of cloudy patches on the normally crystal-clear lens of the eye. It may affect one or both eyes and causes general blindness. It usually affects people over sixty-five and can be successfully treated by surgery.

Self-health

- Good antenatal care will prevent mothers getting such illnesses as German measles (rubella) which can cause congenital cataract in children. Occasionally cataracts run in families.

- Diabetics are prone to cataracts, but careful control of blood sugar levels may slow or prevent their development.

- Patients taking steroid drugs should be wary of cataracts.

- Anyone noticing their sight getting worse should consult their doctor immediately.

CATARRH

Catarrh is an unscientific term which means different things to different people. Most people, though, think of it as a blocked nose accompanied by a thick discharge. Children are prone to catarrh because they have not developed strong defences against colds and flu, the commonest causes of catarrh.

Self-health

- Stopping smoking will make you less prone to catarrh.

- Keep children away from people with colds and flu.

- Try to identify and avoid allergic causes such as house-dust mites, pet fur or pollen.

CAT SCRATCH FEVER

Cat scratch fever is a rare disease caused by the scratch or bite of a cat. A few days after the injury a blister develops over the wound and a few weeks later it becomes swollen and obviously infected. Glands round the injury may also become swollen and even form abscesses.

Other symptoms include feeling unwell, a slight fever, tiredness and headache. These may last for several months, but usually they gradually disappear after about one month. Sometimes the glands need to be drained surgically.

Self-health

- The most obvious precaution is to keep away from cats. The trouble is that to keep away from all cats would be overly cautious, but on the other hand there is no way of knowing which cats are likely to cause the illness. Most families therefore accept this small risk of having a pet.

- If a cat does injure you, clean the wound with a mild antiseptic and make sure you have up-to-date tetanus coverage (see **Tetanus**). You should watch the wound carefully until it heals. If it blisters or becomes infected, and especially if local glands become swollen, you should consult your doctor immediately.

CERVICAL CANCER

Women have about a one in eighty chance of developing this growth at the neck of the womb (where it joins the vagina). The symptoms are bleeding from the vagina between periods, bleeding after sex or after the menopause, or an unexpected strong-smelling discharge.

This cancer may prove fatal if left untreated, but if treated early with surgery and/or radiotherapy the outlook is excellent, which is why early detection is so important.

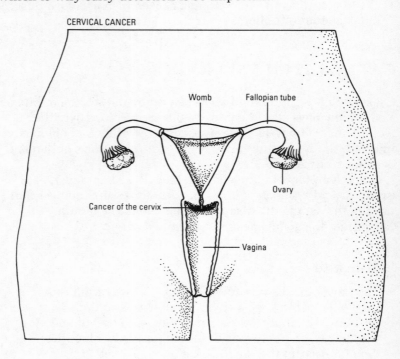

CERVICAL CANCER

Self-health

- The papilloma (wart) virus has been linked with cervical cancer. This virus does not cause the type of warts people get on their fingers, but is caught during sex. A woman's chances of getting this virus (and therefore possibly the cancer) increases not only with how many different sexual partners she has had but also with how many her partner has had.

  No one who develops cervical cancer should be labelled promiscuous. It takes only one partner for a woman to be infected with the wart virus, and the link with cervical cancer is still far from proven.

Screening

- Every sexually active woman should have a cervical smear test at least once every three years. The test detects abnormal cells before they turn into cancer, and treatment is easy at this

CERVICAL SMEAR TEST

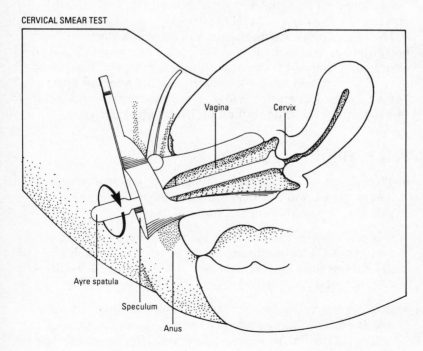

Vagina

Cervix

Ayre spatula

Speculum

Anus

stage. The test is available from your GP or local family planning clinic. The doctor does an internal examination and removes a few cells from your cervix using a wooden spatula. It may be slightly uncomfortable, but certainly not painful.

The cells are examined under a microscope and you should have the result within a few days. Make sure you get your result and never rely on 'no news is good news'. Finally, make sure you know when your next smear test is due.

CHICKENPOX

This mild infectious disease is caused by the virus *herpes zoster* (sometimes called *varicella*), the same virus that may months or years later cause shingles. It is usually a childhood infection but adults (especially those whose immunity system is not working well) may also catch it. There is usually a period of one to three weeks between being in contact with someone with the illness and developing the symptoms yourself.

The most dramatic symptom is a rash, which starts on the body and spreads to the limbs. The rash starts as small, red spots which may change to watery blisters that burst and then crust over. You may also have a slight temperature and feel as if you've got flu. Generally, though, a full recovery is made within five to ten days and the rash rarely leaves any scarring.

Self-health

- There is no vaccine against chickenpox, but once you have had an attack you are most unlikely to have another because you will have developed an immunity to it.

- It is probably sensible to keep your children away from others with chickenpox but do not be too upset if they catch it. It is not a dangerous illness, although just occasionally a sufferer may develop encephalitis.

- Do not scratch the spots because it may introduce infection into them, causing them to become pussy, and even need antibiotic treatment. You may find applying a soothing cream such as calamine helps reduce the itchiness.

- Paracetamol helps reduce fever and any flu-like symptoms.

- Your doctor should be contacted to diagnose the chickenpox. He or she will not normally be needed further, except in some countries where a new prescription medicine, acyclovir, is sometimes used early in the illness to reduce symptoms. If you (or your child) find yourself becoming more ill for no reason and especially if you are drowsy, have a severe headache and feel nauseated you should contact your doctor immediately because it is just possible encephalitis may be developing.

CHILBLAINS

Chilblains are patches of reddish-blue skin usually affecting the fingers, toes or calves in cold weather. Normally, arteries narrow when it gets cold so that less blood reaches the skin and the body conserves heat. But in just a few people this process does not work properly and the result is red, itchy, swollen, often painful and broken skin.

Self-health

- Wear plenty of clothing to keep the body, hands and feet warm. Two thin layers are better than one thick one because the air trapped between them acts as insulation.

- Wear a hat that covers your ears. Children in particular lose a lot of heat through their heads.

- If you have diabetes you should take special precautions because you will be more prone to chilblains.

- Keep the house warm. Special heating allowances are available from the DSS so if you are on a low income check to see if you are eligible.

CHIROPRACTIC

Chiropractic is a system of healing based on the belief that most of the body's ills are due to misalignment of the joints (subluxations) of the spine, especially the joints between the vertebrae.

The founder was the American Daniel David Palmer (1845–1913) who believed these ills could be cured by manipulating the alignment of the spine. This manipulation can be quite violent and in unskilled hands is dangerous. Sometimes a single manipulation is all that is necessary; more often a longer course is recommended.

Self-health

- There is no doubt that many chiropractors are very skilled at manipulating the back and can help many people with back problems. Whether they can successfully treat other illnesses is much more a matter of doubt. There is very little research to back up their claims.

- Because manipulating the back is dangerous and can lead to permanent damage it is important that the practitioner is skilled and experienced. In the UK there are about 200 chiropractors registered with the British Chiropractors Association, 5 First Avenue, Chelmsford, Essex, CM1 1RX, all of whom have had to complete an approved course. There may be another 3,000 practising without having completed a course, and it is probably unwise to contact these. Some doctors and physiotherapists are now beginning to use similar techniques to those recommended by chiropractors.

- There are many reasons why it may be dangerous to manipulate a back (e.g. osteoporosis, cancer, fractures, infections such as tuberculosis) so many experts believe a back should not be manipulated without a thorough examination and X-rays first. You may wish to discuss this point with a chiropractor when you visit.

CHOLERA

Cholera is caused by the bacterium *vibrio cholerae*, which is present in the faeces of infected patients and carriers. It is spread in areas where there is poor hygiene by the faeces contaminating water, raw vegetables and fruit. Six to forty-eight hours after drinking or eating the contaminated water or food, the affected person develops usually painless diarrhoea which is so serious that there is a real danger (up to sixty per cent chance) of death from dehydration if it is left untreated. There may be vomiting and muscle cramps too.

Self-health

- Everyone should practise good personal hygiene, but in affected countries this must be scrupulous. During major disasters such as earthquakes, floods or war there is always a risk of cholera.

- Travellers to affected countries should be immunized against the disease (see **Travelling Abroad**). Immunity lasts up to six months in theory, but it is not completely effective so vaccination should not be an excuse to neglect good hygiene.

- Great care should be taken over selecting food in affected countries. Water should be boiled and food cooked thoroughly to kill the bacteria.

- As soon as symptoms begin you should start drinking non-alcoholic fluids such as bottled water or fruit juice to combat the dehydration. On no account stop drinking in the mistaken belief that this will dry up the diarrhoea. Inform your doctor of your suspicion immediately. He or she will arrange hospital admission and intravenous fluids if necessary as well as prescribing antibiotics to kill the bacteria. Treated this way almost everyone makes a full recovery over one to two weeks, without any long-term problems.

CHOLESTEROL

Cholesterol is a type of fat. It is a normal part of many tissues of the body (especially the brain, liver, nerves and blood) and is essential for health. It comes partly from food, e.g. eggs and milk, but eighty per cent of the body's requirements is made by the body itself in the liver.

The problem is that in some people the level of cholesterol in the blood rises so high that it begins to coat the inside of the arteries. The resulting narrowing of the arteries increases the chances of many diseases, particularly heart disease and strokes. This tendency for cholesterol to gather in the arteries is increased if you eat a high-fat diet with a high proportion of saturated fat (see chapter on Healthy Eating).

Self-health

- Because only twenty per cent of the body's cholesterol is absorbed from food it might be thought that changing your diet would do little to reduce the risks. However, the type of fat you eat does affect the way cholesterol is processed in the body, and it is for this reason that the DHSS Coma (1984) report made the following recommendations:

  1. Everyone should reduce the amount of saturated fats they eat by one-quarter.
  2. Fats should provide no more than thirty-five per cent of the energy (measured in kilocalories) provided by the diet.
  3. More than half of all fats should be monounsaturated and polyunsaturated.

- Take moderate exercise, e.g. swimming, tennis, cycling or walking, for thirty minutes three times a week.

- Eat a high-fibre diet (see chapter on Healthy Eating).

- Do not drink too much alcohol (see **Alcoholism**).

- Eat plenty of green, leafy vegetables, because the vitamin C they contain reduces the amount of cholesterol in your blood.

Screening

- The following groups are at special risk and should have their blood cholesterol measured:

  1. People with high blood pressure
  2. Diabetics
  3. People with angina (see **Heart Disease**) or pain in the legs after exercise (claudication)
  4. Anyone under sixty years old who has heart disease
  5. Anyone who has a close relative under sixty with heart disease

6. Women on the contraceptive pill who smoke

- Measuring the level of cholesterol in your blood is a fairly accurate way of estimating whether it is too high. There is no one level above which every doctor will agree you are at risk, but most will become concerned if it is above 350–400 mg/dl and will probably put you on a special diet. If this is not successful there are medicines that reduce the amount of cholesterol in the blood.

CIRRHOSIS OF THE LIVER

Cirrhosis is a slow-moving but usually progressive disease of the liver in which the useful, active liver cells are replaced by useless fibrous tissue. These changes make the liver less able to carry out its many vital functions. The person may lose appetite and weight and feel sick and weak. Later the body becomes jaundiced, small spidery marks (spider naevi) may appear on the face and body, men lose their sex drive and women stop having periods. Eventually the body retains so much fluid that the ankles and abdomen swell, and the person becomes confused and drowsy, with trembling hands and no memory or concentration. At this stage the outlook is very serious.

Self-health

- Cirrhosis is rare except among heavy drinkers. So if you are regularly drinking more than 2½–3 pints of beer a day (or 5–6 measures of spirits or glasses of wine) you are at risk of developing cirrhosis. Take notice of warning signs and see your doctor and local self-help groups for practical advice.

- Occasionally hepatitis may cause cirrhosis. Do not drink alcohol while you have hepatitis or for about six months afterwards (ask your doctor for a precise timetable). You may always be prone to cirrhosis and less able to drink alcohol.

- Any doctor or dentist prescribing medicines for you will want to know if you have cirrhosis because some medicines may be dangerous for you.

CLAUSTROPHOBIA

Claustrophobia is an abnormal fear of confined, enclosed spaces.
Sufferers are unable to travel in lifts, cars or trains and some may
even have problems confined at home.

Self-health

- Avoiding enclosed spaces is one way of preventing
  claustrophobia, but this limits your social life and is not a
  long-term solution.

- Try gradual exposure to the situations that bring on your fears.
  On each occasion take a further step towards mastering your
  fears without going so far as to bring them on, because this
  will undo your good work. Look at pictures showing the
  places you fear and imagine yourself coping. Lessen your fears
  by discussing them with friends and relatives who will
  appreciate your problem and help you cope.

- If none of this works, see your doctor, who will arrange
  professional help. Sometimes a short course of tranquillizers
  or anti-depressants may be all you need. Occasionally a
  technique known as 'flooding' is used. This means you are
  forced to confront your fears in a situation from which it is
  impossible to escape. This causes severe anxiety (and so
  should never be attempted without medical advice), but once
  you realize your fears are groundless, you will learn to
  overcome them.

COELIAC DISEASE

Some babies and children, and occasionally adults, are allergic
to gluten, a protein found in many cereals. When the lining of
their small bowel comes into contact with gluten it loses its
healthy, fluffy appearance and becomes flat so that it does not
absorb food so well. The baby starts to lose appetite and weight,
and passes frequent pale, loose, nasty-smelling faeces, often with
a lot of wind. In its mild form the disease may slow growth and
development; in more severe cases it can be life-threatening if
the cereals are not stopped.

Self-health

- A gluten-free diet will rapidly stop symptoms and prevent them developing in the future. Exclude all wheat and rye and avoid breakfast cereals, gravies, bread, cakes and biscuits made with wheat flour.

- Substitute rice, corn or soya flour for wheat flour. It is perfectly possible to enjoy tasty and varied food on this diet. Many manufacturers make special gluten-free foods. Lists are available from big supermarkets such as Sainsbury's.

- When eating out in restaurants stick to fresh fruits and plain meat or fish dishes without sauces.

- When travelling take a good supply of gluten-free bread, biscuits and cereals.

COLD

A cold is an infection caused by a virus. It usually affects the nose and throat (a 'head' cold) but it can also spread to the larynx (laryngitis) or lungs (bronchitis). It lasts two to three days, or longer if bacteria invade the infected part (e.g. the throat), causing a secondary infection. Babies and toddlers are prone to colds because they have not yet developed resistance or immunity to them.

Self-health

- Keep away from people with colds. Similarly, if you have a cold, do not breathe or cough over other people.

- Wash your hands frequently if you have a cold, as research has shown that viruses are passed on by contact as easily as being carried in droplets.

- Avoid getting cold or wet (catching a chill) as this will reduce your resistance to viruses.

- There is no purpose in taking antibiotics to prevent yourself getting a cold as these do not have any effect on viruses. Your doctor will prescribe antibiotics only if he or she thinks you have developed a secondary bacterial infection.

- The American Dr Pauling published research in 1970 that showed that taking large doses (1–2 g per day) of vitamin C could reduce the number of colds people get. However, this has never been confirmed by other researchers, and the general view now is that vitamin C in even larger doses (200–500 g per day) can make the symptoms better but not prevent a cold.

- Do not smoke. Smokers catch more colds and suffer worse than non-smokers.

COLD SORES

Cold sores are painful ulcers of the lip, cheek, gums and tongue caused by the virus, *herpes simplex*. Most people (eighty per cent of the population) carry the virus, usually having caught it as children from infected parents or relatives. The virus passes through the child's skin to a nerve where it travels up to hide in a nerve junction. Here it may stay never causing a cold sore. Or a stimulus like flu, a cold, stress, a menstrual period, strong sunlight or emotional problems may encourage it to travel back down the nerve to the skin causing a cold sore.

Self-health

- Viruses from the cold sore can be easily passed on to other people or other parts of your body so some basic precautions are worthwhile, especially for nursing mothers. For example do not test drink or food (for temperature or taste) with an infected mouth or tongue before feeding it to a baby or toddler.

- Make sure you wash your hands after touching a sore because you could easily spread the infection to other parts of the body, especially eyes and genitals. You need to be particularly careful after applying treatment like ointment. Women putting on eye make-up are at particular risk.

- Avoid breaking the blister and picking the scabs. Not only can you infect your fingers with the virus, but you may also allow bacteria to infect the cold sore and make it worse.

- Avoid kissing if you have a cold sore on your mouth or tongue, or having sex if your genitals are infected. Once the sore has disappeared you can enjoy both kissing and sex again.

- If you have a cold sore make sure you don't share crockery, cups or glasses with other members of the family – also avoid using the same towels, bathmats and face towels as these provide the perfect climate for the viruses to grow.

- A new prescription medicine, acyclovir, is helpful if used early.

COLIC

Colic is pain caused by the gut going into spasm. It is often troublesome in young babies (three-month or evening colic) who cry a lot, arch their backs and kick their legs.

Self-health

- Your baby might be taking in too much wind when feeding. If you are breast-feeding you may have too much milk or it may be coming too fast, so try expressing the first milk by hand before allowing your baby to feed, or confine the feed to one breast only. Use your other breast for the next feed, but if it becomes uncomfortable you may need to express it meanwhile. If you are bottle-feeding, the hole in the teat might be too large, allowing your baby to gulp down air as well as milk. Change the nipple to one with a smaller hole.

- Feed your baby in a more upright position, try not to bounce him or her during feeds, and always 'wind' the baby at the end.

- If you are bottle-feeding try a different type of milk.

- If you are breast-feeding cut out dairy foods from your own diet as these may cause colic in your baby. Onions, leafy vegetables like cabbage, beans, pulses, garlic and alcohol can also make some babies windy.

- Try to feed your baby in as calm and contented an atmosphere as possible. Any anxiety or haste on your part will be quickly transmitted to your baby.

- If all these suggestions fail, see your doctor. It is most unlikely there is a serious cause for your baby's colic, but it is worth reassuring yourself that it is just a stage which will pass in time.

CONFUSION

A mental state in which the person, usually elderly, is unable to make sense of the situation he or she is in. It may vary from a mild loss of memory and muddled feeling to a total loss of contact with reality, verging on dementia (see separate entry).

Self-health

- Avoid putting elderly people in unfamiliar, stressful situations with which they will find difficulty coping. Elderly people need routine and familiar surroundings.

- A well-balanced diet with plenty of vitamins served regularly on time is important for elderly people. Occasionally vitamin deficiencies can cause confusion.

- If an elderly person gets very cold (body temperature falls below 35°C) it is likely he or she will become confused. See **Hypothermia** for ways to prevent low temperatures.

- Do not assume all elderly people become confused. Some may have developed a physical illness such as diabetes (see separate entry) or thyroid disease (see **Thyroid Gland, Overactivity** and **Thyroid Gland, Underactivity**) and will need to see their family doctor.

CONJUNCTIVITIS

Conjunctivitis is inflammation of the conjunctiva, a thin, clear layer that lies over the white of the eye. The eyes may look red and congested, and feel gritty. They become sticky and crusted, especially on waking. It is caused by a viral or bacterial infection, or an allergy (for example to grass pollen, tobacco or house-dust mites).

Self-health

- The commonest way the infection is caught is by rubbing the eyes with contaminated towels or flannels, or with fingers that have become infected. It is most important you use clean or disposable towels in public places, and at home someone with conjunctivitis should have their own towel and flannel.

- If the conjunctivitis is allergic, try to identify what brings it on. Beware of cosmetics, and some ointments, eyedrops or eyewashes which themselves might cause the inflammation.

CONSTIPATION

Everyone has different patterns of bowel movement. Some have two or three movements a day, others have only two or three each week. It is not the frequency that matters. What matters most is that the faeces are soft and not painful to pass. Only consider yourself constipated if you pass small, hard, infrequent stools or if there has been a change in your normal bowel routine.

Self-health

- Eat a high-fibre diet (30 g a day) to make sure your stools are bulky and easily passed.

- Drink plenty of fluid to keep the faeces soft. In babies small, hard stools are a sign that they are not getting enough to drink.

- Avoid laxatives; they can cause constipation themselves by making the bowel inactive.

- Some medicines cause constipation (e.g. iron pills and cough mixtures). If you notice that you have become constipated since starting a medicine, tell your doctor.

- You may have become constipated because you have a painful condition like piles (see **Haemorrhoids**) or an anal fissure which makes it uncomfortable to pass a stool. See your doctor for treatment for the condition and your constipation.

- One of the first signs of depression is constipation. Improving your mood may well prevent further bowel problems.

- Take plenty of exercise appropriate to your age, and try to achieve a regular pattern of bowel movement.

Screening

- A change of bowel habit could be an important sign of a serious illness. If it persists for longer than two or three weeks you should see your doctor.

CONTRACEPTION

Every day about 200,000 babies are born into a world where there will be double the present population in about forty years. Not only will these babies have an enormous impact upon their environment but the sadness is that up to one-third may be unwanted.

There is therefore clearly an urgent need for contraception. The fact that there are so many different types, however, suggests that so far there is no perfect one. Some of the common methods are described below.

The calendar/rhythm method

- This method takes advantage of the days when a woman is infertile, i.e. for a short time after the end of her period before her ovaries produce an egg ready for fertilization (known as ovulating), and also for a longer time after ovulation and before her period begins. The difficulty is being certain exactly when these times are.

- For the most accurate guide to when you are 'safe' keep a record of your longest and shortest menstrual cycles over twelve months. Day one of a cycle is traditionally the first day of bleeding and the day before bleeding begins again is the last day of the cycle.

  Subtract twenty from the length of the shortest cycle (e.g. 26 − 20) to give you the first day of the fertile period (i.e. day six). Since many women may bleed for four to five days, during which time intercourse is avoided by some, this may give you

only one to two days for 'safe' intercourse before ovulation.
Subtract eleven from the longest cycle (e.g. 30 − 11) to give
you the last day of your fertile period (i.e. day nineteen). After
day nineteen intercourse is 'safe' until you may wish to stop
again with the start of your next period.

- Ovulation can be timed more accurately if you are aware that
  up to thirty-six hours after ovulation the body temperature
  rises by 0.2–0.6°C. Using this information you can measure
  your temperature accurately every day and resume 'safe' sex
  three days after the rise in temperature.

- With experience you can refine the rhythm method still
  further by observing the mucus from your cervix. In general
  terms it is safe to have sex during the early part of your cycle
  while the mucus is thick and cloudy. However, as soon as it
  becomes thin and clear you should stop until three full days
  after the 'peak' time of thin mucus when you can start again.
  Obviously it will take time for you to recognize the different
  types of mucus. You can also be confused by the fluids you
  produce in your vagina when you are sexually aroused, by
  semen, and by menopausal changes.

- Finally there are now urine testing kits which measure how
  much luteinizing hormone is in your urine. The level
  increases just before ovulation. The test can be done at home,
  is simple, reliable and takes only thirty minutes.

ADVANTAGES

1. No known side effects
2. Acceptable to many religious groups
3. Cheap, with no medical follow-up needed once the method is
   working well
4. Under the user's control

DISADVANTAGES

1. There is a very real chance of pregnancy. Average figures
   suggest that you will conceive once every six years but they
   do not say when in those six years it will be. However, you
   can reduce the chance of pregnancy further if you confine sex

to after ovulation as described above, and not before when risks are much greater.

2. There are restrictions on when you can enjoy sex, which some couples find irksome. It may also push them towards alternative sexual activities which one of the partners may not find acceptable.

The Combined Oral Contraceptive Pill (COC)

The COC first became available in the USA in 1960 and in the UK in 1961. Usage now varies between less than one per cent in Japan and about forty per cent in the Netherlands. In the UK, the COC is used by one-quarter to one-third of sexually active women.

The COC works by blocking the release of eggs (ovulation) ready for fertilization. Back-up effects include making the cervical mucus less receptive to the passage of sperm and the womb less receptive to the fertilized egg.

ADVANTAGES

1. The COC is almost 100% reliable if taken exactly as prescribed. If you forget one tablet take it as soon as you can, even if it means taking two within a few hours of each other. If you go for longer than thirty-six hours without taking a tablet you could become pregnant and must take other precautions. Continue to take the remaining tablets for the month and you can stop other precautions when you start a new course.

2. The regular withdrawal bleed at the end of each course reassures you about the success of contraception.

3. It is very convenient. You can have sex at any time without preparing or worrying.

4. It does not affect or spoil the act of intercourse.

5. It can help many period problems such as heavy, irregular, or painful bleeding.

6. It may help alleviate premenstrual tension (see separate entry).

7. It provides some protection against pelvic inflammatory disease (see separate entry) by making the cervical mucus hostile to germs passing through it. Pill-takers have fifty per

cent less chance of being hospitalized for pelvic inflammatory disease than non-takers.

8. Because it prevents ovulation it also prevents ectopic pregnancies (pregnancies outside the womb, e.g. in the Fallopian tubes).
9. It protects against benign breast disease (see **Breast, Lumpy**) – but not breast cancer.
10. It helps some patients with rheumatoid arthritis (see **Arthritis**).
11. It reduces the risk of cancer of the ovary by forty per cent overall, and the longer you have taken the COC the better the protection. Protection may last up to fifteen years after stopping.
12. It reduces the risk of cancer of the womb by fifty per cent overall, again the benefit increasing with time 'on the Pill'. Protection may last up to ten years after stopping.
13. It improves the condition of some women's skin, particularly those prone to spots during their period.

DISADVANTAGES

1. Circulatory diseases have been shown to be more common in COC users. These include deep vein thrombosis (see **Thrombosis**), heart attacks (see **Heart Disease**) and strokes (see **Stroke**).

   The COC does raise blood pressure (see separate entry) in a few women, so if you smoke, or have a family history of any of these disorders, you should consider whether the COC is right for you.
2. The COC may increase the risk of cervical cancer (see separate entry) and heart disease (see separate entry). Regular cervical screening and heart examination may help prevent this problem.
3. The COC may cause a slightly increased risk of jaundice, gallbladder disease and a very rare liver cancer.
4. Some women find the COC causes them to retain fluid, swell and put on weight. This swelling may explain why some women have difficulty with contact lenses and others suffer from nausea and headaches. Occasionally the COC makes women feel very depressed and lose interest in sex.

The Mini Pill

The mini pill (MP) contains only the hormone progestogen. It is used by about three per cent of contraceptive users (eight per cent of oral contraceptive takers).

It works by making cervical mucus hostile to sperm and by changing the lining of the womb to make it difficult for the fertilized egg to settle. It may also affect ovulation in some women.

ADVANTAGES

1. If used correctly it is very effective.
2. It can be useful for older women for whom the combined pill (COC) might be dangerous.
3. There is as yet no evidence that the MP increases your risk of either cancer or circulatory diseases (such as stroke or heart attack).
4. It has fewer side effects than the COC – less nausea, headaches, weight gain, or loss of interest in sex.
5. Many of the advantages of the COC also apply to the mini pill, e.g. protects against menstrual disorders and pelvic inflammatory disease.

DISADVANTAGES

1. You need to be extremely careful about taking the pill at the same time each day, so it is not suitable if you are disorganized.
2. It alters the duration and volume of blood flow during your period. Some women bleed at unexpected times. Cycle irregularity is the most common reason for stopping this method. In fact, the more irregular the cycle the more effectively the MP is working and vice versa.
3. Some women may develop painful ovarian cysts.
4. There is an increased risk of ectopic pregnancies (those outside the womb).
5. It provides no protection against ovarian and cervical cancer or non-cancerous breast disease.

The Morning-After Pill

The morning-after pill (MAP) contains large doses of hormones and is effective up to seventy-two hours after unprotected sex. Depending on when you take it during your cycle it works by preventing ovulation, making cervical mucus hostile or preventing implantation in the womb.

ADVANTAGES

1. It provides you with an opportunity to avoid an unwanted pregnancy after unprotected intercourse has taken place, so it is ideal for an emergency.
2. It is 96–99% effective in preventing conception.
3. It has no known serious side effects provided it is used only occasionally.

DISADVANTAGES

1. Nausea and vomiting are common.
2. The failure rate is 1–4% – quite high compared to other methods.
3. You should avoid MAP if you have had a deep vein thrombosis in the past.
4. It should only be used for emergencies.

Intra-uterine device (IUD or coil)

An IUD or coil works by stopping the fertilized egg settling in the womb and beginning to grow. There are several different types and your doctor will discuss with you which one suits you best. Worldwide, about sixty million women use IUDs, of which forty million are in China. In the UK and USA about four per cent of women taking contraceptive measures use them.

ADVANTAGES

1. An IUD is more effective than the 'cap' or condom (but less effective than the Pill).
2. It has no effect on other body systems, e.g. it does not make you feel sick or gain weight.

3. It needs no special preparation before sex and most couples are unaware of it during sex.
4. It does not need any daily action, like taking a pill, apart from monthly checks that the tail or string is still there. If it is not, take other precautions and see your doctor.
5. It can be safely used by women who are smokers or who are at risk of circulation diseases or cancer.
6. It is not associated with any kind of cancer.

DISADVANTAGES

1. An IUD should generally not be used by women who want to have children in the future because it can cause pelvic infections which reduce fertility. Furthermore, unlike the condom or the Pill, it does not have a protective effect against infections.
2. Expert medical care is needed to insert an IUD, and occasionally the device is accidentally pushed through the wall of your womb. It also needs to be removed by a doctor.
3. It can sometimes come out of your womb without you knowing it and then you are at risk of pregnancy.
4. It may cause unusually heavy, irregular or painful periods.
5. It can cause pelvic pain.
6. Because it prevents implantation of the egg in the womb it can cause pregnancies to implant elsewhere (e.g. in the tubes, which may have serious consequences such as heavy bleeding or damage to the tubes).

The diaphragm (cap)

The diaphragm or cap is a dome-shaped latex sheath which is placed across the entrance of the cervix at the top of the vagina. It works by holding spermicide (sperm-killing jelly) against the entrance of the cervix so that sperm are killed on their way through, also by keeping sperm in the acidic vagina (which kills them) rather than in the alkaline cervix (which encourages them) and by preventing sperm being drawn in to the cervix and womb.

The cap's popularity has been declining since the 1950s; now only about four per cent of women use it in the UK.

ADVANTAGES

1. If used correctly the cap is an effective contraceptive.
2. It has no effect on other body systems.
3. It is used only when needed.
4. It gives some protection against sexually transmitted diseases, pelvic inflammatory disease (see separate entry) and cervical cancer (see separate entry).
5. It can be used during your period to hold back the blood and help make lovemaking more enjoyable.

DISADVANTAGES

1. It is less effective as a contraceptive than the Pill or IUD, although the failure rate is very low.
2. Some women dislike having to handle their genitals when putting the diaphragm in before sex and taking it out afterwards.
3. There is some loss of spontaneity because the diaphragm has to be put in before sex. Some women dislike such premeditated preparation (but some find it sexy).
4. There may be some loss of vaginal and cervical sensation. However, there should be no pain if the cap is fitted properly.
5. Some couples find the spermicidal cream messy.
6. It needs to be fitted initially by a doctor or nurse, there is usually a week of training when other protection must be used, and checks are made every six to twelve months afterwards to make sure the fit is still good and the cap still in good condition.
7. A few women develop vaginal irritation or allergy, mainly due to the spermicidal cream but occasionally from the rubber.
8. Occasionally it is possible to forget to remove the cap and this may cause some vaginal abrasions or ulcers.

Spermicides

Spermicides are preparations that kill sperm as they try to swim through the vagina into the cervix and womb. They must be put into the vagina before sex and generally work for up to three hours.

Spermicides are not recommended for women for whom an unplanned pregnancy would be a disaster, but they can be useful for 'spacing' children, and for menopausal women in whom fertility is reduced.

ADVANTAGES

1. Spermicides are easy to buy and use.
2. There are no health risks, and no medical supervision is necessary.
3. They need be used only when required.
4. They give some protection against sexually transmitted diseases and pelvic inflammatory disease.
5. They can be used as a lubricant of the vagina.
6. They work well with other barrier methods (e.g. the cap, see p. 156).

DISADVANTAGES

1. Spermicides are not reliable except when used with a barrier method.
2. They are messy, need some premeditated preparation before sex and may interfere with lovemaking.
3. They can cause irritation or allergy in the vagina.
4. It has recently been discovered that there may be some risk of spermicide absorption from the vagina into the bloodstream.

The Sponge

The contraceptive sponge is made of foam impregnated with a spermicide and has a depression in the middle to fit over the cervix and a tape to remove it. It is moistened with tap water a few seconds or up to twenty-four hours before sex and then inserted high in the vagina, where it should be left for at least six hours after sexual intercourse. It is about as effective as spermicidal cream on its own.

ADVANTAGES

1. It has most of the advantages of spermicides (see above) plus it is not messy.

DISADVANTAGES

1. It has similar disadvantages to spermicides (see above) plus some women find it breaks up and can be difficult to remove.

See also **Sterilization, Female**.

The condom (sheath)

About four million couples worldwide use the condom. Japanese couples add up to a quarter of all condom users in the world (seventy-five per cent of Japanese couples who practise contraception use condoms). By contrast use is low in the Middle East, Latin America and Africa (which may partly explain the rapid spread of AIDS in this continent), accounting for only four per cent of worldwide use. One 1983 survey suggested that about twenty per cent of all couples in the UK use the sheath – mostly those under twenty-one and over thirty – making it the second most popular contraceptive after the Pill.

ADVANTAGES

1. The sheath is effective if used correctly, as follows:
   a. There should be no genital contact before you put the sheath on because sometimes fluid containing sperm leaks from your penis before ejaculation.
   b. Always use a new sheath for each act of intercourse.
   c. Do not damage the rubber (e.g. with long fingernails).
   d. Always make sure air is squeezed out of the tip of the condom to leave room for the sperm.
   e. Do not wait until the penis is soft before removing the sheath or you may spill semen within the vagina.
   f. Do not use an oil-based grease like Vaseline for lubrication because it may quickly perish the rubber – use KY jelly instead.
   g. Many doctors recommend that the woman uses a spermicide as well as a sheath but the Family Planning Association no longer considers it essential, because of worries about spermicidal absorption into the bloodstream and concern that its messiness may reduce condom use.
   h. If the sheath breaks or slips off, the woman should see her

doctor within seventy-two hours about the morning-after pill (see p. 155).
2. It is easily obtained and relatively cheap.
3. There are no medical side effects and no medical supervision is needed.
4. It provides protection against most sexually transmitted diseases and may protect against cancer of the cervix.
5. It is good for men who ejaculate prematurely (see **Ejaculation, Premature**) because it reduces sensation. This is particularly true of thick condoms.
6. Can be ribbed or textured, which some women may find more pleasurable.
7. It reassures the woman that a contraceptive is being used and that the man is taking responsibility.

DISADVANTAGES

1. It has to be bought and remembered in advance and may interrupt spontaneous sex. It is seen by some couples as a psychological and physical barrier to true closeness.
2. It reduces male sensation, although less so with modern products.
3. It is ineffective if not used properly and so is not recommended for long-term use in sexually active couples. The most common mistake is failure to leave enough space at the end of the condom to accommodate the sperm during ejaculation.

Withdrawal method (coitus interruptus)

The withdrawal method is when the man withdraws his penis from the vagina before he ejaculates.

Despite being described by Marie Stopes as 'harmful to the nerves as well as unsafe', the withdrawal method is a lot better than no method at all.

ADVANTAGES

1. It is free.
2. It doesn't have to be remembered in advance.
3. It has no medical side effects.

DISADVANTAGES

1. It is considerably less effective than most conventional contraceptives. Some men have semen in fluid which escapes from the penis before ejaculation and is impossible to prevent. Others forget to withdraw.
2. Some women may not trust the man to withdraw and so will not be able to relax and enjoy themselves. Surprisingly, research has shown that this is a less common problem among regular users than might be expected.
3. Some women may find themselves left short of an orgasm because the man has to withdraw just when he is at his most passionate. This problem can, however, be overcome by a skilful and considerate lover (see **Orgasm, Lack of, Female**)
4. Some lovemaking positions will have to be abandoned because the man needs to be able to withdraw quickly.

THE MALE PILL

There have been technical advances in the last few years that make a male Pill within the next five to ten years a real possibility.

One of the obstacles to research in the past has been manufacturers' concern that women would not trust men to take the Pill as instructed. However, attitudes to shared responsibilities for contraception are changing and many women would now be comfortable with this thought.

See also **Sterilization, Male (Vasectomy)**.

CORNS

Corns and calluses are areas of thickened skin, usually on the toes and soles of the feet. They tend to develop over bones, due to constant friction from new or badly fitting shoes, particularly high-heeled ones. They may become painful.

Self-health

• Wear comfortable shoes (e.g. sandals) which avoid putting pressure on the feet.

- Corn pads remove pressure from corns and so may encourage them to disappear. Corn-removal plasters are sometimes effective.

- If you suffer from diabetes mellitus (see separate entry) be wary of calluses because deep ulcers can form without you knowing.

- Go to a chiropodist for treatment if you are not succeeding in removing corns yourself.

COT DEATH

A cot death is the death of a baby, while sleeping in its cot, for no known reason. It happens in about one in 5,000 babies usually between three to eighteen weeks old.

Self-health

- Breast-fed babies appear to be less at risk of cot death than bottle-fed ones.

- Try to prevent your baby coming into contact with colds and coughs because many parents of cot deaths have noticed that their babies have had a sniffy nose or cough shortly before their death.

- Don't overheat your baby with bedclothes as this has been linked with cot deaths.

- Put your baby on its back to sleep. Recent research suggests this position reduces its chance of a cot death. A pillow is usually not advisable until the baby is at least a year old.

- If you have already lost one child from cot death or think your child is particularly at risk, discuss the problem with your doctor. A special alarm that monitors your baby's breathing might be advisable.

COUGH

Coughing is designed to rid the breathing passages of material such as mucus or even blood which may be blocking or irritating them. Coughing is 'productive' if mucus or blood comes up, and 'unproductive' if nothing comes up. There are very many causes, including smoking, lung diseases (such as asthma and bronchitis), some digestive disorders, and anxiety.

Self-health

- Since there are so many causes of coughing, only general advice can be given.

- On the whole a 'productive' cough is a good thing, which should not be prevented since it is ridding the body of possibly dangerous material. In fact, many physiotherapists spend much of their time persuading people to cough more to clear their lungs, for example after an operation.

- A dry 'unproductive' cough is not helpful and may be exhausting. It may be associated with a cold (see separate entry), in which case it should disappear after three or four days. Meanwhile expectorants, which loosen phlegm in the nose, throat and upper breathing passages, cough suppressants (which should not be used by people with bronchitis or asthma) and decongestants bought from the chemist can sometimes be helpful. However, these medicines should not be taken for longer than two weeks and if the cough persists beyond this you should see your doctor.

- Some coughs are due to allergies. See **Hayfever** and **Allergic Rhinitis** for ways to prevent them.

- Children are prone to coughs, especially if they have a cold. The temperature of their room at night is important. If it is too cold the air will irritate the throat. If it is too warm the air will make the throat dry. It should be about 67° C. Always make sure the child has plenty of warm drinks while suffering from a cough. Occasionally a humidifier is helpful.

Screening

- A cough that persists for more than two to three weeks should not be ignored. Tell your doctor so that he or she can examine you as necessary.

CRAB LICE

Crab lice are harmless lice which infest pubic hair and are usually caught during sexual contact. They are pinhead size and can sometimes be seen holding on to the base of a hair near the skin. They often cause intense itching.

Self-health

- Celibacy is the only certain way of avoiding crabs. The fewer your sexual partners the less chance you have of catching them.

- There are no medicines which can prevent you getting crab lice, but treatment from your doctor or hospital special clinic is usually successful.

Screening

- If you have caught crabs, you may also have caught a more serious sexually transmitted disease. If you notice any unusual symptoms see your family doctor or hospital special clinic immediately.

- You should tell all your sexual partners as soon as you discover that you have crabs so that they can get themselves treated and do not pass on the crabs to other people.

CRADLE CAP

Cradle cap is a type of seborrhoeic eczema (see **Eczema**) which affects infants. It varies from a few scales on the scalp (like dandruff) to a thick, white cap.

Self-health

- The appearance of cradle cap does not suggest a mother has been neglecting her baby.

- It cannot be prevented, but mild forms will respond to dandruff-like scalp preparations (see **Dandruff**). Consult your

doctor about a more serious outbreak, but feel reassured that it
will disappear within a few months.

CRAMP, CALF

The muscles of the calf occasionally go into spasm without you
being able to control them. It may happen during or just after
exercise or at night. For reasons we don't fully understand
pregnant women are particularly prone to cramp. It is not a
serious symptom unless it happens often.

Self-health

- Before exercise warm up gently and then 'warm down' gently
  afterwards.

- If the weather is very hot or humid be sure to include plenty of
  salt in your diet (in tablet form) because too little salt in the
  bloodstream can cause cramp. This is particularly important if
  you are going to exercise hard.

- If you are prone to night cramps, keep your legs up during the
  evening and try raising the foot of your bed by four to six
  inches. If this fails see your doctor. He or she may prescribe
  medicine to prevent the cramp or find that the cause is poor
  circulation in your legs.

CRAMP, MENSTRUAL

These painful spasms are due to contractions of the womb
muscles, usually on the first day of bleeding but sometimes a few
hours before the blood starts or continuing for two or three days
afterwards. They are usually felt in the lower abdomen but
sometimes in the whole pelvis, the back and inner thighs.
Symptoms are usually worse in women under thirty and may
improve thereafter, although everybody is different and there are
no rules.

Self-health

- There are a number of home remedies and it is a question of finding which works best for you.

- Heat helps to relax the spasms. Use a hotwater bottle or heating pad on the lower abdomen. Sometimes a deep heating oil (such as tiger balm) rubbed into the painful area helps. Some women find a hot bath useful but do not make it so hot you feel faint or sick.

- Warm drinks, especially herbal teas or broth, can help. Some women find a strong alcoholic drink does the trick.

- There is no need to avoid exercise; in fact some find jogging, stretching exercises or tennis helpful.

- Back massage can be wonderfully relaxing, and some women find lovemaking and orgasm take the pain away.

- A good balanced diet is important. Eating plenty of fibre will prevent constipation which makes the cramps worse, and there are some reports that 500 mg calcium and 250 mg magnesium daily as tablet supplements for one week before the pain starts are helpful.

- If home remedies do not work tablets that help prevent the pain are available. Since the symptoms are thought to be due to a chemical substance, prostaglandin, these tablets contain anti-prostaglandin medicines. The best known is aspirin, which works for many women. Consult your doctor or pharmacist if you need stronger types. With this kind of medicine be a little wary if you suffer from asthma, stomach ulcers or indigestion.

- The contraceptive pill works by stopping the cyclical menstrual changes which bring on the symptoms. It is helpful for the few women in whom all other preventive efforts have failed.

CROUP

Croup is a harsh wheezing or grunting noise made by children, usually under five and at night, trying to breathe through a larynx (voice box) that has been narrowed by a viral infection. Older children and adults suffer from laryngitis rather than croup because their air passages are bigger and so the narrowing does not affect them enough to cause croup.

Self-health

- The usual precautions against viral infections are necessary, particularly if your child is prone to them (see **Colds**).

- Sometimes bacteria infect the surfaces of the breathing passages when they are already damaged and inflamed by a virus. This can itself cause croup. So if your child is prone to croup your doctor may prescribe antibiotics to be taken at the start of an infection to prevent this secondary bacterial infection and the resulting croup.

- If your child is prone to bad attacks of croup be sure you know what to do in case of sudden breathing difficulties, and take your child to hospital sooner rather than later. Most such children need no more than close observation, but a few become very distressed and may need a tube passed through the mouth into the windpipe to help their breathing.

CRYING, BABIES

First-time parents are often astonished by how much their baby cries; experienced parents with a new baby may be surprised how quickly they had forgotten how much babies cry. Some experts quote two to three hours of crying every day within the first few months as being normal. That said, no parents like to hear their baby cry and will do all they can to stop them.

Self-health

- There are various different reasons for crying, and to a limited extent it is possible to give general guidelines about how to diagnose the cause from the nature of the cry and the circumstances. Generally, though, every parent needs to become familiar with how their own baby reacts and behaves.

PAIN

The cry of pain is usually a long, very loud screech. The knees may draw up, the face go red and nothing will comfort the baby. First check there is no obvious cause for the pain, such as an injury, insect bite or cat scratch. Then use the general measures suggested below.

HUNGER

A hungry baby's cry is softer than a 'painful' cry and the knees are not drawn up. It happens if a feed is missed or delayed or if you are not feeding your baby enough food.

THIRST

Hot weather or a fever will make a baby sweat more than normal. Offer milk or water.

COLIC (see separate entry)

The cry caused by colic is very similar to that for pain. It is loud and accompanied by drawing up of the knees and a red face. Colic most commonly occurs when babies are ten weeks to three months old. Usually no cause is found, and the colic has generally settled by the age of six months.

Holding babies in a position which puts a little pressure on their stomach may help stop them crying. So try carrying your baby over your shoulder, in the crook of your arm, so his or her legs can draw up, or stomach-down over your arm. Try walking with your baby in a rhythmical, calm way, or patting, or rocking in a cradle, or take him or her for a drive in the car. Check your feeding technique, and if you have just started solids stop for a while because this may be the cause.

WET NAPPY

Some experts think the act of passing water alone causes some babies to cry. Most agree that few babies like a wet nappy.

Change your baby's nappies regularly. This may stop your baby crying and will have the added benefit of preventing nappy rash.

PERSONALITY

Babies have their own distinct personalities from the earliest age. Some are active, bright little things who will scream if they are left unattended and bored lying on their back in a cot. Others are tense and easily frightened by loud noises, too much handling, bright lights or being suddenly undressed. Yet others are quiet and calm and only scream when their routine is interrupted.

Active babies need the action they demand. This can be demanding but at least it avoids the screams! Prop them up and use baby bouncers and walkers as much as you can.

Tense babies need a calm, relaxed atmosphere, dim lights, quiet music and a regular routine. They like to be firmly held for dressing and feeding and often enjoy close physical contact with their mothers.

Calm babies like to be left in peace.

TIREDNESS

Tired babies have a grumbling, meaningful kind of cry.

Avoid disruption to the sleep routine if possible. If this is unavoidable try to build a 'bank' of sleep in advance. If all else fails settle the baby with a feed, rhythmical movement and sound (see below).

TEETHING

About six months after birth the first teeth (the incisors) begin to appear. This may make the surrounding gums painful, causing your child to grizzle, and to dribble because extra saliva is being produced. It may also change the consistency of your baby's faeces and possibly cause a rash but it does *not* cause vomiting, fits, fever or bronchitis as has sometimes been claimed.

Offer a sugar-free rusk or teething ring (bought from a chemist). Teething drops and solutions can help but often contain sugar or even a local anaesthetic, so they should not be used often. Sometimes paracetamol can be effective. Make sure you stick to the recommended dose for your baby.

WIND

Some babies take in a lot of wind while they are feeding (especially bottle-feeding) and need a 'wind' after they have finished. Experiment with your child to find what works best for you both. Patting on the back while the baby lies over your shoulder is usually successful. Some experts, though, think wind is an overdiagnosed cause of crying and that there is often another explanation.

ILLNESS

Most babies cry when they are ill, and it is a good thing they do because it is the best way of signalling something is wrong. In fact doctors are more worried by an ill child who is not crying than one who is yelling lustily. So if there are other signs of illness such as fever, vomiting, diarrhoea or refusal to feed and if

---

Some tips to comfort a crying baby

1. **Position**
   Experiment to find the position your baby likes best.

2. **Movement**
   Most babies like to be rocked – some gently, others more vigorously. Try a rocking chair or stroller, or walk slowly round the house. Many babies find the movement of a car soothing.

3. **Sounds**
   Low, rhythmical singing and lullabies (or even humming if you can't sing!) can have a magical effect on your baby. Our eldest child responded instantly to Tina Turner's music, perhaps because he was exposed to a great deal of it while warm and comfortable in his mother's womb.

4. **Swaddling**
   Some babies, especially in the first few weeks, like to be wrapped up firmly (but not so firmly they cannot breathe!).

5. **Sucking and dummies**
   Many babies are soothed by sucking the breast, bottle, finger or dummy. You may find some people disapprove of dummies – but they don't have to put up with your crying baby every day! However, do try not to put the dummy in your baby's mouth at the first whimper.

you are uncertain of the cause of these symptoms you should see
your family doctor immediately.

WHEN ALL ELSE FAILS

Enlist the help of relatives or friends to give you some time off.
The fact that you are close to breaking point may communicate
itself to your baby and make the crying worse. A change can
make all the difference.

If you have no one close who can take responsibility for your
baby, it may occasionally be necessary to put the baby in the
safety of his or her cot, shut the door and move out of earshot.
No parent likes to do this often but provided you are confident
there is nothing seriously wrong with your baby, it may
occasionally be best for you both. And if you find you need to do
this more often than you would like, get professional help from a
doctor, nurse, or counsellor. They will certainly not blame you
and will be delighted you have sought help sooner rather than
later.

CURLY TOES

This describes toes that no longer lie straight and may become
twisted so they do not lie flat on the ground. Sometimes they are
called hammer, mallet or claw toes.

Self-health

- If you have close relatives with curly toes and notice that your
  toes are beginning to curl, try to wear comfortable, roomy
  shoes which will not make the condition worse.

- If there is still some movement in the toes, strengthen the
  muscles by stretching your toes out straight. Gentle
  manipulation may also help.

- Prevent yourself getting sore patches of skin or ulcers by
  wearing pads (e.g. corn pads) over areas at risk.

- Surgery may occasionally be needed to prevent curly toes
  becoming worse.

CYSTIC FIBROSIS

This is a hereditary condition that affects about one in every 1,500 newborn babies. The disease is due to several types of the baby's glands not working properly – for example, the pancreas does not produce enzymes for digestion, so food passes straight through the baby without being absorbed properly. The glands of the tubes in the lung produce a thick, sticky mucus that blocks the tubes instead of a thin mucus that traps germs and can then be coughed up. So the child is prone to nasty chest infections.

In the past, affected children rarely lived more than a few years but nowadays we know so much more about how to prevent serious problems that children often live into adolescence or even their twenties.

Self-health

- Carriers of the disease have a one in four chance of having an affected child. If you know it runs in your family you should consult a doctor for genetic counselling. At the moment there is no way of definitely preventing your child inheriting the disease, though it may be possible in the future.

- If cystic fibrosis runs in your family you should have your baby tested for the disease shortly after it is born. The sooner it is diagnosed, the better chance you will have of preventing serious complications.

- Artificial enzymes and a low-fat diet often help the baby put on weight and have near-normal stools.

- Special lung exercises, physiotherapy and drainage of the sticky mucus help prevent chest infections. Doctors may also prescribe long-term, low-dosage antibiotics.

- Parents should give great emotional and physical help but not overprotect the child unnecessarily.

CYSTITIS

Cystitis is inflammation of the lining of the bladder. This inflammation is usually due to bacterial infections, but a few women have sensitive bladders which react to certain chemicals or are allergic to some substances. The symptoms are pain or stinging when you pass water, strongly smelling urine, a need to pass urine frequently and sometimes uncontrollably, or occasionally bleeding from the urethra (the tube that drains urine from the bladder to the outside) when you pass water. Sometimes you may notice backache or a low pelvic pain, or notice you have a temperature and feel terrible. It is common in women (more than half of all Western women suffer from it at some stage in their lives) because the urethra is short and allows germs to get into the bladder easily.

Self-health

- Drink at least two to three pints of fluid a day, more if the weather is hot. This volume flushes out the germs from the nooks and crannies of the bladder.

- Don't wait until the last possible moment before passing water, and don't rush away before your bladder has had a chance to empty itself completely.

- After you have opened your bowels get into the habit of wiping your bottom from front to back so that you do not transfer germs from your back passage to your vaginal area.

- Some women find they need to wash their bottom and genital area every morning and evening, even if they have not had sex. Soapy water should be applied to the bottom but not to the sensitive genital area, where warm water is sufficient. Avoid perfumed soap, vaginal deodorants or talc.

- Consider whether the timing of your cystitis is related to sex. If it is, there are things you can do to help:

  1. Pass water before and after sex.
  2. Make sure you are aroused and well lubricated before intercourse begins so that your partner does not bruise your urethra, giving the germs a better chance of getting into the bladder. Many women find a mild lubricant like KY jelly helps.
  3. Don't practise anal petting or intercourse.

4. After intercourse, washing your bottom and genital area with tepid water may help.

- Some women find coffee, tea and alcohol cause cystitis. Others, though, find these drinks useful, because they stimulate the kidneys to produce urine to flush the germs away.

- Many women know the times they are likely to get cystitis and find that a very short course of antibiotics (for example, two or three tablets) or a level teaspoon of bicarbonate of soda diluted in a drink prevents them developing the symptoms. Consult your doctor if you think you need this treatment. In a few cases, long-term low-dosage antibiotics are the only effective method of keeping cystitis at bay.

CYTOMEGALOVIRUS INFECTION

This virus causes an illness like glandular fever (see separate entry) from which almost everybody recovers, often noticing little more than that they felt slightly unwell. Occasionally, however, infection may be passed from a mother to her unborn baby, causing congenital problems. One or two per cent of babies are affected in this way and of these about one in seven may have permanent eye or hearing problems or even be mentally retarded.

Self-health

- There is no specific vaccine yet that can prevent this infection.

- Depending on how the virus has affected them, children who have been damaged by cytomegalovirus will need to be encouraged to make the most of their lives, despite their handicaps.

- In theory it would be a good idea to avoid any chance of conceiving a baby when you have this infection. The problem is that the symptoms are so vague it is usually impossible to tell you have it, and there is nothing you can do to prevent yourself developing cytomegalovirus once you are pregnant.

D

DANDRUFF

Dandruff consists of scales of dead skin from the scalp. It may be 'dry', when it showers on to clothing, or 'greasy', when it sticks in the hair. Sometimes greasy dandruff gets worse and the scalp becomes red, itchy and inflamed (seborrhoeic eczema).

Self-health

- No one knows what causes dandruff but it is made worse by emotional upsets or hormonal changes.

- 'Dry' dandruff may be prevented by a shampoo suitable for dry hair. If not, ask your chemist for sulphur and salicylic acid cream BP, which has an extra dislodging effect. Dampen your hair first so it parts easily, making a parting on one side of the head and rub the cream in generously. Repeat this process with new partings, working across the head. Leave the cream overnight and then wash it out with a tar shampoo. You may have to do this two or three times a week to start with. Later you can work out how often you need the treatment to prevent dandruff.

- If you have 'greasy' dandruff start with a medicated shampoo such as Head and Shoulders or ZP11. If the dandruff is still bad try a tar-based shampoo such as Polytar or Genisol. Sometimes a shampoo with selenium sulphide (e.g. Selsun or Lenium) helps, and if all else fails the sulphur and salicylic acid cream treatment described above may do the trick.

- If your dandruff does not respond to treatment, see your doctor for further advice.

DEAFNESS

About ten million people in the UK suffer some loss of hearing, mostly elderly people – the average age for attending a hearing aid clinic for the first time is seventy. About two million people use hearing aids and about 100,000 people have virtually no hearing at all, so hearing aids are of little help. Hearing loss usually comes on gradually; if it happens suddenly go to the nearest casualty department because immediate treatment may restore it.

Self-health

- The simplest cause of hearing loss is a build-up of wax in the outer ear. Some people need regular syringeing of the ear by a doctor or nurse to prevent hearing loss.

- Do not push things (e.g. cottonwool) into the ear, as this may cause deafness, particularly in children.

- Repeated ear infections may cause some hearing loss. This may not be noticeable when you are young but will make the hearing loss of old age worse. Be sure to seek treatment for infections or earaches.

- If a pregnant woman catches German measles (rubella), particularly in the third month of pregnancy, her child may be born deaf. Every girl should be immunized against rubella.

- A difficult birth, in which the baby suffers loss of oxygen, may cause deafness. The only way to guard against this is to make sure you look after yourself during pregnancy and attend all your antenatal checks.

- Deafness may run in some families. If it does, see a doctor for genetic counselling before starting your family.

- Some drugs (e.g. some antibiotics, or even aspirin in very large doses) can cause deafness. If you notice hearing loss, ringing in the ears or giddiness shortly after starting a new medicine, stop taking it immediately and see your doctor.

- Excessive prolonged noise will cause deafness. Always wear earplugs or muffs if they are provided at work. If they are not and the noise is louder than that inside an underground train (about ninety decibels), insist on your health and safety officer or local environmental health officer finding out whether it is a danger.

- Guard against single very loud noises which can be particularly harmful. For example, wear earguards when firing a powerful rifle.

- Discotheques and rock concerts are dangerous only if you go to many and are within one or two feet of the speakers. Most people are not at risk, though the musicians and staff often are.

- Personal stereo-cassette players have worried some authorities. Generally, though, if used with common sense they are not a problem.

- Once hearing loss is established, most people can prevent themselves becoming completely deaf by using a hearing aid. These are worn either on the body or behind the ear and there are many different types to suit your particular needs.

- Occasionally an operation may prevent your deafness from getting worse.

- There are many 'aids to living' which can make your life easier. These include special doorbells, televisions, alarm clocks, telephones and baby alarms. You will be encouraged, too, to learn how well you can manage by lip-reading alone.

Screening

- If you have difficulty hearing the doorbell or telephone, or want the TV louder than other people, or complain that people 'always mumble these days', you may need treatment. Consult your doctor early rather than late – it will make treatment easier.

DEMENTIA

Dementia is the steady deterioration of a person's personality, intellect and physical condition without any detectable underlying cause. Of course, all people over sixty start to lose their physical and mental agility, and the borderline between such a decline and mild dementia may be a narrow one. However, dementia is usually a more serious condition in which the sufferer goes relentlessly downhill until friends and relatives can no longer recognize this new person.

Symptoms include loss of memory for recent events, inability to think clearly or carry on a conversation, and loss of initiative and interest in old pastimes and friends. Later there will be unstable moods and emotional swings, varying from extreme apathy to violent aggression. The person may become totally uninhibited, often sexually and in their behaviour towards other people. Eventually sufferers may become bed-bound, developing urinary and faecal incontinence, unable to feed themselves and unaware of their surroundings.

Dementia is a common problem affecting one in ten people over sixty, and one in five over eighty. Dementia can also affect people under sixty when it is known as pre-senile dementia. In these people the disease seems to progress faster and often proves fatal within five years.

Self-health

- True dementia without a known cause cannot be prevented. The best that can be done is to slow the progression and prevent unnecessary illness or injury to the person.

- Try to keep the person at home in familiar surroundings for as long as possible. As soon as there is a move away from home, quick deterioration is inevitable. It is essential to make the home as safe as possible. Pay particular attention to the kitchen and bathroom. Make sure the rooms are well lit, there are no open fires, the electricity supply has been made safe and there are no trailing leads.

- Make sure the person has the benefit of all the community services available. Ask the advice of the GP and physiotherapist, and arrange for health visitors or community nurses to visit regularly. Food may be provided by a meals-on-wheels service, and there are often local day centres where the person can go to enjoy companionship and a good meal.

- Dementia may have an underlying and treatable cause like

pneumonia, cystitis, strokes, shortage of thyroid hormone (myxoedema), depression, alcoholism or vitamin deficiency (see separate entries where appropriate). It is important that the person is examined for these illnesses to try and discover a treatable cause of the dementia.

- Do not feel guilty if it is finally decided that the demented person can no longer live at home. You will be doing your best for the sufferer by agreeing to him or her being cared for elsewhere.

DENTAL CARE

Teeth are covered by enamel, which is the hardest substance in the body. However, it can be eroded by acid produced by bacteria which live in dental plaque, a layer of mucus, food particles and bacteria which gathers mainly between the teeth and gums. The bacteria break down sugar in the food to create the acid, which then erodes the enamel to form tiny cavities. These cavities become larger until the acid erodes into the layer below, the denture, and finally the pulp of the tooth. If this decay is not stopped, you will suffer abscesses, toothache and finally the tooth will die.

Self-health

- Brush your teeth at least twice a day and preferably after each meal. There are no hard and fast rules about how to brush your teeth except that you should do so thoroughly and reach all those awkward crevices.

- Use a nylon brush with a small head for maximum manoeuvrability. Rinse the brush well after use so it does not become a source of infection to your gums. Replace old, limp brushes which are no longer effective. Each member of the family should have his or her own toothbrush.

- There are special 'disclosing' tablets which stain plaque so that you can see where your brushing has failed.

- Wooden points are available to clean between your teeth, but be careful not to spear your gums and make them bleed. A safer alternative is dental floss, available from most chemists.

- Check the fluoride content of your water if you have children. There should be at least one part per million for it to be effective in hardening enamel and preventing decay. Fluoride toothpastes are especially helpful for children.

- There is some dispute about how frequently you should visit your dentist. Some experts believe that small enamel cavities can heal spontaneously so that some cavities may be filled unnecessarily if you visit the dentist too often. However, a good rule of thumb is every six months for children and every year for adults.

- Avoid foods with added sugar. Discourage your children from developing a taste for sweet foods, and offer them fruit or savoury snacks rather than sweets.

DENTURES, PROBLEMS WITH

Surveys have shown that about fifteen per cent of denture wearers are unhappy with them. The main problem is the base plate (false gum) which rubs on the real gums, causing inflammation and mouth ulcers.

Self-health

- Ask your dentist to check your dentures (if full) every two years. Partial dentures or false teeth should be checked six-monthly.

- Dentures will last between six months and five years, depending on how fast your mouth and jaw change shape. If they become loose and ill-fitting see your dentist before it develops into a serious problem. Some researchers believe that 900 mg calcium a day helps the jaw keep its shape better by preventing bone loss.

- Remove your dentures at night to rest your gums. Clean them and put them in a glass of water so they do not dry out and bend.

- Clean your real gums and teeth (see **Dental Care**). If they become sore and inflamed, clean your dentures with a mild antiseptic.

- Some people with dentures suffer from persistent fungal infections of the mouth. Better-fitting dentures or anti-fungal lozenges may prevent problems.

DEPRESSION

Everyone feels in low spirits sometimes, but if it lasts longer than three or four weeks it becomes depression. There are so many different types that doctors have divided them into two categories. Endogenous depression is the type in which there is no obvious cause, it seems to come from within the person. Exogenous is the type in which there is an obvious cause, such as a death in the family, illness or unemployment. The symptoms of both types include poor concentration, listlessness, lack of interest in anything, a feeling of worthlessness or being persecuted, frequent crying for no reason, eating problems, constipation and loss of interest in sex.

Self-health

- Prevention is best started in childhood, as babies and young children should be brought up to feel loved and wanted. Such children will be less prone to depression in later life.

- The next vulnerable time is during adolescence, when hormonal and emotional changes make many adolescents depressed, a few even considering suicide. It is vital that parents anticipate such problems and use sympathy and understanding to prevent them becoming serious.

- Some reports suggest that as many as eight out of ten mothers experience some 'blues' after the birth of a child. Such depression is more common in those who have had their baby induced, or had a forceps or caesarian delivery. It is important that her partner, relatives and friends provide support for the mother at this time, both emotionally and physically, such as by doing the housework and cooking, and making sure she does not spend long hours alone. An exhausted mother will quickly become a depressed mother.

- Older people are the most likely group to become depressed and commit suicide. The causes are often social and only society can prevent them. Yet loneliness (see separate entry) is described by many depressed people as the single, most important cause and all of us are responsible for that.

- Suicide (see separate entry) is the most terrible consequence of depression. Many suicides cannot be prevented, but vigilant, caring relatives and friends could prevent some. In particular, any mention by the depressive of suicide should be taken seriously and the person persuaded to consult his or her GP – failing this, tell the GP yourself.

- Anyone with a personal or family history of depression is at risk. Symptoms should be noted early and action taken quickly to prevent the illness getting worse.

- Any physical illness (especially glandular fever, flu or stroke) can bring on depression. Women going through the menopause (see separate entry) are at risk, as are those with too little thyroid hormone (see **Thyroid Gland, Underactivity**).

- Many medicines cause depression. The most common are steroids and medicines to reduce blood pressure, but any medicine taken over a long period (e.g. the contraceptive pill) can be responsible. Do not take medicines unless they are necessary.

- Pain (see separate entry), particularly long-term, is a frequent cause of depression. Treat the pain successfully and the depression will disappear.

- Drinking too much alcohol (see **Alcoholism**) is another preventable cause of depression.

- Some people do not have an external cause for their depression, and are unable to cope with it themselves. For them skilled psychotherapy, medicines (e.g. tricyclics and monoamine oxidase inhibitors) or even electroconvulsive therapy (ECT) may be needed to treat the condition and then on a long-term basis to prevent it returning.

DIABETES MELLITUS

Someone with diabetes tends to have too much sugar circulating in their blood. This is caused by the pancreas's failure to produce enough of the hormone insulin to regulate blood sugar levels. In mild forms it may not be recognized or, if it is, needs treating only with a special diet. In more serious forms tablets or insulin injections may be needed to reduce the amount of sugar in the blood. Occasionally it can be so serious that it is life-threatening. About two per cent of the population have diabetes.

There are two main types. One mild form, often not recognized, affects people over thirty-five (often overweight) in which the pancreas produces some, but not enough insulin. This can usually be treated by diet and tablets. The other, more serious form usually affects younger people and occurs when the pancreas is not working at all, so they need tablets or insulin replacement by injection.

Because diabetics have too high levels of sugar in their blood the sugar overflows into their urine. This causes them to pass a lot of water, feel thirsty and lose weight.

Self-health

- Diabetes cannot be prevented, except perhaps by avoiding becoming overweight, but its complications can be reduced by understanding the problems and keeping your sugar levels normal.

- The most serious problem is that diabetics can go into a coma due to very high levels of sugar in the blood. To prevent this make sure you stick to your diet – eat regular small amounts of carbohydrate, avoiding sweets, sugar, biscuits and puddings but eating plenty of fibre in the form of wholemeal bread, cereals, fruit and vegetables. If you have been prescribed tablets or insulin, take them regularly as instructed.

- Be careful if you catch any illness, especially infections, because you may need higher doses of your medicine or insulin. If you are unable to eat·because of illness, you will still need to take some insulin. You should contact your doctor for advice about adjusting the dosage in the event of *any* illness or infection.

- Diabetics can also go into a coma due to very low levels of sugar in the blood. To prevent this, make sure you take no more tablets or insulin than you have been prescribed. Eat regular meals and remember to eat more if you exercise unusually hard. You should recognize the early symptoms of coma (dizziness, trembling, blurred vision, slurred speech, tingling, headache, and sweating) and always have some sugar lumps or biscuits at hand to eat until you feel normal again (usually within a few minutes). Your friends and relatives should know about the symptoms too so that if you become confused they can give you something with sugar in it. An alternative to food is an injection of the hormone glucagon, which will temporarily raise the amount of sugar in the blood. Your relatives and friends can be taught how to give this injection, but it should only be done in an emergency and you should see your doctor afterwards.

- You should check your blood sugar levels or check your urine for the presence of sugar regularly, depending on what type of diabetes you have. If you are a mild diabetic it may not be necessary more than two or three times a week. If you have severe, 'brittle' diabetes with big swings in your blood sugar levels, you may need to do so three times a day. The blood test is more accurate than the urine tests and now that kits are available free on prescription they should be used in preference.

- Diabetics are at risk of developing damage to the back of the eye (retinopathy) and to the kidneys, which can occasionally result in kidney failure. Keeping blood sugar levels within normal limits will help reduce your chances of developing these problems.

- Diabetes can damage small arteries, reducing the circulation to hands and feet. It can also cause loss of sensation in these areas (peripheral neuropathy). The combination means that diabetics are poor healers and are prone to infections, ulcers and even gangrene in extreme cases. To prevent these you should not smoke, because smoking also damages arteries, you should treat cuts carefully and see your doctor at any sign of infection. Wear well-fitting shoes and have corns or ingrowing toenails treated by a chiropodist, as the feet are particularly prone to these problems.

- Wear a bracelet or carry a card explaining you are a diabetic and what to do in an emergency.

- Always warn every doctor or dentist who looks after you about your diabetes because it may affect their treatment.

Screening

- Urine or blood testing for diabetes is easy and everyone should be tested, the younger the better. Certainly every mother should be tested during pregnancy because diabetics need special care at this time.

- If you have a close relative with diabetes you have about a one in twenty chance of developing it yourself so you have good reason to get yourself tested as soon as possible.

DIARRHOEA

Scientists describe diarrhoea as passing more than 200 g of faeces a day. But that information doesn't help most people worried about their bowels! The important point is that diarrhoea is an unusual looseness or frequency of passing stools for you. In other words what may be diarrhoea for you may be normal for someone else; it is the change in habit that matters.

Diarrhoea is a symptom of an illness, it is not an illness in itself. In many cases it lasts less than forty-eight hours and no cause is ever found, although an infection of some sort is suspected. Occasionally, though, it may last longer and be the sign of a more serious illness like irritable bowel syndrome (see separate entry) or thyrotoxicosis (see **Thyroid Gland, Overactivity**).

Self-health

- When travelling abroad (see separate entry) take precautions to avoid infections. If you do get diarrhoea it is important to drink plenty of fluids and avoid solid food until the diarrhoea has settled.

- Some people, particularly elderly people, with a tendency to constipation sometimes get what they think is diarrhoea. In fact what has happened is that the bowel has become so overloaded with faeces that it is no longer able to work properly and so fluid leaks round the side of the faeces appearing as 'diarrhoea'. As you can imagine, the worst course of action is to take anti-diarrhoea medicine! The best thing is to prevent the constipation in the first place (see **Constipation**).

- Be warned that some medicines may cause diarrhoea (see chart). Sometimes this is an unavoidable side effect but often your family doctor will be able to prescribe alternatives.

- Stress is known to cause diarrhoea. See chapter on Stress and Mental Health.

- If your diarrhoea lasts for more than forty-eight hours or if it contains blood you should consult your family doctor without delay.

Screening

- Persistent diarrhoea may be a sign of serious illness, so consult your doctor, who will examine you thoroughly. Possible investigations include blood tests, barium studies of your gut, or passing a telescope up your back passage to view the inside of your bowel (sigmoidoscopy or colonoscopy).

Some medicines that can cause diarrhoea

- Antacids for indigestion or heartburn (e.g. magnesium trisilicate, cimetidine)

- Medicines for raised blood pressure (e.g. propranolol)

- Antibiotics (e.g. penicillin)

- Asthma medicines (e.g. theophylline)

- Drugs for treating heart failure (e.g. digoxin)

- 'Water' pills for getting rid of too much fluid (e.g. frusemide)

- Iron for treating or preventing anaemia

- Medicines for treating arthritis (e.g. indomethacin)

- If diarrhoea is accompanied by other symptoms such as loss of appetite or losing weight without explanation there is even more reason for you to see your family doctor immediately. Blood in the diarrhoea is another important sign that you should be carefully screened.

DIPHTHERIA

Diphtheria is a serious infection caused by the bacterium *corynebacterium diphtheriae*, which, if untreated, kills about one third of its victims. Since the immunization programme began in the UK in 1940 it has been almost completely eradicated; for example in 1978 there were only two cases. In less developed countries, though, it remains common. Symptoms include a sore throat, a greyish film on the tonsils, swollen glands in the neck and, in severe cases, inflammation of the heart.

Self-health

- Diphtheria can be prevented by immunization during childhood. Three injections of diphtheria toxoid (with whooping cough and tetanus, known as DPT) are given in the first fifteen months of life followed by a booster at five years old.

- Any of the immunization injections should be delayed if your child has a cold, infection or fever. Your doctor will also want to know if your child has had fits because occasionally this affects the immunization programme.

DIVERTICULAR DISEASE

Diverticulae are small, sac-like swellings which develop outwards in the lining of the last part of the bowel. They are virtually unknown in Africans, who eat a high-fibre diet, but affect as many as one in three Westerners over the age of sixty. This is because the Western diet is highly refined with little bulk, so the bowel has to strain hard to push the faeces along. Symptoms include pellet-like constipation, excessive wind, cramping pains, even tenderness in the left side of the abdomen. If the pouches become infected the person develops diverticulitis which is more serious and may need antibiotics and/or surgery as treatment.

Self-health

- Eat a high-fibre diet. This means wholemeal rather than white bread, plenty of cereals containing bran, and fruit and vegetables.

- Remember, though, that a high-fibre diet can itself cause bloating and excessive wind, so find a balance for your body.

DIZZINESS

Dizziness (or vertigo) describes the sensation that you are spinning about while everything else is still, or that you are still and everything else is spinning about you. The sensation is often unpleasant and may cause you to vomit, fall or faint.

Self-health

- If you feel dizzy, lie down immediately. It will help the symptoms and prevent you falling or fainting.

- If it happens more than once you should see your doctor, who will try to find the cause of the dizziness – for example wax, ear infection, head injury or disturbances of the inner ear. If the cause is found and treated the dizziness will disappear.

- Dizziness may be a sign of high blood pressure so get it checked.

- Often the cause of dizziness is not diagnosed. However, there are medicines which can prevent attacks – see your doctor.

DOWN'S SYNDROME

This condition occurs when a baby is born with too many chromosomes – forty-seven instead of forty-six. This causes a mental retardation which can vary from mild to severe, and a characteristic appearance including a flat face and back of head, a broad ridge to the nose and slit eyes which slope upwards at the corners. It affects about one in 1,000 children.

Self-health

- Women over thirty-five have an increased risk of giving birth to a child with Down's syndrome. If it is their first child the risk is increased to approximately one in fifty, and by the age of forty-five the risk is one in twenty-five. For many couples this risk is great enough to prevent them trying to have a child. Others take the risk, particularly if the mother is screened early.

- If a young woman with normal chromosomes has a baby with Down's syndrome the risk of having another one is tiny.

- The age of the father does not significantly alter the chance of having an affected baby.

Screening

- Screening makes sense if you intend to take action (i.e. have an abortion) if the results are positive. If not, many would argue it is valueless.

- There are two main ways of screening:
  1. Amniocentesis is performed between the sixteenth and eighteenth week of pregnancy. Under anaesthetic a needle is inserted through the abdominal wall into the sac surrounding the baby and some fluid is taken. This is then tested for chromosomal abnormalities. This test carries a half to one per cent chance of causing a miscarriage.
  2. Chorionic villus biopsy is a new technique in which a sample of sac round the baby, the chorion, is taken under anaesthetic. Using ultrasound waves the instrument is guided either through the abdomen (like amniocentesis) or through the cervix, to the correct point where the sample is taken. The advantage is that it is done in the ninth to the eleventh week of pregnancy so abortion can be early and therefore less risky. The disadvantage is that there is a two to three per cent chance of a miscarriage after it.

DRUG DEPENDENCE

A drug addict is someone who depends on a drug substance, so that they need to take it in order to feel well or in control of themselves. This dependence shows itself in two ways:

1. Physical dependence happens when a person's brain or body has been temporarily (or permanently) changed by a drug in some way. If it is not available to them they suffer unpleasant withdrawal symptoms such as sickness, trembling or panic.
2. Psychological dependence occurs when a person feels emotionally disturbed without a drug but does not show obvious withdrawal symptoms. The strength of this sort of addiction should not be underestimated.

Some people can become very dependent on non-drug activities like gambling or even work. Habits and expectations of all types can be hard to break.

Drug users are not necessarily 'junkies' living only for the next 'fix'. Many appear to live normal lives. And it is worth remembering that alcohol and cigarettes cause far more damage to the health of people in this country than that caused by all other forms of drug abuse combined.

Self-health

• The best form of help is prevention. Even the happiest families can suddenly be faced with a drug abuse problem, but the chance of it being serious is likely to be reduced by a home life in which people have been able to learn about the benefits and risks of drug usage of all types, legal and illegal. It is best that questions about drugs are discussed within the family in a balanced, supportive way, preferably before problems arise.

A 'preventive environment' is also one in which both children and adults are able to gain an understanding of the causes and symptoms of mental illness or distress, in part so they can talk about any problems they may have themselves without shame, embarrassment or fear. They are then less likely to have to turn to drugs to try to cope with life, or to fail to notice when they are in danger of developing a problem.

There are telltale signs and symptoms of drug abuse which can be recognized (see below). Generally speaking the most important sign is when someone behaves in an unusual way for which there is no obvious explanation. The earlier the abuse is discovered, the better the chances of reducing the harm it can cause.

Ways of helping, once drug abuse is suspected or confirmed, have to be carefully planned. The purpose is always to reduce harm to and increase support for the affected person and his or her family in the most effective and least distressing way possible. It is not merely to 'clamp down' on drug use. Anger, blame, guilt or fear born of ignorance will only make matters worse and further undermine the self-confidence and self-respect of those who fall into drug abuse as a way of coping with life.

Sometimes underlying problems such as loneliness, failure to be able to meet others' expectations, or unhappiness in marriage cannot be easily resolved. But often just discussing them can, in time, open the way to better understanding and better ways of dealing with them. Seeking the advice and help of independent agencies (see p. 468) — and caring individuals such as your family doctor or an experienced local social worker — may well be the most sensible thing to do.

- The first step to helping people avoid or give up undesirable drug-use habits is to understand why they may have become dependent on them in the first place. The possible reasons include:

  1. **Social pressures**.   If people find themselves in a group where drug taking is normal they feel they have to join in. This applies to drinking alcohol and smoking cigarettes (the biggest single killer in Britain today) as much as it does to activities like glue sniffing, smoking cannabis or injecting heroin. Not everyone has the confidence to say 'no' when their friends say 'yes'.
  2. **Rebellion**.   Taking drugs upsets people in authority. So it is a way for people lacking self-confidence or a clear idea of their own worth to seek attention and assert their independence.
  3. **Parental example**.   Young people who see their parents drinking regularly, smoking or habitually taking tablets in

moments of stress may be led to believe that taking drugs is a normal way of coping with life.

4. **Overwork**.   Both stimulants like cocaine and amphetamines and depressants like alcohol can be abused because of people's attempts to cope with overwork, which itself may be a symptom of not facing up to other problems in life. Middle-aged men are perhaps most at risk of abusing drugs for this reason, although young people facing the stresses of housework and caring for young children may also try 'coping with chemicals'.

5. **Lack of a role in society**.   Lonely people and those who do not enjoy their work or home lives, or who are worried about the future, are naturally often mentally distressed because they do not know what to do or how to fit in. Some young people say that they resort to drug taking as a way of gaining self-knowledge. Older individuals may turn to alcohol to try and cope with being alone.

6. **Poor medical care**.   This can increase the risk of individuals abusing medical drugs. For example, if medicines like tranquillizers are prescribed for too long people can be exposed to needless risks of dependence.

7. **Mental illness**.   Some people who take illegal drugs may be trying to ease the symptoms of serious mental illnesses, such as schizophrenia and depression.

8. **Shyness and fear**.   Drug taking, from tobacco smoking to the abuse of substances like LSD or heroin, may come from people's attempts to overcome feelings of insecurity and lack of self-worth. Rather than criticism or blame, they need encouragement to see themselves in a better light.

- So a calm, constructive approach is needed first to provide a home atmosphere which makes drug abuse and dependence less likely, then an understanding approach to why someone is seeking refuge in drugs, and finally the use of professional help early rather than late if the family finds it is not coping.

- Make time for your children and build a close relationship with them. Happy children with a positive future are less likely to turn to drugs. If there are difficult times children will more readily turn to caring parents for help than to drugs. However, there are no rules in this difficult area; many excellent parents have children who abuse drugs and they

Signs of Drug Abuse

Smoking and alcohol, see separate entries.

Solvents

- The smell of glue on the breath
- Finding hidden tubes of glue
- Inflammation round the nose
- Personality changes such as unusual tiredness, irritability, fears and poor concentration
- Poor performance at school

Cannabis, cocaine and heroin

- There may be physical signs such as half-smoked cigarettes, silver paper, even syringes and needles.
- Often more readily noticed are the personality changes such as irritability, loss of social confidence and interest, tiredness, unexplained fears and phobias, loss of weight and interest in food, loss of interest in sex, and difficulties with relationships and work.
- Unexplained furtiveness and stealing may be an indication that someone is on drugs which need financing.

should not feel personally guilty. Try not to make drug taking a 'no-go' area, as this might make it seem more attractive to a youngster. Instead discuss the advantages and disadvantages calmly and sensibly, without at any time appearing to accept it. Be sure your children realize the legal consequences. In the West this may vary from a few months to thirteen or fourteen years in prison. In some Eastern countries the penalty for trafficking in drugs can be death.

DUPUYTREN'S CONTRACTURE

This is a condition in which the fingers (usually the ring finger and little finger) become increasingly bent forwards because fibrous tissue grows in and under the skin of the palm and prevents the tendons to the fingers moving properly.

Self-health

- Dupuytren's contracture often runs in families so nothing can be done to prevent it.

- Occasionally it is linked with drinking alcohol. Stopping drinking may help but usually it is too late.

- If you notice your fingers bending up uncontrollably see your doctor soon so that a surgeon can decide whether surgery is necessary. The longer you wait, the stiffer the joints of your fingers become, the more difficult the surgery and the less satisfactory the outcome.

DYSLEXIA

Dyslexia is a condition in which a child has great difficulty in learning to read and write despite being of normal intelligence and receiving normal teaching. Many educationalists now prefer to call such difficulties 'learning difficulties'. It may affect up to one in twenty-five children, and boys are three times more commonly affected than girls.

Self-health

- The most important point about this condition is that it should be recognized early so that appropriate tuition can be arranged immediately. It is not a condition that will simply respond to trying harder using conventional teaching methods. You may suspect dyslexia if:

    1. Your child had speech problems before school.
    2. There is a family history of learning and speech difficulties.
    3. Your child is slow to read and spell (and may therefore be

reluctant to try) while appearing to cope well with other areas such as mathematics, oral classwork or puzzles.

4. Your child finds particular difficulty with learning sequences such as maths tables, days of the week and long instructions. Other difficulties include confusing letters like b and d or q and p whose shape is similar.

5. Your child gets confused over right and left. It seems also that ambidextrous people (people who can use their right and left hands with equal skill) are prone to dyslexia.

- Avoid frequent changes of school, classroom and teacher because these contribute to the difficulties. Stress at home and lack of parental help and support are also contributory factors.

- Special tuition will make all the difference to your dyslexic child so embrace it with enthusiasm. Your child may need to attend special classes at school in addition to normal schoolwork, and you may be shown exercises (which can be fun) to do at home. Your child will quickly make up lost ground and, although he or she may always be a poor speller, will have an equal chance of a good education and satisfying job.

E

EAR, INFECTION

Infections of the ear are caused by bacteria, viruses or fungi and affect the outer ear (otitis externa) and the middle ear (otitis media). Both conditions have to be taken seriously because they may cause permanent deafness. The symptoms include fever, feeling unwell, pain when moving or touching the ear, and discharge from the ear. It is generally children who are affected by ear infections.

Self-health

OUTER EAR

- Children who swim a lot are more likely to suffer from ear infections (swimmer's ear). Make sure the ear is dry after swimming but be careful not to damage the lining of the canal (e.g. with a rough towel) because this will let the germs in and start an infection.

- If your child gets many infections (children with eczema are prone to them) keep water away from the ear by using earplugs, cottonwool soaked in oil or a bathing cap. If you put something in the ears, though, be careful not to damage the delicate lining or germs will spread and cause an infection.

- At the first sign of an ear infection see your doctor immediately and ban further swimming until it is cured.

MIDDLE EAR

- The middle ear is the cavity surrounding the delicate mechanisms of the ear behind the eardrum. It is kept ventilated by the Eustachian tube, a narrow canal that runs

EAR INFECTION

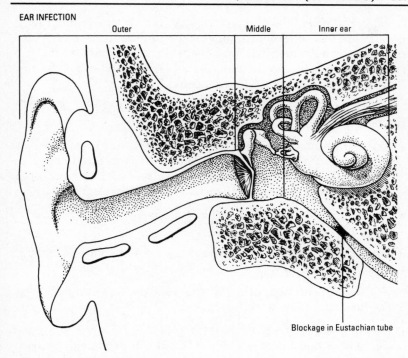

Outer   Middle   Inner ear

Blockage in Eustachian tube

from the middle ear to the throat.

One problem with this tube is that in children it is very short, which allows germs to travel easily from the throat into the ear. So beware of colds, coughs and sore throats, which will be a source of infection.

- The other problem with the Eustachian tube is that it can be blocked by inflammation. This means that no fresh air reaches the middle ear, and germs then have the opportunity to reproduce quickly and cause an infection. To prevent this, suck mentholated pastilles if you have a cold or sore throat and see your doctor who may prescribe vasoconstrictor drugs (nose drops or spray) to unblock the Eustachian tube.

EAR, RINGING (TINNITUS)

In the UK as many as 300,000 people suffer from ringing in their ears (also called tinnitus) so badly that it severely affects their lives. In the USA it has been estimated that six per cent of the population has suffered from it at some time in their lives. The ringing may have many different causes and can vary from a gentle hum to a violent hammering all the time which occasionally drives the sufferer to suicide.

Self-health

- Try to find the cause. This may be ear wax, an ear infection or catarrh, some drugs, hardening of the arteries, raised blood pressure, Menière's disease or loud noises (such as gunfire). If action is taken to remove the cause, the ringing may stop.

- Avoid stimulants such as coffee, tobacco or, in some cases, exercise.

- Use a ticking clock to mask the ringing when trying to sleep in quiet surroundings.

- Try sleeping on high pillows. This may prevent congestion in the head and help stop the ringing.

- Do not become overtired, and try to avoid stress and anxiety. Remember that tinnitus will not cause you to go deaf, or lose your reason, nor is it fatal.

- Use a tinnitus masker on the advice of your GP. A hearing aid may also be necessary and will improve the quality of your life.

- Medicines are available which prevent tinnitus in some people. Consult your GP.

EAR WAX

Wax is produced by small glands of the lining of the outer ear to protect it against infection. Some people produce a lot of wax which may harden in the ear, causing deafness and a feeling of fullness.

Self-health

- There is no way you can slow the rate at which you produce wax, but you can prevent it hardening in the ear and causing symptoms. First put two or three drops of wax softener (which can be bought from the chemist) or olive oil into the ear twice a week and keep it in overnight with cottonwool. The wax will soften and you may avoid the need for syringeing. If not, see your doctor or nurse about syringeing.

ECZEMA

Eczema is an inflammation of the skin. It is usually itchy and red, and there may be flaking or blisters which weep a clear fluid. It is often called dermatitis especially when there is an external cause (e.g. allergy). There are many different types and treatment depends on the cause.

Self-health

- **Contact eczema.** This eczema occurs when the skin comes into contact with substances to which it is allergic. Symptoms may develop within a few hours of contact or slowly over days. The only method of prevention is to avoid direct contact with the irritant by wearing protective clothing, gloves or goggles, and to avoid articles which you come to learn cause symptoms (e.g. the nickel on wristwatch straps).

- **Atopic eczema.** This eczema runs in families prone to such conditions as asthma (see separate entry) or hayfever (see separate entry). It may start in children as young as two months (infantile eczema) and last into late adolescence or even adulthood. In infants it affects the head, face, forearms and lower legs. Later it affects creases, such as behind the knees and on wrists. As many as ten per cent of children are affected by eczema at some time in their lives but most recover completely. There is no certain way of preventing this eczema but as cow's milk can be an allergen, some reports suggest that breast-feeding for the first four to six months may help prevent it.
  Should your child develop this type of eczema you can help by dressing him or her in cotton clothing and avoiding using creams or ointments without first consulting your doctor.

Sometimes antihistamine tablets prevent the itching and occasionally steroid creams or ointments help. The other important preventive measure is to avoid the *emotional* problems which are known to bring on an attack.

- **Seborrhoeic eczema.**   This eczema occurs wherever the sebaceous or grease glands of the skin are numerous, for example the scalp, chest, armpits, groin. The cradle cap (see separate entry) of infancy is the earliest form and many people are affected by the mild form, dandruff (see separate entry).

  Regular washing will reduce the chance of the skin becoming infected. Coal-tar soap is particularly recommended and shampoos with either zinc pyrithione (e.g. Head and Shoulders) or selenium sulphide (e.g. Selsun or Lenium) will help prevent the condition recurring.

- **Hand eczema.**   'Hands that do dishes' are prone to eczema. It is the alternate wetting and drying that does the damage rather than immersing them in water for long periods. The skin's water-holding capacity becomes reduced, minor scratches quickly become major and the skin is always vulnerable even if it appears to have recovered fully.

  Avoiding washing up is the ideal preventive step, but this is not practical for most people. A dishwasher will help. Wash your hands as infrequently as possible, and use lukewarm water and mild, unperfumed neutral pH soaps (e.g. Simple Soap, Purely Soap or Neutrogena). Aqueous cream as a soap substitute is useful and can be used liberally between hand washes. Always wash soap off with clear, running water and pat your hands dry with a soft towel to avoid damage to the skin. Be sure the skin under rings is kept clean and dry (and the rings themselves because they can easily start a rash).

  Make sure your hands do not come into direct contact with strong detergents or cleaning agents, and be wary of picking up bottles containing these as they are often contaminated. Wear gloves for housework but use plastic rather than rubber ones, which can cause an allergy. Use cotton undergloves and keep a good supply so you can change and wash them often. After your work is finished and your hands are clean and dry, apply a moisturizing cream or lotion to trap water in the horny layer of your skin so it does not dry out.

Tips for coping with eczema

1. Use hot water liberally. It soothes the itch and used with soap will clean off dirt and irritants. Daily baths are a great help. Too much bathing may make eczema of the hands worse, however.
2. Choose your soap carefully. Some are harsh and dry out your skin, giving it a stretched feeling. Baby soap is often best. Experiment to find the most suitable for your skin. Emulsifying ointment can be used as a substitute.
3. Use a bath oil (e.g. Alpha Keri, Oilatum, Emulsiderm) to help prevent your skin drying out after a bath. Also apply plenty of emollient, such as Vaseline or Nivea, throughout the day if necessary.

- **Discoid eczema.**   Discs of red, flaking, itchy skin may appear on the arms and legs. There is no known cause so prevention is impossible, but fortunately it usually disappears within a few months. Symptoms can be eased as for atopic eczema.

- **Varicose eczema.**   People with varicose veins (see separate entry) may develop this dark-brown eczema on the lower third of their legs. You should have varicose veins treated by injection or surgery, or by improving the circulation to your lower leg. This is done by exercise, keeping your feet up when sitting, avoiding standing for long periods, and using special elastic stockings.

EJACULATION, PREMATURE

Some men are unable to control ejaculation of their sperm (or orgasm) so that they may 'come' before their penis is erect, at the moment they penetrate a woman or very shortly afterwards. This can cause great distress to both partners but it can be prevented.

Self-health

- Do not worry if premature ejaculation happens at the beginning of a relationship or after a long period of abstinence. Control will improve with familiarity and regular sex.

- Premature ejaculation sometimes has a psychological cause.

This may be a deep-rooted fear of women or the sexual act, or the man may feel hostile towards his partner and this is the only way he knows to 'punish' her. Sometimes a couple can get to the root of such problems by talking it through together; often a professional such as a GP, marriage counsellor or sex therapist is needed.

- The partner should show she enjoys sex (including her fantasies) to give the man confidence and make him realize he is not defiling her. But she must also be careful not to show she expects too much from him or this will shatter his confidence further.

- A well-proven method to help prevent premature ejaculation is for the man to masturbate to orgasm (or the woman to help him) before intercourse. This often allows both to enjoy controllable orgasm later.

- Using a sheath or anaesthetic cream reduces the sensation in the penis and may help delay ejaculation.

- 'Stop-start' intercourse often helps and many women enjoy this type of intercourse. The man thinks about boring things like work or washing-up during the 'stop' period.

- The 'squeeze' technique is the best way of learning to delay orgasm. The couple abandons intercourse for a while, substituting other ways of stimulating each other. Just as the man is about to 'come' the woman squeezes his penis firmly just below the tip which will quickly make it go limp. This process is repeated several times and on sufficient occasions for the man to gain confidence in his control. Then intercourse starts again and each time the man feels he is about to 'come' the woman squeezes his penis as before. Gradually the time taken to reach this point increases until the couple can enjoy satisfying sex.

EPISIOTOMY

During labour it is sometimes necessary to cut part of the vagina to let the baby out quicker or prevent the mother tearing uncontrollably, which could cause problems in later life with

painful sex (see **Sex, Painful, Female**) or difficulty controlling
the bowels.

Self-health

- There are one or two steps you can take to make an episiotomy
  less likely, but do not feel you have failed if you do have to
  have one. The chances are that it could not be avoided, and
  guilt will only prevent you making a full recovery.

- Make sure that your doctor and midwife know that you feel
  strongly about not having an episiotomy unless it is absolutely
  necessary. Some units perform episiotomies more readily than
  others so they need to know your feelings.

- Some experts believe episiotomy is less likely if you labour
  upright, not on your back. If it is necessary for you to be on
  your back you may be less likely to need an episiotomy if your
  legs are only about a foot apart (and not widely spread as often
  happens) because this puts less pressure on the pelvic tissues.

- Ask your midwife or doctor about perineal massage. This
  softens and stretches the skin of the vagina to make childbirth
  easier.

- Pelvic floor exercises (see separate entry) are valuable. They
  will not specifically prevent an episiotomy but they will help
  your muscles recover from the stretching they underwent
  during childbirth.

- Any episiotomy takes about six weeks to heal so do not try to
  have sex too early or it may prove very painful. Explore gently
  how quickly you are healing and take it one step at a time. It
  may help to use a lubricant during sex to start with.

ERECTION, FAILURE OF

A man who is impotent cannot have, or maintain an erection –
unlike a sterile man, who is capable of an erection but whose
sperm are not fertile. There are many causes for impotence,
mainly psychological but also physical, such as stress, alcohol,
tiredness or illness.

Self-health

- Some men take a sexual failure badly, believing it casts doubt on their masculinity. But there is no need to. Most men have the occasional failure and the best thing is to shrug it off and enjoy next time even more.

- Deep-rooted anxiety, fears or uncertainty about their role may cause some men more serious erection problems. Often discussions between the couple may help, particularly if the problem is seen as something for both partners to solve, not just the man. Sometimes, though, it may be necessary to get expert help from a marriage counsellor, GP or sex therapist.

- Some men may blame their sexual failures on their partners, either because they do not stimulate them or because they are not attractive. Certainly a couple should learn together what gives each partner most satisfaction, but attaching blame is never helpful and usually creates further anxiety, antagonism and tension, making a further failure more likely.

- If a man starts having repeated sexual failure the couple should consider his lifestyle. Reducing stress and/or alcohol may solve the problem. If not, a doctor should be consulted because occasionally a physical illness such as diabetes may be the cause.

EYE CARE

Sight is a very precious gift and it is only right that you should do everything you can to preserve it.

Self-health

- Wear safety goggles if your job involves any substances (e.g. sparks or metal splinters) that could damage your eyes.

- Consider whether you should take safety precautions when playing sport, e.g. goggles against squash balls which are nicely designed to enter the orbit of the eye.

- Beware of dangers at home, e.g. boiling fat.

- Wear spectacles or contact lenses if they are prescribed for you. There is little reason for the widespread belief that doing so will weaken your eyes. Quite the contrary, if you don't wear them you may suffer headaches and other symptoms and there is no other certain way to correct faulty eyesight.

- Do not use ointments, drops or solutions unless prescribed for you by your doctor.

- Do not ignore symptoms like a red eye, new difficulty seeing in the dark, blindness looking straight ahead or round the edges, or any unexplained change in your vision.

- Do not read or do other close work in poor light, especially if you are over sixty, because this strains the eyes.

Screening

- Examine your baby's eyes for obvious defects like a squint and tell your family doctor if you notice anything that worries you.

- Check your child's eyesight regularly to make sure he or she

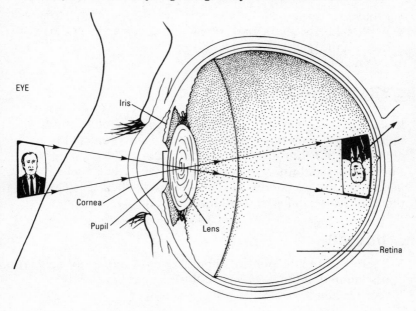

EYE

Iris

Cornea

Pupil

Lens

Retina

can see well enough to read, play sport, read the blackboard etc. Poor sight (along with poor hearing) is a major cause of doing badly at school.

- Have your eyesight checked regularly by an optician, especially once you are over fifty. Once every two years is sufficient for most people. At these checks other conditions such as cataract, glaucoma, diabetes or raised blood pressure (see separate entries) may be noticed.

EYE, DRY

Lacrimal glands at the side of the eye produce fluid to keep them moist. Normally they keep up a regular supply of fluid but some conditions such as rheumatoid arthritis (see **Arthritis**) affect the glands and dry up the eye. Strong emotion has the opposite effect, causing the glands to overflow with fluid, known as tears.

Self-health

- Protect your eyes carefully in very hot, dusty, sandy climates.
- Artificial tears can be prescribed by a doctor to keep the eyes moist if the glands are not working.

EYE, SQUINT

If one eye looks in a different direction from the other it is known as a squint. It is the most common eye problem in childhood, affecting about three per cent of children, but it is uncommon in adults who have not previously had one. A squint usually suggests a condition elsewhere in the body (e.g. high blood pressure, diabetes or an inflamed artery in the forehead).

Self-health

- Squints cannot be prevented but it is most important they are not ignored or the 'lazy' eye will become permanently damaged and unable to work or see properly.

- If your child has a squint beyond the age of three months, see your doctor so the eyes can be assessed. An eye patch, glasses or even surgery may be needed to correct it.

- Any adult who develops a squint should see a doctor so that the cause of the squint can be found.

EYE, STICKY

A bacterial or viral infection may cause the eye to become red, crusted and sticky. Untreated, it clears within two to three weeks but treatment is usually recommended.

Self-health

- Sticky eyes can be caught from other people, particularly children. If your child has a sticky eye keep his or her towels, sheets and flannel separate from the rest of the family's. Bathe the eye in warm water and apply treatment, making sure all contaminated materials are either thrown away or cleaned before other children touch them. Wash hands after contact.

- Avoid irritants such as tobacco smoke and cosmetics.

EYE STRAIN

All eyes, even those with perfect vision, need to be looked after to prevent strain and deterioration.

Self-health

- Eat plenty of green, leafy vegetables, carrots, fruit and liver to provide the vitamin A your eyes need, especially so you can see better in the dark.

- Make sure lighting is good enough for you to see without strain. As you grow older, the lens in your eye clouds up so that less and less light gets to the back of the eye. Research has found that by the age of fifty, as little as fifty per cent of the light may be getting through the lens, falling to forty-four per cent by the age of sixty. So it is very important that you use better lighting as you grow older. Increase the wattage of your bulbs, have more light sources, paint your walls lighter so there is more reflected light, and don't have sharp contrasts between dark and light places because your eyes will not be able to cope with them.

- Don't expose your eyes to too much sunlight or glare as this will cause eyestrain and headaches. Turn away from strong sources of light at work and wear sunglasses to protect your eyes.

- Rest your eyes regularly, especially if you are working with VDU screens. Make sensible routines and stick to them.

- Wear glasses or contact lenses you have been prescribed, because straining to see without them, especially for reading or VDU work, is bad for the eyes. However, this does not mean you have to wear them all the time and you may like to do eye exercises to keep your eyes healthy. Ask your optician about these.

EYE, WATERING

A watering eye is usually due to a blockage in the canal that drains away the fluid that moistens the eye. The blockage is commonly caused by inflammation from a cold or flu, or in babies because the canal has not opened up. Often, though, the cause is not found.

Self-health

- If you catch a cold or flu, a decongestant bought from the chemist may help your eyes.

- Avoid irritants such as smoke.

- If your eyes water continuously without an obvious cause see a doctor. It may be that the canal needs syringeing or even a small operation.

F

FAINTS

Fainting occurs when the blood flow to the brain is reduced, causing the sufferer to fall to the ground unconscious. Once the person is lying flat and the blood flow to the brain is restored, he or she often makes a quick recovery. If not, you should seek expert help quickly.

Self-health

- Many causes of fainting, such as a fright, strong emotion, an accident, severe pain or bleeding cannot be prevented, but other causes can.

- Avoid hot, stuffy rooms if you are prone to fainting.

- Do not stand in one place for long periods either on an empty stomach or without walking about or stamping your feet to keep the circulation going.

- Don't stand up suddenly, especially if you have been unwell, in bed for a long time, or in a hot place.

- Some people faint if they look up sharply (e.g. to take a jar down from a high shelf) or move their neck in a particular way. Learn to avoid these movements.

- If you are pregnant you are more likely to faint because your heart has to pump round a lot more blood and your blood pressure may be low.

- If you have heart disease, beware of fainting because your heart cannot pump the blood to your brain so easily.

- If you continue to faint for no obvious reason, see your doctor because there are causes (e.g. anaemia) that can be diagnosed and treated to prevent you fainting.

FALLS

Falls are serious for elderly people because their bones are brittle and may break. It has been estimated that in the UK there are about three million falls each year needing medical attention – equivalent to one fall for every three elderly people. Many of these people will die, as much from the problems of being immobile in bed as from the breaks themselves, so it is vital that every precaution is taken.

Self-health

- Guard against falls by keeping fit, exercising and eating a healthy diet. Even a few days in bed can make you weak and shaky when you start walking again.

- If you feel unwell or more shaky than normal see your doctor to make sure there is not a preventable physical cause (e.g. anaemia or Parkinson's disease).

- Make sure carpets and floor coverings are secure round the edges. Avoid using slippery floor materials in the kitchen or bathroom. Rugs should never be put on highly polished floors.

- Make sure your house is well lit, especially on the stairs. Light-coloured paint and high-wattage bulbs help.

- Fit a strong banister rail along all steps and stairs.

- Fit secure handrails to baths and near lavatories. Use non-slip bathmats.

- Make sure electric wires are fixed to skirting boards or walls and not running loose.

- In your bedroom use a night light or a bedside lamp that can be easily reached. Do not stumble about in the dark. A high percentage of falls amongst people over seventy occur in the bedroom.

- Try to keep rooms tidy so you do not fall over books, toys, ashtrays, etc.

- Use glasses if you need them and do not walk about wearing a pair designed for reading.

- Use a stick or walking frame if it makes you feel steadier. Make sure your shoes and slippers have non-slip soles, and do not use long shoe laces which could trip you up. Do not go out in icy conditions unless you have to.

- Elderly people who live alone should wear an alarm so that they can alert others if they have an accident. Less sophisticated systems, such as a whistle, telephone call or daily sign for neighbours, may work just as well.

FEEDING PROBLEMS, BABIES

Do not feel guilty if you and your baby have feeding problems. They are common, even for experienced parents. Some problems you can solve yourself but get professional help if your baby starts to lose weight, cries continuously, or is tired and listless with no appetite.

Self-health

- Most experts agree that breast-feeding is generally better than bottle-feeding for both mother and baby. However, there may be perfectly good reasons why you cannot or do not wish to breast-feed, so do not feel guilty if you decide to bottle-feed instead. You have not failed as a mother, and your baby will grow up perfectly healthy.

- Do not bury your baby in your breast or your clothes because his or her nose will become blocked, making suckling difficult.

- If your breasts are engorged (see **Breast-feeding, Engorgement**) or your nipples do not naturally stand out, it may be difficult for your baby to 'latch on'. A warm bath before breast-feeding may encourage the milk to flow.

- Do not be surprised if your baby does not feed well when tired (rather than hungry) or upset.

- Illnesses such as colds, ear infections or thrush (see separate entries) may make your baby reluctant to feed. See your doctor if there is no obvious cause for your baby being unwell.

- Do not become upset if your baby falls asleep while suckling.

He or she may even need waking to start sucking again. Some feeds can take as long as an hour.

- If your baby seems hungry soon after a feed, simply increase the number of feeds you are giving. If you are breast-feeding this will stimulate your breasts to produce more milk.

- Some babies regurgitate quite large amounts of milk – this is known as posseting. There is no need for concern, provided you are sure your baby is not vomiting. If there is a lot of air mixed up with the regurgitated milk, try feeding in a more upright position with no bouncing. If you are bottle-feeding check the size of the hole in the nipple to make sure it is not so small that your baby has to suck hard or so large that your baby is flooded with milk.

- A baby who cries after feeding can be very wearying for parents. One cause is the evening or three-month colic (see **Colic**) when your baby refuses to be comforted by cuddling, feeding, rocking or any of your usually successful remedies. There is not much you can do except to check with your doctor that something more serious is not wrong and be reassured that it will usually pass by the age of six months.

- If you are bottle-feeding make sure you are mixing the feeds according to the manufacturer's instructions. If they are too diluted your baby will cry because of undernourishment. If they are too concentrated the baby will cry because he or she may be taking in too much salt and therefore feels thirsty.

- Many mothers believe that wind in the stomach causes crying and that 'winding' prevents it.

FEEDING PROBLEMS, CHILDREN

Most parents have feeding problems with their children at some stage but the worst conflicts can be avoided if you follow the advice below.

Self-health

- Make meal times a happy routine for children early on. Feed them nutritious foods they like and set an example by showing them you enjoy your own food.

- Never force children to eat. A battle will make them even more determined and there may be times when a child wants a fight to 'punish' you or show independence.

- Don't stick to adult mealtime routines. If your child prefers yogurt before the main dish, for example, serve it this way.

- Introducing new foods in small portions between favourite foods will give you the best chance of success.

- Try not to let your child notice your worries about feeding. If you do it may be used as an attention-seeking opportunity.

FEET, ACHING

Surveys show that nearly eight out of ten people suffer from aching feet at some stage in their life.

Self-health

- The greatest single cause is badly fitting footwear, so buy shoes that are at least 0.5 cm longer than your feet and wide enough not to crush them. Ideally the heel should be no more than 5 cm high, and the sole and upper made of flexible natural materials.

- Wear insoles, inserts or supports if necessary to support your feet.

- If you are overweight, try to lose weight.

- Look after your feet by wearing the appropriate shoes when playing sports. Remember that just running increases the weight on your feet by three to four times.

- Do exercises to strengthen the muscles of your feet – for example, standing on tiptoe, making circles with your toes in the air, walking on the inside and outside edges of your feet.

- Put your feet up at any opportunity and persuade a friend or lover to give them the occasional massage!

FEET, FLAT

A flat foot is one in which the normal arch does not exist.

Self-health

CHILDREN

- Babies have flat feet because the muscles of the feet have not developed and the arches are filled with fat. One or two years after a child begins to walk, the arches will start to develop and by the age of sixteen they will be fully developed. So do not worry about flat feet in young children unless they feel any pain, in which case consult your doctor.

- Plenty of walking will help prevent flat feet – especially as it will help prevent obesity which is another cause of flat feet.

- Make sure shoes are well fitting.

ADULTS

- Try not to spend long periods standing, but if you do have to, wear shoes with good arch supports.

- Try to keep to the normal weight for your height – being overweight puts a severe strain on the 'bridge' that is the arch of your foot.

- An arch support placed inside your shoes may help.

- Do exercises to strengthen the muscles of your feet. For example, alternate standing on tiptoe with standing on your heels and lifting your toes for two minutes three times a day. Or draw as large circles as possible in the air with your feet. A chiropodist or physiotherapist will be able to advise you.

FEET, SWOLLEN

There are many causes of swollen feet. In young people it is usually due to accidentally damaging the soft tissues, such as the ligaments or tendons, or breaking the bones. In older people it is more likely to be due to circulation problems.

Self-health

- Wear loose shoes that do not restrict circulation.

- When playing sport make sure your footwear is suitable and will support your feet.

- Do not wear socks that are very tight below the knee.

- If you have to stand for long periods, stamp your feet up and down regularly to get the circulation going.

- If your feet tend to swell, rest with them propped up so gravity helps to drain the fluid away. Exercise your calf and foot muscles at the same time.

- Sometimes wearing support stockings (on prescription from your doctor or available from your chemist) prevents swollen feet.

- If you have varicose veins see your doctor, who will arrange for them to be treated if necessary.

- If despite your efforts the swelling remains, see your doctor. You may have a medical condition that needs treatment.

FITS

Fits are spasms caused by abnormal electrical signals from the brain to the muscles. They can last just a few seconds, in which case they may not be apparent to anyone except the sufferer, or they can last for minutes, even hours in bad cases.

Self-health

- A high temperature (e.g. over 30.5°C) may bring on a fit in susceptible children – generally those aged one to five with a relative who is prone to fits. As soon as the fever starts dress the child in cotton clothes, treat with paracetamol and start sponging with tepid (not cold) water to bring the temperature down (see **Temperature**).

- Some fits are brought on by flashing lights, television, alcohol, or tiredness, so avoid these wherever possible.

- Always see your doctor, who may be able to prescribe medicine to prevent fits recurring.

FOOD POISONING

If you eat food containing bacteria or toxins (poisons produced by the bacteria) you risk making yourself ill, especially from diarrhoea and vomiting (gastroenteritis). A few people, particularly the young and the elderly, even die.

Self-health

- Good personal hygiene is important. Make sure you wash your hands after going to the lavatory and before meals. Never use the kitchen sink. Never cough, sneeze or spit over food. Make sure any cut is clean and covered with a waterproof dressing (or gloves) when preparing food.

- Don't prepare food if you are ill, especially if your symptoms include diarrhoea or vomiting.

- Store food in clean, covered containers. Keep cold food cold, and hot food piping hot. Do not store raw meat alongside cooked meat in the refrigerator, and avoid leaving cooked meat out for long periods. Follow manufacturers' storage instructions and do not keep food longer than the recommended date.

- Throw away food if you notice unexpected discoloration, white-coloured patches, slime or mould.

- Try not to handle food more than you can, and don't dip your fingers into food to taste it.

- Keep cooking utensils clean and dry. Chopping boards can easily spread germs so wash them regularly with hot, soapy water, especially after cutting meat or poultry. Beware of dirty washing-up or tea-cloths.

- Be particularly careful with milk foods, especially cream, ice-cream, cream fillings and custard which must be thrown away quickly if not eaten.

- Always thaw poultry completely before cooking then make sure it is fully cooked. Follow thawing instructions carefully without short cuts. A large bird can take up to forty-eight hours to thaw out. Warm food is the most likely breeding ground for bacteria, so eat poultry either cold (below 10°C) or piping hot (over 60°C).

- Rotate your food stock so supplies do not become old and stale. Once opened, bottled goods usually need refrigeration. Do not use swollen, badly rusted or dented cans. Once canned foods have been opened transfer them to a clean container and treat them as fresh food.

- Microwave ovens are a convenient way of thawing and cooking food. Follow the manufacturers' instructions carefully. In particular rotate food during cooking and don't ignore the standing time for food afterwards.

- Make sure your refrigerator, freezer and oven are working properly, and buy a fridge thermometer if necessary to ensure it is running at the correct temperature. Good maintenance could prevent illness.

FORESKIN, INFLAMMATION

Inflammation of the foreskin is common, so have no hesitation in seeing your doctor about it. The foreskin will be red, inflamed, painful, sometimes itchy. There may be a discharge and occasionally it hurts to pass urine.

Self-health

- Retract the foreskin to clean beneath it. Avoid strong or perfumed soap because it may irritate the skin.

- If the foreskin is difficult to pull back you may wish to consider circumcision, a small operation which removes the foreskin. Consult your doctor.

- Wearing a sheath (condom) during sexual intercourse reduces your chances of getting a sexually transmitted disease such as herpes (see separate entry). It will also prevent an allergy to contraceptive creams developing. Just occasionally, though, men are allergic to the condoms themselves so beware of this if your inflammation persists despite all efforts.

- Some clothing (e.g. nylon) may cause inflammation so try cotton underwear. Sitting about in damp clothing will also make the problem worse.

FORESKIN, UNRETRACTABLE

A foreskin that you cannot pull back (also called phimosis) is normal in babies so there is no need for concern until the boy is about three to five years old.

Self-health

- Never try to force the foreskin back. It will happen of its own accord in most boys.
- Sometimes a tight foreskin may cause difficulties passing urine or pain on erection. A small operation may be necessary. This could either be a dorsal slit to make the hole in the foreskin larger or a circumcision to remove the foreskin altogether. Both are done under anaesthetic and should cause discomfort for no more than two or three days.

FRACTURES

A fracture is a broken bone. Most are caused by accidents that cannot be prevented, but it is possible to take sensible precautions to make you less likely to have a fracture.

Self-health

- Look after children, especially near stairs and roads. If you suspect a bone has been broken, take your child to your doctor or to hospital immediately. Don't put it off because you fear you will be accused of neglect or, worse, battering.
- Make sure your children eat food with plenty of calcium (e.g. milk) to build strong bones.

- If you are a menopausal woman suffering from osteoporosis (see separate entry), consider having hormone replacement treatment.

- If you are on medicines, particularly tranquillizers, remember that they may make you giddy, sleepy or sluggish, and more likely to fall. If you take steroids for a long time you will be prone to weaker, more brittle bones.

- Stress fractures occur in some athletes when they change their shoes, increase their mileage schedule or train on a new, harder surface. Beware of the very real danger of these fractures and do not ignore pain from the lower leg (tibia or fibula bones) or feet (metatarsal bones).

- Elderly people should take special precautions against falling (see **Falls**).

DIFFERENT TYPES OF FRACTURE

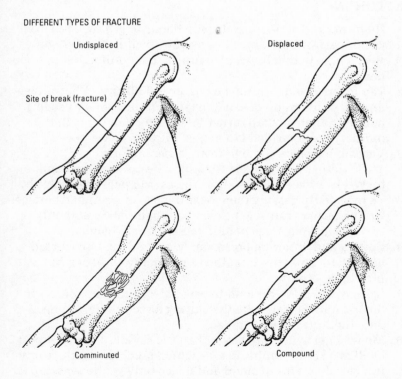

Undisplaced

Displaced

Site of break (fracture)

Comminuted

Compound

G

GADGETS FOR DISABLED AND ELDERLY PEOPLE

Disabled people may suffer needless problems and frustrations because they cannot perform everyday tasks. Here is a selection of aids which can prevent those frustrations and enable them to continue living a normal, independent life.

KITCHEN

1. High-friction, non-slip mats help hands to grip wide-necked jars or narrow bottle tops to unscrew the lids. Screw-tight steel bands will help people with good co-ordination but poor power.
2. Tap levers make turning the tap on and off easy. They either replace or fit on top of existing taps. For temporary use (e.g. holidays) there are tap turner hooks which fit beneath the ordinary cross-headed tap to give extra leverage.
3. Vegetable peelers come in many different forms:
   a. Broad-handled peelers to fit into the palm of the hand.
   b. Work-surface peelers allow the user to peel vegetables by repeatedly passing them over the peeler's serrated surface. The peelers can also be clamped to the surface so only the vegetable has to be held if you are single-handed.
4. Cutting and buttering bread can be a problem. Use a bread board with spikes to hold the bread or any L-shaped block to prevent it slipping.
5. Scissors are often difficult to use, but sprung versions with broad handles distribute the cutting force evenly and need only light pressure to operate.
6. Modern jug kettles are better than the standard type but best of all is a kettle-tipping device which holds the kettle firmly in place on a hinged stand and needs only gentle pressure to tip the kettle forward for pouring. A spiral spring will return

it to the horizontal. Similar devices also exist for teapots.

7. Cutlery may be easier to use with the addition of large-diameter foam or 'soft-grip' handles which slip over the existing handles. For permanent use specially designed, broad-handled cutlery is available.

8. Food can be stopped from sliding around the plate by divided crockery or by a plate guard which snaps on to the edge of the plate.

9. Specially designed handles make cups and glasses easier to hold. However, don't forget the humble straw, which is particularly useful for people lying in bed or half propped up. Elegant ones with non-return valves help people with poor sucking ability.

BATHROOM

1. There are many adaptations now, including seat raisers and handrails, which should make your lavatory safe and comfortable to use. Many are lightweight and easily removed to save embarrassment.

2. Non-slip mats are worth their weight in gold. They may be needed beside handbasins, lavatories and next to the bath as well as in it. Handrails within the bath are also very useful.

3. You should talk to your doctor and occupational therapist about hoists and lifts if you think you need them.

4. Toothbrushes can be held much more easily using specially adapted handles. Electric toothbrushes can be a great help.

5. Two main devices exist to help squeeze toothpaste out:
   a. A handle can be attached to the tube and turned to squeeze the toothpaste out.
   b. For single-handed use there is a device which sticks to the wall with self-adhesive pads and also squeezes out toothpaste by means of a handle.

6. Brushes can be extended with long, flexible handles to make washing the feet and back easy.

7. Hairwashing can be difficult for people confined to wheelchairs or unable to stand. Now there is a special hairwash stand which consists of a lightweight basin with an optional tub to catch the suds.

8. A pill dispenser is useful for those who forget their tablets. It holds a week's supply and has space for four different tablets.

BEDROOM

1. Putting on stockings and socks can be a problem. Now there are aids that hold stockings open so the foot can be placed in them and then pull the stockings up to within reach.
2. Long shoe horns make it easier to put shoes on and shoe removers will help take them off.
3. Button hooks allow buttons to be fastened using one hand only.
4. Jackets and shirts can be pulled over a disabled arm or shoulder using a device with a long, wooden handle and wire loop.
5. All sorts of 'reachers' – long, scissor-type grabbers – are now available. Some have a magnet on the end to help pick up metal objects. Others have pistol-grips with a wrist support to help carry whatever is being picked up.

TELEPHONES

1. Telephones with jumbo-sized buttons and electronic push-button keyboards are now available.
2. Loud-speaking telephones mean people with limited muscle power do not need to hold the receiver up to their head.
3. Telephones with 'pips' on the buttons to help recognition are useful for visually handicapped people.
4. Cordless telephones are easy and light to handle.
5. Phone cards are easy to use in public telephones.

ELECTRICITY

1. Most houses are not designed with disabled people in mind. However, rewiring is not necessary. Switches with large contact plates and an easy rocking action to make or break contact can be applied to many devices e.g. light switches, immersion heaters.
2. Sockets can be raised from floor level by a simple device which fits to the wall.
3. Remote-control switches that can be operated from a single infra-red hand unit are now available to control up to four sockets.

WALKING AIDS

1. Difficulty getting up from a chair can be prevented by raising a favourite chair on blocks, or by buying a spring-loaded chair which gently raises the sitter to a standing position at the touch of a button.
2. Walking sticks should always have a rubber cap at the bottom, and are now adjustable to ensure they are the right height. Many can also be folded for greater convenience. Don't forget a reflective band placed round the stick which helps it to be seen at night in traffic.
3. All sorts of walking frames are now available. Some fold so they can be fitted into the boot of a car; others are open at the front so they can be used over a lavatory.
4. Shopping baskets on wheels are a great help both in shops and around the house. Some have a fold-down seat which allows the user to sit down and rest.

GALLSTONES

Gallstones are pebblelike masses which form in the gall bladder, the part of the body that collects bile. About one in five people over forty have gallstones but it is only when they cause inflammation or get stuck in the tube (the bile duct) leading from the gall bladder to the intestine that they cause symptoms such as abdominal pain, a bloated feeling, wind and vomiting.

Self-health

- Eat a low-fat diet because it is fat that stimulates the gall bladder, causing pain.

- Eat a low-sugar, high-fibre diet because research has shown that people who do so are less likely to develop gallstones, perhaps because they have less cholesterol, one of the main constituents of gallstones, in the gall bladder. Eating a low-cholesterol diet, though, does not seem to help.

- Keep your weight down.

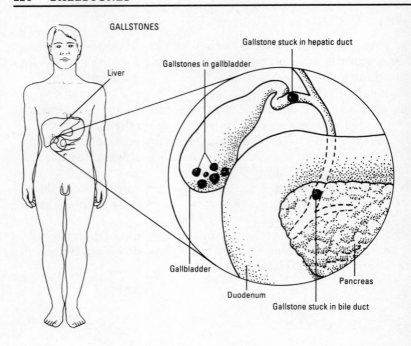

GALLSTONES

Liver

Gallstones in gallbladder

Gallstone stuck in hepatic duct

Gallbladder

Duodenum

Gallstone stuck in bile duct

Pancreas

GANGRENE

Gangrene is flesh that is dead or dying due to lack of oxygen. Toes and fingers are commonly affected because their blood supply may easily become blocked.

There are two types. If there is no infection it is called dry gangrene (e.g. after a blockage of the artery or frostbite). If there is infection it is called wet gangrene (e.g. a wound gets infected).

Self-health

DRY GANGRENE

- Do not smoke, especially if your family is prone to gangrene, because smoking narrows the arteries and makes them more likely to become blocked.

- Keep body extremities warm.

- Avoid tight-fitting clothes or shoes.

- If you are diabetic, keep your blood sugar levels well controlled.

- See your doctor as soon as you notice any discoloured flesh appearing. It may be possible to prevent it spreading by medicines or surgery.

WET GANGRENE

- Clean wounds carefully. If there is any sign of infection, see your doctor immediately. Antibiotics and/or surgery may prevent it spreading.

GASTRITIS

Gastritis is inflammation or irritation of the lining of the stomach. There are two types:

Acute gastritis is caused by something specific (e.g. drinking alcohol, certain medicines and eating too much), has nasty symptoms like severe pain in the upper abdomen and vomiting, and usually disappears within a few hours or days once the cause has been removed.

Chronic gastritis is low-grade inflammation of the lining of the stomach which persists for a long time (months, even years), causing vague discomfort in the abdomen, nausea and generally feeling unwell.

Self-health

- Gastritis may be the penalty you pay for a night out. Symptoms are difficult to control but see **Hangover**.

- Avoid over-eating. Some, but not all, people find spicy foods particularly bad. Others find small, bland, frequent meals help.

- Avoid drinking too much alcohol. If necessary, experiment to find out what brings on the symptoms. A few people find just one drink, especially spirits, will do so. Particularly avoid drinking on an empty stomach.

- Some medicines may cause gastritis. Aspirin and anti-arthritis drugs are common causes but be careful with any medicine.

- If changes to your lifestyle do not prevent the gastritis, see your doctor, who may prescribe medicines. These are usually effective and have no or few side effects.

GERMAN MEASLES

This is a common infectious disease (also called rubella) which develops fourteen to twenty-one days after contact with an infected person (usually child). The symptoms are usually hardly worse than a bad cold and include a rash of tiny, pink, slightly raised spots, a raised temperature, swollen glands, often behind the ears, and occasionally joint pains.

Self-health

- Prevention is very important because if a woman has German measles within the first three to four months of her pregnancy it is quite likely it will permanently damage her child (for example it may cause deafness or blindness). Everyone should be immunized against German measles so it cannot spread among the population and infect pregnant women.

  At about eighteen months to two years old all toddlers should receive the MMR (Measles, Mumps, Rubella) vaccine by injection (see **MMR Vaccine**). Doctors believe the risk of serious side effects from this vaccine is small, and certainly far less than the risks of side effects from one of these diseases.

- Girls aged eleven to thirteen who have not had German measles should receive the vaccine. Some doctors, though, think all girls should receive the vaccine because the original diagnosis of German measles may have been wrong, so unknown to them they might still be susceptible. As far as possible, keep your children away from others with German measles, particularly if they have not been vaccinated.

GLANDULAR FEVER

This infectious disease (also called infectious mononucleosis) is caused by a virus and affects mainly adolescents and people in their twenties. It develops one to six weeks after contact with an infected person. It is often called the 'kissing disease' but many people develop it without close contact. The symptoms are often vague, and include feeling generally unwell, tiredness, poor appetite, headache, swollen glands, occasionally a rash.

Self-health

- There is no vaccine to prevent this illness.

- Most people would think refusing to kiss much too drastic a step to take to reduce their chances of getting glandular fever!

- Most people recover from glandular fever within a few weeks but occasionally it lingers on for months. One serious problem it can cause is depression.

GLAUCOMA

Glaucoma is a serious eye disorder which affects about one in 100 people over forty and causes blindness in about 20,000 people each year in the UK. The main problem is that the pressure of the fluid inside the eye builds up to such an extent that it starts to damage the structures of the eye, causing deterioration of the eyesight and then blindness. There are two types:
   Acute glaucoma occurs when the pressure suddenly builds up and you notice blurring, haloes around lights, pain and redness in the eye.
   Chronic glaucoma is a gradual build-up of pressure within the eyeball. It is not as serious as acute glaucoma but unless diagnosed and treated it will gradually cause blindness.

Self-health

- There is no specific way you can prevent glaucoma except by taking the medicines your doctor prescribes or undergoing surgery once it has been diagnosed. So it is important you tell your doctor or optician if you notice any change in your vision or the appearance or feel of your eyes.

- Medicines and/or surgery can prevent the serious complications of glaucoma.

Screening

- Everyone over forty should have their eyes tested every two years to check for glaucoma (and other eye conditions).
- If someone in your family has had glaucoma you should be examined every year because it may be hereditary.

GONORRHOEA

Gonorrhoea (also known as 'the clap') is caused by the bacterium *neisseria gonorrhoea* caught by sexual intercourse or other types of sexual contact. Symptoms start appearing about one or two weeks later.

Men may notice pain when passing urine, a discharge from the penis, or swollen glands in the groin. Later the symptoms may disappear so you think you have never had it or are cured, but you will still be infectious unless you have been treated.

Women may well have no symptoms at all. Sometimes they have pain passing urine, or pass urine more frequently than normal. There may also be a strong-smelling discharge from the vagina or urethra (the tube running from the bladder to the outside).

Both sexes can develop arthritis as a result of gonorrhoea and for women the most serious long-term problems are pelvic inflammatory disease and infertility.

Self-health

- Chastity is very effective but may be too drastic a step for most people! Restricting yourself to one partner who sticks to you is more enjoyable for most.
- Men should wear a condom, even if there is only a small risk of giving or receiving infection. This usually (but not always)

prevents a man giving gonorrhoea to a woman and vice versa.

- If your partner tells you that he or she has gonorrhoea see your doctor immediately. If the contact was recent, antibiotics will prevent you developing the illness. If it was some weeks or months previously antibiotics will treat the illness and perhaps prevent problems such as infertility and arthritis.

- Never have sex with someone if you know you have gonorrhoea. Always tell everyone you have had sex with as soon as you discover you have gonorrhoea, even if it causes you terrible embarrassment. Other people's health is not something you should take liberties with.

GOUT

Gout is a type of arthritis (see separate entry) in which the body fails to break down and eliminate purines, substances found in high-protein foods. As a result, uric acid builds up in the blood and joints causing great pain, swelling and inflammation. The big toe is affected in seventy per cent of cases but the knees, hands and elbows may also be affected.

Self-health

- You are more at risk of getting gout if other members of your family have had it. Tell your doctor about family gout if you develop symptoms in your joints because it may speed diagnosis and prevent you suffering unnecessarily.

- Some people find that certain foods (e.g. seafood) or alcohol bring on attacks. They do not cause the gout but they may make it worse. You will need to experiment yourself to find out what to avoid.

- Medicines are available which prevent gout. If you have been prescribed them take them regularly or the gout will return – painfully.

- Some people with gout do not need regular medicines. But be sure to have your anti-attack pills at hand so that you can take them immediately symptoms start. The earlier you take the pills the better.

- Some people believe that eating cherries regularly may prevent gout. There is very little scientific evidence for this but it is entirely harmless, very enjoyable and may help you.

GRIEF

After the death of someone close to you, you may go through several grieving stages. Generally there are a few days or weeks of numbness during which you almost appear to be behaving normally. This is followed by about six weeks of intense grief which will gradually lessen during the next six months. Finally there may be a feeling of emptiness, apathy and gloom. By the end of the year most people are beginning to build new lives, though it is quite normal to experience short periods of grief for the loved one for the rest of your life.

Self-health

- It is important that you progress through each stage of grieving and do not become stuck in one. The period of intense grief is most traumatic but most important and if you do not express your feelings at this stage you may be troubled by depression and other problems all your life. So acknowledge your loss to other people, and do not try to keep a 'stiff upper lip'.

- Talking about your loved one, going through possessions and enjoying the memory of happy times will all help.

- Many people find comfort and help by turning to their religion.

- Others turn to spiritualism, but the problem with this is that by denying reality and encouraging a desire for the presence of the dead person it may prolong grief.

- Some people's grief is so intense and distressing that tranquillizing pills may be necessary. However, most people don't need tranquillizers, which may, in fact, prevent the normal grieving stages.

- Many people find bereavement counsellors very helpful. These people, often volunteers, have special skills which will help you to come to terms with your loss and the necessary changes to your life. Ask your doctor or social services department how to contact these counsellors.

- If someone close to you is grieving there are many practical things you can do to prevent their misery becoming unbearable.

  1. Help in the home with cooking and cleaning.
  2. Help with difficult decisions, because the person may not be thinking clearly.
  3. Do not be afraid to talk about the dead person and encourage your relative or friend to do so.
  4. Continue to give your support once the first weeks are over. Loneliness often coincides with the worst stages of grieving and makes life much harder. Remember anniversaries and Christmas because these are often difficult times for newly bereaved people.

- Do not ignore talk of suicide (see separate entry). Consult a doctor or social worker immediately.

Special Situations

MISCARRIAGE

- Many people do not realize how desolated parents, particularly mothers, feel after a miscarriage. They need to be encouraged to go through the grieving stages as for a dead person.

- There are no hard-and-fast rules on whether to try for another baby straightaway. It suits some couples, not others.

STILLBIRTH

- The grief after a stillbirth is often as intense as that for a baby who has died. It may also be made worse by a feeling of guilt and/or anger. It is important that all emotions are expressed and full support given.

CHILDREN

- Children should be allowed to grieve in their own way. It will not help to impose an adult pattern upon them. They may appear to recover more quickly than an adult, particularly if they can attach themselves to someone else.

- Questions should be encouraged and answered simply and honestly.

- Children often think the death of a loved one is their fault. They should be reassured gently.

- Try not to impose too many major life changes on a child shortly after a bereavement.

- Do not hide your own grief from a child. It will help the child to feel involved and teach him or her that grief can and should be expressed.

PREMATURE GRIEVING

- Sometimes, illness can cause someone's personality to change so greatly before death that friends and family no longer recognize the person they loved. Dementia (see separate entry) is the most common cause of this unhappy situation. As a result, friends and relatives start grieving for the person before they have physically died. It is a special problem that often needs expert help.

GUM DISEASE

Just as tooth decay is the enemy of children's teeth, gum disease is the enemy of adult teeth. Research suggests that ninety per cent of people over thirty-five with natural teeth have gum disease.

The problem starts when a sticky coating of food and bacteria (known as plaque) forms on your teeth along the gum line. The bacteria attack your gums which become inflamed, bleed and pull away from the teeth. This creates ideal pockets for bacteria to breed further and eventually the teeth loosen and fall out.

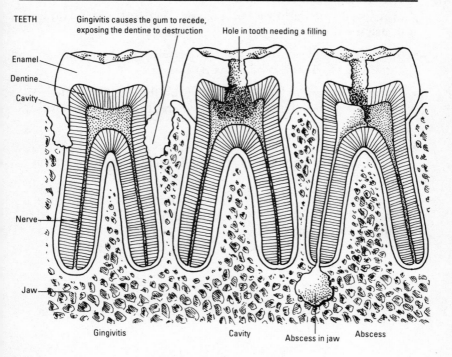

TEETH

Gingivitis causes the gum to recede, exposing the dentine to destruction

Hole in tooth needing a filling

Enamel

Dentine

Cavity

Nerve

Jaw

Gingivitis   Cavity   Abscess in jaw   Abscess

Self-health

- Adults need to concentrate as much on keeping their gums healthy as their teeth.

- Theories about how to brush your teeth change as often as the weather. The important principles are to use a nylon brush with medium-soft bristles, to be gentle, to brush in sweeping movements away from the gum so you do not force bacteria into the gums, and to brush regularly. Many dentists suggest brushing after every meal but twice a day thoroughly is probably enough.

- Children should use a fluoride toothpaste. Fluoride has very little effect on adult teeth but nevertheless may have some benefit.

- Using dental floss or tape between your teeth once a day helps prevent plaque building up. Ask your dentist to show you how to use the floss.

- Toothpicks will remove food from between teeth, but be careful not to damage the gums with them.

- There are harmless dyes, available from the chemist, which colour plaque so that you can see where it is collecting and remove it.

- The more often you eat, and the more sugar the food contains, the more likely you are to create ideal conditions for bacteria to attack your gums.

- Even if you have no symptoms, see your dentist at least once a year, and more often if you have gum disease. He or she will remove the plaque and help prevent your teeth falling out.

H

HAEMOPHILIA

People with haemophilia bleed very easily because they do not
have enough of the clotting substance Factor VIII in their blood.
The illness affects only males, though females can be carriers.
About eighty per cent of cases are inherited.

Self-health

- If you have haemophilia it is important you look after your
  general health in order to avoid the complications of the
  illness. The severity of haemophilia varies greatly, so only you
  will learn what activities you should avoid and when the
  clotting processes of your blood may need boosting. Generally,
  violent activities like rugby and football should be avoided,
  but swimming, cycling and running are good for you. You may
  also need to make special preparations for procedures like
  going to the dentist, where you do not want your gums to
  bleed excessively.

- The Factor VIII you are missing can now be safely collected
  from other people's blood donations and injected into your
  blood without the risk of AIDS. This helps your blood clot
  normally, but only for about forty-eight hours. So you can use
  it as a precaution when you know you are at risk of bleeding
  (e.g. having a tooth removed) or to treat bleeding which will
  not stop (e.g. bleeding into a joint). You should be particularly
  careful to prevent repeated bleeding into joints because
  otherwise they may become stiff and sore.

- Avoid certain medicines such as aspirin or anti-arthritis
  medicines because they are likely to cause stomach bleeding.

HAEMORRHAGE

The body has three main ways of coping with bleeding from a damaged blood vessel (vein or artery). First the blood vessel narrows immediately to reduce the amount of blood flowing through it. Then special blood cells called platelets gather round the wound and join together to plug the hole in the vessel. Finally blood itself starts to clot in the hole until eventually no more escapes and the bleeding stops.

Most everyday wounds stop bleeding in this way (sometimes with a little help from you), the blood vessel is repaired and everything returns to normal. However, more serious wounds can bleed very fast and if you lose more than one and a half to two pints of blood you are in danger of becoming unconscious and even dying. Children have less blood in their bodies and so are in danger if they lose smaller amounts.

Self-health

MINOR HAEMORRHAGE

- The most important thing to do if you receive a minor injury (such as cutting your finger or catching your forehead on a sharp object) is to press firmly over the wound with a bandage, clean towel or even your finger if nothing else is available. If you think there may be a foreign body (like a piece of glass) in the wound be cautious about pressing too hard because you may make the bleeding worse. But do not poke about in the wound looking for the foreign body – just take a quick look, remove anything obvious and seek medical help.

- Next raise the affected part above the level of your heart to reduce the amount of blood flowing to the wound, while continuing to press firmly over it.

- Sometimes putting a cut finger under running cold water is effective because the cold causes the blood vessel to narrow further.

- Once the bleeding has stopped, press on the wound for a few minutes longer to give the 'repair' every chance of working. Then put on a clean bandage and keep an eye on the wound to make sure it doesn't start to bleed again.

SERIOUS HAEMORRHAGE

- If a medium-sized or large vein or artery is cut or damaged there may be serious bleeding which, if not stopped, could be life-threatening.

- Stopping serious bleeding is similar to stopping minor bleeding except that you have to act quicker, more forcefully and get medical help immediately. In particular you need to place a clean bandage or piece of clothing over the wound and press firmly on it. If the cloth becomes soaked in blood do not remove it, simply place another bandage over it and keep pressing firmly.

- If the bleeding is particularly fierce, comes in spurts, and is a bright pinkish-red colour it is almost certainly coming from an artery. This type of bleeding can be temporarily controlled by placing a finger (or occasionally tourniquet) over pressure points. But do not press for much longer than fifteen minutes or you may damage the limb from lack of oxygen. So stop pressing for a minute or so and then start again.

  1. In the arm the brachial artery can be controlled by placing a firm finger over the inner border of the upper arm.
  2. The femoral artery of the upper leg can be controlled by pressing a finger into the groin just where it meets the upper leg.
  3. The popliteal artery to the lower leg can be controlled by a finger pressed firmly into the middle of the back of the knee.

Screening

- Some people naturally bleed more readily than others. However, if you think you bleed much more easily than others or you notice that you have started to do so, you should see your doctor. There are one or two rare illnesses (e.g. haemophilia, see separate entry) that may be causing it.

HAEMORRHOIDS

Haemorrhoids (or piles, as they are better known) are stretched and swollen blood vessels in the rectum (the last part of the bowel) which result in one or more swellings. Sometimes the swellings remain inside the anus, sometimes they appear outside. Piles are common – there is a saying that people are divided into two groups: those that admit to having piles and the liars! Bright-red bleeding, a mucous discharge, irritation and itchiness are common symptoms. Pain develops later, especially if a blood clot forms in the haemorrhoid. Constipation is the most common cause.

Self-health

- If piles are common in your family, be particularly careful not to become constipated, because the tendency to piles is partly hereditary.

- Eat a high-fibre diet of fruit, vegetables, brown rice and wholemeal bread to prevent yourself becoming constipated.

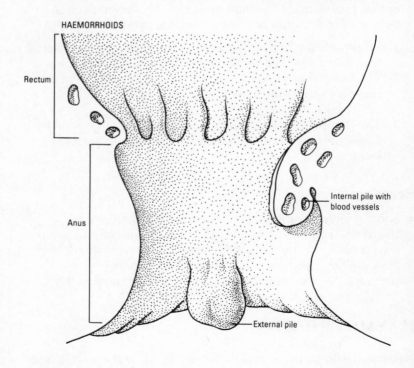

HAEMORRHOIDS

Rectum

Anus

Internal pile with blood vessels

External pile

This will also help prevent you becoming overweight, which is another cause of piles.

- Sadly there seems to be no truth in the old wives' tale that avoiding sitting on cold floors or radiators will prevent piles.

Screening

- Bleeding from the back passage is the most common symptom of cancer of the bowel. Consult your family doctor immediately if you notice any such bleeding. If he or she discovers piles it may be that no further action will be taken; however, in many cases you may be referred for specialist diagnosis and treatment.

HAIR, EXCESSIVE

Many women worry about excessive hair, but only you can decide whether you have too much on your face, and body. The main thing is not to become so obsessed that you start noticing every tiny hair. You are no less feminine if you have more hair than the fashionable ideal.

Self-health

- If other members of your family have a lot of hair you may be affected too.

- The amount of hair you have is probably controlled by the various hormones in your body, but it is not known how. Research shows that people with a lot of hair have similar levels of hormones to those who do not. It may simply be that their hair is more sensitive to the effect of the hormones.

- The most effective way to prevent hair growing is electrolysis, in which the hair follicle is destroyed by the electric current so it cannot grow again.

- Fine, not too dark hair can be successfully bleached with six per cent hydrogen peroxide (20-volume peroxide).

- Shaving is effective for a short time but does not prevent hair regrowing. Equally, it does not make hair grow faster or thicker. Using a pumice stone afterwards helps keep the hair away a little longer.

- Plucking is effective for small areas but hair will regrow. Waxing works on the same principle over a larger area.

- Depilatories (cosmetic hair removers) work by destroying the protein in hair. Because they destroy protein they all irritate the skin to a greater or lesser extent. The sulphide-based ones work most effectively but cause the most irritation and have an unpleasant smell. The thioglycolate ones (e.g. Immac, Sleek and Nudit) do not smell so strongly and are less irritating to the skin.

HAIR, HEALTHY

There are three main areas you need to think about if you want a healthy head of hair.

GOOD HEALTH AND LIFESTYLE

- Eat a healthy diet (see chapter on Healthy Eating) with plenty of protein and iron (meat, eggs, cereals, peas and beans are good sources) plus plenty of fruit and vegetables to provide the vitamin C needed to absorb the iron.

- Your hair will reflect your mental state. If you are tired and tense your hair will appear dull and lifeless. Planning your life to cope with stress better (see chapter on Stress and Mental Health) will also make your hair more healthy.

- Flaky scalps may be helped by a diet low in dairy products but high in foods containing vitamin B (see chapter on Healthy Eating).

CLEANLINESS

- How often hair should be washed varies from person to person but a good guide is once every two or three days if your hair is short and once every five to seven days if it is longer. Long hair will split if you wash it very often.

- Hair can be washed with soap but it produces a poor lather and is difficult to wash out. Shampoos are better but remember that many have additives to which your scalp may be allergic. Expensive shampoos are not necessarily better than cheap ones except they may make your hair shine brighter for a short time. One lather is usually enough for each wash.

- Use warm water and rinse the hair thoroughly after lathering until it squeaks as it is pulled through the fingers (this shows the shampoo has been removed).

- Do not rub hair roughly but pat dry and then comb into place. Use gentle heat to dry it – not your hairdryer at full blast!

- Conditioners may help if the outer layer of your hair – the cuticle – is damaged.

- Cutting the hair regularly does not stimulate it to grow faster or stronger but it does prevent split ends.

COSMETIC TREATMENTS

- Combing your hair rather than brushing it causes less damage.

- There are several ways of perming the hair. None is harmful if done by an expert hairdresser or if the instructions are carefully followed. Give hair time to recover between perms.

- Synthetic dyes have largely replaced the harmless but messy vegetable dyes. The temporary ones cause no problems because they simply coat the hair. Permanent ones can be more destructive because they penetrate the hair. Some people are allergic to them. You can be tested for allergy by putting a small amount of the dye on the skin (e.g. the arm) and waiting for a reaction within forty-eight hours. If the skin goes red, painful or blistered you should avoid that dye.

- Repeated bleaching with hydrogen peroxide may make the hair brittle and prone to thinning and split ends.

HAMMER TOES

Hammer toes are those in which the joint closest to the foot becomes fixed at an angle, often as much as a right angle. This prevents the toe straightening when walking so the top of the toe or its tip may develop a corn or even an ulcer.

Self-health

- There is no way hammer toes can be prevented, so the best that can be done is to prevent problems like corns or ulcers.

- Wear comfortable, roomy shoes so the toes are not rubbed. Sometimes insoles, pads or felt can help prevent corns or ulcers.

- Occasionally surgery is needed to prevent the problem getting worse. The rigid joint is removed and the toe straightened.

HANGOVER

Hangovers are caused by alcohol; the more you drink, the worse they will be. But they are also made worse by substances in alcoholic drinks called 'congeners', which are the byproducts of distillation or fermentation or both.

Self-health

- Some drinks such as vodka, gin and white wine contain few congeners, but others such as red wine and beer have plenty to give them their special taste, so these are the drinks to avoid.

- Mixing drinks will not cause a worse hangover except that it is more likely to expose you to congeners and is often associated with heavy drinking.

- Alcohol stimulates the kidneys to produce more urine than usual. This causes the body – and particularly the brain – to dry out. To prevent the resulting unpleasant symptoms drink plenty of non-alcoholic drinks while you are drinking alcohol, and afterwards drink as many glasses of water as you can.

- Many people find that a bad headache can be prevented by taking a painkiller before going to bed. Choose paracetamol rather than aspirin, which may cause bleeding of the stomach.

- Sleep is a good way of preventing a hangover, the longer the better.

- Stress and tiredness make hangovers worse. The alcohol may give you a boost for a short while but as soon as its effects wear off your exhausted body will suffer worse symptoms. Try to learn a method of relaxation (see chapter on Stress and Mental Health), you are less likely to drink so much and your body will be in better shape to deal with it.

- Removing alcohol from the bloodstream is done by the liver, which works steadily removing about half a pint of beer or a single whisky each hour. The liver is a remarkable and resilient organ but if you insult it by becoming an alcoholic (see **Alcoholism**) or if it is injured by an illness such as hepatitis (see separate entry), it will no longer be able to process alcohol efficiently.

HAYFEVER

Hayfever is neither caused by hay nor associated with a fever. 'Grass pollen sensitivity' would be a better name to describe it. It affects about one in ten people.

The main symptoms are sneezing, a runny or blocked nose, itchy eyes and sometimes an itch at the back of the throat. These symptoms can vary enormously in severity in each person, so sufferers often cannot judge from one moment to the next how badly they are going to be affected. In the UK, June and July are usually the worst months for hayfever sufferers, but it is later the further north one goes.

The difference in weather from year to year also affects sufferers, and what most of us think of as a good summer is a bad one if you have hayfever. Hot, dry weather with a breeze to blow the pollen about are the perfect conditions for hayfever.

On average, people tend to suffer from hayfever for eight to ten years, though it frequently lasts longer. If it is very bad, skin tests, normally carried out in the autumn, can show exactly which pollens are responsible for the symptoms, so you can try to avoid them.

Self-health

- Avoid exposing yourself to high pollen counts.

  1. Check the pollen count in newspapers. Counts over fifty may be troublesome. If figures are high try to avoid going out, or at least be sure to take your medication and keep it with you.
  2. On warm, sunny days a lot of pollen will be released in the morning but by midday it will have been carried upwards by the warm air, so this is the safest time to go outside. Later the air will cool and the pollen will descend again, floating through open bedroom windows (so keep them shut). On rainy days less pollen is released and the count may be low.
  3. Mow your lawn in the morning while the grass is still damp and the pollen cannot escape. Children should not roll about in grass (especially newly mown).
  4. You may need to avoid camping or holidays in the countryside. Go instead to the sea where there are few plants, or to mountains and moorland where the wind blows the pollen away.
  5. Keep car windows closed if possible.

- Certain medicines will prevent or reduce attacks. These include tablets, nose drops or sprays, capsules or liquids. Many of these can be bought from a chemist, but if your symptoms are not helped see your doctor. Remember that these medicines may cause drowsiness, which is dangerous if you are driving or working with machinery.

HEADACHE

Headaches vary from a minor annoyance to such a bad problem that your whole life can be affected. Before you can prevent them you (with your doctor if necessary) will need to find the cause. Persistent severe headaches may occasionally indicate a more serious problem; always consult your doctor.

Self-health

- The most common cause is stress. See the chapter on Stress and Mental Health for tips on prevention.

• Any illness, particularly an infection, can cause headache. Often a mild painkiller such as aspirin or paracetamol will take the pain away.

• Migraine (see separate entry) is a common cause of headache.

• Certain foods may cause headaches in susceptible people. Coffee (or coffee withdrawal), and chocolate are well-known causes. Monosodium glutamate (often found in Chinese food) can cause headache, plus nausea, stomach pain, cramps, and dizziness. Very cold food, such as ice-cream, causes headaches in some people. Some cured meats contain additives called nitrates which can cause headache. Tyramine-containing foods such as yeast extracts and yeast products, pickled herrings, cheese, liver, sausages may cause headaches. So may histamine-containing foods such as sauerkraut, sausagemeat and salami. Experiment and avoid the foods that give you a headache.

• Have your eyes checked by an optician because poor eyesight can cause headache.

• If you are over thirty-five, or if high blood pressure runs in your family, have your blood pressure checked regularly (every year or so). Headaches can be brought on by raised blood pressure.

• Don't drink too much (see **Alcoholism** and **Hangover**).

• Be sure you are not exposed to excessive noise or fumes at work. Get advice from your local health and safety officer if you are worried.

HEARTBURN

Heartburn (also called indigestion or dyspepsia) is not a disease like measles or bronchitis but a collection of different symptoms, such as discomfort in the stomach, feeling sick, burping, wind, and waterbrash (bringing up sour-tasting stomach contents into the mouth or throat). These symptoms usually occur after eating and suggest that something is wrong with the gullet or stomach.

Self-health

- Eat sensibly. Avoid foods and drink that upset you. Chew well before swallowing. Establish a regular meal pattern. Some people benefit from frequent, small, milky meals. Others find these meals stimulate too much acid and they do better with infrequent meals. Particularly avoid large, heavy meals shortly before going to bed.

- Smoking irritates the lining of the stomach, making you more prone to ulcers, gastritis and indigestion. If you are a smoker, try to give up (see **Smoking**).

- Control your weight. Overweight people are more prone to indigestion.

- Change your lifestyle so that you learn to cope with stress better (see chapter on Stress and Mental Health). Stress stimulates acid in the stomach which may irritate the lining and cause indigestion.

- Cut down your alcohol consumption or give it up altogether, because alcohol irritates the lining of the stomach.

- Discuss any medicines you are taking with your doctor because some (e.g. aspirin and anti-arthritis medicines) may cause heartburn.

- Raise the head of your bed on a few bricks or books by 15 cm. This often prevents heartburn at night. Sleeping on more pillows may not be good enough because it raises your neck and head only.

- Avoid stooping; instead kneel to pick things up.

- Don't wear tight clothing and corsets. These force the contents of your stomach upwards, causing heartburn.

- You will be prone to heartburn during pregnancy because the baby pushes your stomach upwards into the chest cavity, causing heartburn. You may need to take some or all of the precautions listed above. Remember to be cautious about taking medicines during pregnancy though. Your symptoms will usually disappear once the baby is born.

- Try antacid medicines from the pharmacy. There are several

different types so you can experiment with others if one
doesn't work. It is a good principle to take the medicine when
you expect symptoms (e.g. after a heavy meal) rather than
waiting for them to start.

- If none of the above suggestions work see your doctor. There
  are more powerful medicines to prevent indigestion or else in
  serious cases your doctor may consider surgery.

Screening

- Sometimes heart problems may cause symptoms very like
  heartburn. So if you do not get better after trying the
  suggestions above, your doctor may wish to test your heart.

HEART DISEASE

Heart disease causes one-third of all deaths in the Western
world. Most are due to coronary artery disease or raised blood
pressure (hypertension). This section covers the former; for tips
on coping with high blood pressure, see separate entry.

The heart is a pump which needs oxygen to drive it. The
oxygen is supplied by the coronary (heart) arteries. If the arteries
become narrow or blocked from atheroma (a fatty substance that
lives in the arteries), the supply of oxygen to the heart becomes
reduced or absent. As a result the pumping action of the heart
weakens, causing angina or heart failure, or stops, causing heart
attack.

There are now well-accepted ways of slowing this furring of
the arteries, particularly if you come from a family prone to heart
problems. You should do what you can but do not become over-
anxious because this itself will make you more prone to heart
disease.

Self-health

- The most important single thing you can do is to stop smoking
  (see **Smoking**).
- Eat a healthy diet, based on the following guidelines:
  1. Eat less fat, especially saturated fat which is found in meat

CORONARY HEART DISEASE

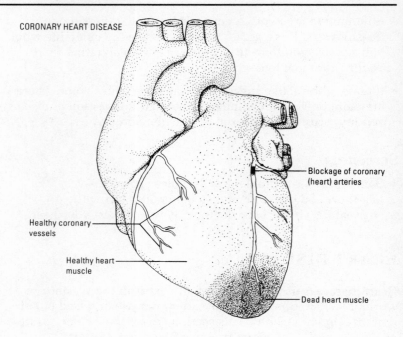

Blockage of coronary (heart) arteries

Healthy coronary vessels

Healthy heart muscle

Dead heart muscle

and meat products, dairy products, some vegetable fats (e.g. coconut and palm oils), and cakes, chocolates, biscuits, cooking fats and some hard margarines.

   2. Eat less sugar. Sugar doesn't give you any valuable vitamins or minerals, so it contains a lot of 'wasted' calories which are stored by the body as fat.

   3. Eat less salt. Most of us consume enough salt from the processed foods we eat. There should be no need to add extra during cooking or at the table.

   4. Eat more fibre. Most experts agree that this contributes to a healthy heart.

   5. Eat more fish oil (in fish such as mackerel, herring, salmon). It now appears that this will protect your heart.

• Women are better protected against heart disease because of the effect of their hormones. Some doctors are now recommending hormone replacement therapy (see separate entry) to menopausal or postmenopausal women as protection

against osteoporosis (see separate entry), but it may also
protect against heart disease. Further research is needed to
decide on its role.

- There are medicines available which make it easier for the
  heart to pump blood round the body. These can help reduce
  the chances of a fatal heart attack, and your doctor will advise
  if they are necessary.

- If you have narrowed coronary arteries you are at risk of a fatal
  heart attack. Surgeons can now replace the diseased arteries
  with veins (usually taken from your leg) so that a normal flow
  of blood and oxygen reaches the heart. This coronary by-pass
  operation is a big one but it is now more commonly performed
  in the USA than appendicectomy, so it is becoming safe. And
  results show it improves both the quality and length of life of
  people with coronary heart disease.

- Take plenty of exercise (see chapter on Exercise). It is
  enjoyable, makes you feel better, improves your circulation,
  and encourages your heart to work efficiently. Exercise two or
  three times a week for about half an hour at a time. Start gently
  and build up gradually.

- Keep your weight within normal limits for your height and
  build. Being overweight means your heart has to work harder;
  however, being mildly overweight is not an important risk
  factor.

- Alcohol may damage your heart, so limit your intake. Men
  should have a maximum of twenty-one units of alcohol,
  spread throughout a week, and women should drink no more
  than fourteen units. One unit is half a pint of ordinary beer or
  cider, a single measure of spirits, sherry or vermouth, or a
  glass of wine.

Screening

- If members of your family suffer from heart disease you may
  be prone to it too if you do not take the right precautions. Take
  special care of your health and make sure you are tested
  (screened) regularly.

- Have your blood pressure checked at least every three years and more often if your doctor advises it. Raised blood pressure is linked with heart disease.

- Have the level of cholesterol (see separate entry) in your blood checked. If it is too high a suitable diet may bring it down to normal. If not, medicines will do so.

- Have the amount of sugar in your blood tested. High levels (see **Diabetes Mellitus**) are linked with heart disease.

- Some doctors believe that people, particularly men, should be screened for heart disease using electrocardiographs (ECGs). These graphs trace the electrical pattern of the heart and can detect disease, especially during and after exercise. The problem is that they are not always accurate, and there are people who have died of a heart attack shortly after having had an ECG which showed no evidence of disease. The future may lie with other techniques such as echocardiography, but they are very expensive.

HEAT RASH

Sweating a lot may make your skin break out into a rash of red pimples in the sweaty area (e.g. the groin and armpits). This may be due to inflammation of the sweat ducts.

Self-health

- Don't rush about in hot climates because this will stimulate your sweat glands even more.

- Have plenty of cool drinks.

- Wear light clothes made of natural materials.

- Highly scented soaps or shampoos may make your inflamed skin worse.

- It is easy to confuse heat rash and fungal infections, particularly as fungi thrive in hot, humid conditions. If the rash does not improve after following suggestions above, consult a doctor about treatment for a fungal infection.

HEATSTROKE

Heatstroke is a condition in which the body gains heat faster than it can lose it. As a result your temperature goes up, your skin becomes hot, red and dry, you may vomit and even become unconscious and die.

Self-health

- Acclimatize to very hot and humid places slowly, particularly if you are fair-skinned.

- Keep out of the direct sun.

- Wear lightweight clothes made of natural fibres.

- Don't rush about because this will raise your temperature.

- Ice-cold drinks will lower your temperature and replace the fluid you are losing in sweat. Avoid alcohol.

- Take extra salt because you will be losing a lot in sweat. If you become short of salt you will experience headaches, dizziness and nausea.

HEPATITIS

Hepatitis is inflammation of the liver, caused by one of at least six viruses:

1. **Hepatitis A.**   This is the most common type and is caught by consuming food, water or drinks contaminated by infected faeces. It commonly infects travellers in places where hepatitis is present. Symptoms start fifteen to twenty days after infection and include feeling unwell, tiredness, nausea, raised temperature, headache, joint pains, jaundice, dark urine and light-coloured faeces. Virtually everyone recovers completely. Recovery may take from two weeks to six months.
2. **Hepatitis B.**   This is a more serious illness usually caught from contaminated blood or equipment. In developed countries blood transfusions and equipment are carefully sterilized, so the infection is generally caught from dirty

needles used for illegal drug injections or tattooing. In less wealthy countries there may be a risk of hepatitis from contaminated blood transfusion equipment. The infection may also be caught by close sexual contact because the virus can survive in saliva, semen or vaginal discharge. Symptoms start seven or eight weeks after infection and are similar to hepatitis A but more serious. In a small proportion of cases they may lead to death or chronic (long-term) hepatitis.

3. **Hepatitis C.**   Much less is known about this type of hepatitis except that there are at least three viruses involved. It can be caught from contaminated food, water and drinks and from blood. Symptoms are similar to hepatitis A; most people recover completely but some develop chronic hepatitis.

Self-health

- Find out whether there is much hepatitis in the area you are travelling to. If there is you will need to take precautions.

- Don't eat in places where you are uncertain about the standard of cleanliness.

- Wash your hands carefully before eating or preparing food.

- If you develop hepatitis, it is best not to prepare food for others, but if this is unavoidable do take extreme care.

- Isolation of people with hepatitis is not necessary.

- Avoid sexual contact with people you do not know. A sheath (condom) will, however, give you some protection.

- Special measures:

  1. A gamma-globulin injection before travelling to an infected area will give you two to three months' protection against Hepatitis A.
  2. A vaccine is available for those at high risk (e.g. doctors, nurses, laboratory staff) and it gives excellent protection. For those without immunization who have been accidentally exposed to infection (e.g. a needle injury) there is a B globulin injection available. This works provided it is used within one to two days of exposure to infection.

HERNIA

A hernia (also known as a rupture) is a bulge or protrusion of body tissues that forces its way between muscles that are weak, that have been cut (e.g. after surgery), or that are absent (as a result of a congenital problem). Usually the hernia contains only soft tissues like fat but if it contains part of the bowel it is more serious because the blood supply to the bowel may become blocked, causing the bowel to become gangrenous and dead. There are different types of hernias, depending on the site, such as inguinal, femoral, umbilical.

Symptoms usually include the appearance of a painful swelling often made worse by coughing or exercise. Sometimes there is no swelling, which makes diagnosis difficult.

Self-health

- Keep your muscles in good shape so they do not become weak and allow hernias to push through them.

- Do not smoke, because this will give you a cough which may cause a hernia or make an existing one worse.

- Do not become overweight because this will make you more prone to a hernia.

- If you notice a swelling developing see your doctor immediately. It may be that a support (truss) will prevent it getting worse. Most hernias, though, need to be repaired by an operation.

- If you know you have a hernia and suddenly you feel pain at the site of the hernia or all over your abdomen, accompanied by feeling sick, burping or bloating you should call your doctor immediately because it may be that your bowel is 'strangulating' in the hernia.

HERPES

Genital herpes is caused by the herpes virus HSVZ, which is very similar to the viruses causing cold sores of the mouth and shingles (see separate entries). Herpes is caught from having sex (genital, oral or anal) with an infected person. The virus passes from your skin along the nerves to a nerve junction. There it cannot be killed which is why once you have had herpes you may get it again at any time in your life.

Within two to ten days of having sex, if you have caught the infection you may notice an itchy feeling of the penis or vulva (female external genital organ), pain passing water, watery discharge, pain having sex and a general feeling of being unwell. Shortly afterwards a rash of small blisters on the genitals and surrounding area (including thighs and buttocks sometimes) will appear. These burst after about twenty-four hours and are followed by small, very painful blisters which take about two or three weeks to heal. You may also notice that glands in your groin become swollen.

Following recovery, there is roughly a fifty per cent chance of another attack of herpes. No one knows why some people are affected and others are not, but if you are prone, you can reduce the frequency of attacks in the ways described below.

Self-health

- At the moment there is no effective vaccine against herpes, but the fewer sexual partners you have, the less likely you are to get herpes.

- If you have herpes blisters or sores do not have sex with anyone because this is when you are infectious. But as soon as they are healed you can start again. Similarly, never have sex with anyone with open sores.

- Because it is possible to have active herpes of the vagina and cervix without knowing it, it may be sensible for men to wear a sheath when having sex with someone they do not know well. This provides good but not absolute protection because in rare cases the virus can pass through the pores of the latex of the sheath.

- Two simple hygienic precautions you can take to ensure you don't spread herpes are to wash your hands with soap and water after touching the sores, and to make sure no one else uses your towel. The virus can survive easily on damp towels.

- Learn which situations bring on attacks of herpes. Tiredness or stress, sexual intercourse, sunlight, tight or nylon underclothing, or a particular time during your period may all be contributory factors.

• There is now a medicine, acyclovis, which can treat (but not cure) the symptoms of herpes. However, it only works if used within a few hours of the onset of symptoms. Some people know when an attack is coming and can take the medicine immediately. Others only know when the blisters appear. For both groups, though, it may be worth having the tablets or cream ready to use at the time rather than having to see the doctor first, because by then it may be too late.

Screening

• If you have sex with different partners it may be worth going to your doctor or local hospital clinic for check-ups every three to four months. It is possible to have – and pass on – herpes without knowing it.

• If you have a new attack of herpes or an unexpected recurrence, be sure to tell your partners. It will create fewer problems for them in the long run if you do so.

• If a woman has active herpes during childbirth the virus may be passed to the baby, causing inflammation of the brain (encephalitis), blindness or even death. Always tell your doctor if there is any possibility that you have herpes. You may need a caesarian section so your baby is not put at risk.

• Women who are infected by the HSVZ virus are eight times more likely to develop cervical cancer than those who are not. So if you have herpes (or have had it), have a cervical smear test at least every three years, and more often if your doctor advises it.

HOMEOPATHY

Homeopathy is a system of healing based on the ideas of the nineteenth-century German doctor Samuel Hahnemann. He interpreted symptoms as evidence of the body's effort to combat illness (rather than signs of the illness), and so recommended that medicines should be chosen on the basis of their ability to reproduce the symptoms, and given in tiny amounts. His other key belief was the concept of the minimum dose, in other words that many remedies become more effective as you dilute them.

Homeopaths will listen carefully to your symptoms and make judgements about your personality because this is the main basis on which they prescribe the remedies. The remedies themselves are prescribed in tincture given by mouth as drops, tablets, pills or granules. The potency of the remedy is usually shown on the bottle. Many practitioners prescribe just a single dose and wait several weeks to judge how effective it has been. In very serious cases the remedy may be given every five or ten minutes until improvement is seen or, for example, every four hours for twenty-four hours, but the long courses of medicines typical of orthodox treatment are unusual.

Self-health

- Homeopathy is said by practitioners and lay enthusiasts to be helpful in preventing illness and maintaining good health, and they will recommend remedies on a regular basis. There is little proof of their value in this role, however.

- There is more evidence that homeopathic remedies can help some symptoms, although the amount of research done on homeopathic remedies is tiny by comparison with conventional drugs. Consult a standard text book about the areas in which homeopathy can be helpful and which remedies to take. They include bruising and muscular pain (*arnica* and *rhus tox.*), bites or cuts (*hypericum, ledum,* or *arnica*) (but always also make sure the person has received tetanus immunization), sore throats and mild chest infections (*aconite, belladonna* and *mercurius sol.*), measles (*pulsatilla*), chickenpox, (*antimonium tart.*), whooping cough (*drosera*), diarrhoea and vomiting (*arsenicum alb.*), indigestion (*nux vomica, phosphorus, graphites*). In all there are about twenty useful remedies for acute illnesses, but many more for the more complicated problem of long-term illness (e.g. eczema, psoriasis, hay fever, migraine, arthritis, cystitis).

- One of the advantages of homeopathy is that remedies cause few side effects because they are taken in such tiny doses.

However, there have been several recent reports of complications arising because people have exceeded the recommended doses, especially when mixtures of more than one remedy are taken.

- In the past there has been too much emphasis by both conventional doctors and homeopathic practitioners on using either orthodox medicine or homeopathy. Now it is recognized that both may play a complementary role working together for the good of the person. Many doctors are now taking courses in homeopathy, and a number of colleges run courses for lay people who wish to practise (e.g. Faculty of Homeopathy, The Royal London Homeopathic Hospital, Great Ormond Street, London WC1N 3HR).

HORMONE REPLACEMENT THERAPY

Most of the hormones responsible for female characteristics are produced by the ovaries. During and after the menopause this production slows although the body continues to produce some.

For many years now doctors have been researching to see whether it is possible to replace these lost hormones, since this might prevent many of the unpleasant side effects of the menopause and the serious effects of osteoporosis (see separate entry).

It now seems that hormone replacement therapy (HRT) can be safely given to certain women. It is available in different forms:

1. **Tablets.**   The most common form (especially useful for severe or frequent hot flushes) is oestrogen tablets. Low doses of oestrogen are likely to be given together with another hormone, progestogen, in order to avoid the very small risk of cancer of the womb which is associated with oestrogen taken on its own over a long period. If you have had a hysterectomy, and so no longer have a womb, you will not be given progestogen.

   Each month you will be given oestrogen alone for eleven to fourteen days, then oestrogen combined with progestogen for ten to twelve days, then nothing at all for seven days. If you have not had a hysterectomy you must expect regular bleeding between days twenty-two and twenty-eight even if you have stopped having periods. The bleeding is likely to be light and not painful. If you have irregular or breakthrough bleeding during HRT (i.e. at odd times of the month), you must see your doctor.

2. **Hormone implants**.   Oestrogen implants are a useful treatment for osteoporosis and the menopause, especially if you have had a hysterectomy. After a local anaesthetic, an oestrogen pellet is inserted under the skin of the lower abdomen. The hormone is slowly absorbed over the next few months. If the symptoms return, a new implant is inserted. If you have not had a hysterectomy, the oestrogen implant will be combined with progestogen tablets for ten to twelve days each month. This means that you will have a 'period', and that there will be no risk of developing cancer of the womb.

3. **Injections and plasters**.   Sometimes fortnightly injections of oestrogen are recommended, and your doctor will decide whether this treatment is right for you. Oestrogen and, more recently, combined oestrogen and progestogen patches to the skin are proving popular with women, and are generally available.

4. **Oestrogen vaginal creams and pessaries**.   These are useful if vaginal soreness and pain on passing water are the only symptoms.

5. **Progestogen alone**.   This is sometimes used to treat hot flushes and night sweats in women who cannot take oestrogen for medical reasons.

6. **Testosterone implants**.   The ovaries also produce the hormone testosterone, which is important for a woman's sexual responses. An implant under the skin, often combined with an oestrogen implant, can help women who have lost their sex drive as a result of the menopause rather than because of other problems.

A few women may notice side effects from HRT. These include nausea, breast tenderness, fluid retention (e.g. swollen feet), a clear, non-irritating vaginal discharge and leg cramps.

Self-health

• Up to two-thirds of women going through the menopause

suffer no symptoms or only minor ones. But the remainder do
have significant problems and if you are one of them it is
worth seeing your family doctor to decide whether HRT would
be suitable. HRT is not a magic potion and it cannot stop
ageing. It does not help facial wrinkles or sagging breasts.
However, hot flushes, night sweats, sore vagina and pain on
passing water can be dramatically improved.

- The value of HRT in preventing osteoporosis is now accepted,
  and some doctors think that every postmenopausal woman
  should receive HRT. Others, however, are more cautious and
  believe it should be kept for those particularly at risk, for
  example women with two or more of the following risk
  factors: early menopause (before the age of forty); previous
  fracture thought to be due to osteoporosis; white or Asian race;
  thin; small-boned; high alcohol intake; current or recent
  steroid treatment; an illness making osteoporosis likely (e.g.
  any cancer, being bedridden or paralysed, rheumatoid
  arthritis, liver disease, thyroid disease or Cushing's disease).

- You should not have HRT if you have had breast cancer or
  cysts, cancer of the lining of the womb, high blood pressure or
  stroke, or clotting of the deep leg veins or the lungs.

Screening

- Unless you have had a hysterectomy your doctor should carry
  out an internal examination to make sure you do not have
  fibroids or an ovarian cyst, and that you are not pregnant.
    If your periods are heavy, a blood test will show if you are
  anaemic.
    Your doctor will probably check your blood pressure
  regularly and advise you to have a cervical smear test every
  three to five years.
    You should examine your breasts each month, and if you are
  not sure how to do this, ask your doctor to show you, or follow
  the diagrams in the section on Breast Cancer.

HOT FLUSHES

A hot flush is a sudden feeling of heat that usually starts on the chest and floods over the neck and face. These parts may look hot and sweaty (but not always) and the sensation is often followed by chills. Hot flushes last for anything from a few seconds to several minutes and may occur once or twice a year or up to twenty times a day. Hot flushes affect sixty to eighty per cent of women during the menopause, though not all so seriously that they need to see their doctor.

Self-health

- If you are prone to hot flushes there is nothing you can do to prevent them entirely. However, if you take a positive attitude your problem will appear less worrying.

- Wear loose cotton clothes to reduce heat and sweating. Wear your clothes in layers so you can take them off and pile them on again easily.

- There is no make-up available to hide hot flushes but remember that they are far more noticeable to you than to others, who may not notice them at all. Keep a solid cologne stick in your handbag or on your bedside table.

- If your hot flushes are worrying you see your doctor, who may suggest tablets to lessen them. These contain the hormone oestrogen in small doses but there is a small risk of womb cancer if the oestrogen is taken alone so for safety another hormone, progestogen, is added for the last ten days of the month (see **Hormone Replacement Therapy**). The dose of hormones needed to control hot flushes varies from person to person so you will be asked to take a 'hot flush count' each day to help the doctor decide what dose to put you on. If you need hormones for more than one year your doctor may suggest taking a few cells from the inside of your womb to make sure you are clear of cancer (**cervical smear**). This procedure does not need an anaesthetic.

HYDATID DISEASE

Hydatid disease is an infectious disease found only in sheep- and cattle-farming communities that use dogs. It is caused by a tapeworm *Taenia Echinococcus* which is excreted in infected dogs' faeces and then swallowed in contaminated food or water by people or passed on directly from dirty hands. The parasite then passes to the liver where it forms cysts. The symptoms are vague ill-health and abdominal pain.

Self-health

- Avoid close contact with working dogs who may be infected. Children are particularly at risk.

- Always wash your hands before eating.

- There are no medicines or injections available to prevent hydatid disease.

- If you live in a farming community and have any of the symptoms of hydatid disease, consult your doctor.

HYPERACTIVITY, CHILDREN

There is no one clear definition of hyperactivity in children. In the USA minor behavioural problems such as difficulty sleeping, short attention span, or temper tantrums may be described as hyperactivity. In the UK the diagnosis is made less frequently and the symptoms are generally more serious.

Self-health

- Make sure your child has plenty of exercise. Children's energy is amazing.

- Consider whether your child's behaviour is a reaction to a difficult family situation and whether this needs changing.

- Set certain rules and limitations on behaviour which will help to guide your child.

- Make sure you are giving your child plenty of your time. The 'hyperactive' behaviour may be a plea for attention.

- If a short attention span is a problem help your child to slow down and concentrate by giving him or her games, puzzles, drawing or reading on which a certain amount of time has to be spent. A timer or buzzer will reinforce your authority.

- You may wonder whether diet is affecting your child's behaviour (see **Allergy, Food** and **Additives**). Various ideas have been put forward, of which the best known is the American Dr Feingold's attempt to pinpoint the problem as one of sensitivity to certain food additives, such as artificial colouring (azo dyes), artificial flavours, monosodium glutamate (used as a flavour enhancer and in Chinese cooking), some preservatives and sodium benzoate. Tests show that about ten per cent of children improve if these additives are removed from their diet. Some doctors are concerned, however, that sticking very closely to the Feingold diet may deprive your child of certain essential foods. However, no harm can come from providing your child with a balanced, varied diet free from additives as a first step to improving his or her behaviour.

Modified Feingold diet for hyperactive children:

- Eliminate all foods containing synthetic colourings and flavourings (monosodium glutamate, nitrites, nitrates, benzoic acid and the additives listed on p. 87).

- For at least four weeks avoid all foods containing the natural salicylates which may be doing the harm, e.g. apples, oranges, raspberries, strawberries, tangerines, plums, peaches, prunes, cherries, apricots and blackberries. Then gradually introduce each food one by one, watching your child's behaviour carefully to see whether there is a change for the worse.

HYPOTHERMIA

If you become very cold (hypothermia) it is possible you may die. Generally 2°C below the normal body temperature of 37°C is dangerous, and you have only thirty per cent chance of recovering if your temperature falls below 25°C.

Elderly people are most at risk of hypothermia because their bodies are less able to cope with low temperatures. In addition, the body mechanisms that detect a drop in temperature become less sensitive with age, so many old people do not realize they are dangerously cold. Finally they often live alone with little money for clothing, insulation and heating.

Early symptoms of hypothermia include drowsiness, confusion, slurred speech, cold, pale skin and slow pulse and breathing. Later the sufferer becomes unconscious.

Self-health

- Keep your home warm, around 20–21°C. Live and sleep in one room during winter if necessary.

- Make sure you have safe, easy-to-use, economical heating.

- Draughtproof and insulate your living rooms.

- Check for damp from blocked gutters or drains.

- Have at least one good hot meal every day – take advantage of meals-on-wheels if necessary. Have plenty of hot drinks – a thermos flask filled in the morning can be useful.

- Keep warm in bed with a hot-water bottle or electric blanket, which costs only a few pence a night to run. Overblankets are best because they can be left on all night. Don't use a hot-water bottle and an electric blanket together in the same bed.

- Several layers of thin, natural (e.g. cotton or wool) clothing are better than one thick layer because they trap air, which acts as an excellent insulator. Try thermal underwear.

- Wear a hat, woolly cap or nightcap because a lot of heat is lost from the head, especially in people with thinning hair.

- Make sure you get all the social security allowances (e.g. heating) to which you are entitled.

- Be a good neighbour or relative to someone at risk of hypothermia by calling on them frequently, especially during the winter.

- If you find someone you think is suffering from hypothermia call professional help immediately. While you wait, warm them gently and, if they are conscious, give them a warm drink and plenty of comfort and encouragement.

I

ILLNESS, EARLY WARNING SIGNS

Some early warning symptoms of possible serious illness

- Feeling generally unwell with loss of appetite and loss of interest in life, hobbies and family.

- Losing weight for no obvious reason. Any loss over 4–5 kg should be taken seriously.

- Chest pain.

- Sudden shortness of breath for no apparent reason.

- Persistently swollen ankles.

- Fainting for no obvious reason.

- A cough that persists for longer than two or three weeks.

- Bad headaches for no obvious reason.

- Persistent indigestion or pain in the abdomen.

- A sore or scab anywhere on the body that doesn't heal within about three weeks.

- Blood in the sputum, faeces or urine.

- Any unexplained change in normal bowel habit, e.g. sudden diarrhoea or constipation.

- Difficulty or pain passing urine; passing urine more frequently; cloudy, strongly smelling urine.

- Unexplained vomiting, especially blood.

- Black, tarry motions.

- Difficulty swallowing.

- Hoarseness that lasts for longer than two weeks for no apparent reason.

- Eyesight problems such as temporary blindness, seeing haloes around lights, or only seeing objects straight in front of you.

- A skin blemish or mole that changes colour or size, or starts to bleed or itch.

- A lump in the breast, change in its shape, or bleeding or unusual discharge from the nipple.

- Bleeding from the vagina between periods or after the menopause.

IMPETIGO

Impetigo is a highly contagious skin disease which is common enough to make one out of 100 people (mostly children) see their doctor each year. It is caused by bacteria and can be caught from personal contact, food, or objects such as towels. Blisters appear mainly on the face, knees or hands, then soon burst, leaving a patch of wet, weeping skin. It is not a serious illness but it does need treatment from your doctor.

Self-health

- You should have your own towel, flannel, soap and other wash things because the infection spreads easily from person to person, especially via wet surfaces.

- Children should not go to school until their impetigo has healed.

- Wash your hands carefully before preparing food, especially cold food.

- Follow your doctor's instructions for treatment carefully.

IMPOTENCE

An impotent man is one who is persistently unable to get or maintain an erection of sufficient hardness to be able to have sex. No one should be worried by occasional failures; everyone has them and they do not mean you will be permanently impotent.

Self-health

- It is important that children are brought up with a healthy attitude to sex as a normal part of life.

- There are several physical causes of impotence which can be prevented.

  1. Any painful condition of the penis (e.g. tight foreskin) should be treated.
  2. Diabetics are prone to impotence because the disease damages the blood vessels in the penis that are needed for an erection. Good control of blood sugar levels throughout the day and night will slow or even prevent this process in some (but not all) men.
  3. Impotence can be caused by alcohol – both temporary impotence, as a result of an occasional night out with too much to drink, and permanent impotence, which may afflict men who drink heavily and regularly (see **Alcoholism**).
  4. Any illness may cause temporary impotence. Once you recover, your impotence will disappear.

- If you are taking medicines check with your doctor because there are several drugs (for example, ones for high blood pressure or prostate disease) that may cause impotence.

- Some neurological diseases (e.g. multiple sclerosis or traumatic damage to the spinal cord) cause impotence because they damage the nerves needed for an erection. This damage is often permanent, but there are operations and sexual aids which create an 'artificial' erection, so talk to your doctor.

- Keep your sex life interesting and varied. Some impotence is caused by boredom alone (see **Sex, Boredom**). Your partner will need to take an active part so discuss it with her.

- If there are no obvious physical (or social) causes for your impotence, you will have to think about the psychological ones (and they are common). These include doubts about your sexuality, hostility towards women, fear of women and their 'purity', unconsciously thinking of your partner as your mother, and worries about sexual diseases or unwanted pregnancies (common in extramarital affairs).

  The first step is to discuss the impotence with your partner as a joint problem not as 'your' problem. You will be amazed how much better this will make you feel (it may in itself cure the impotence), and your partner may be able to help.

It can sometimes help to stop having sex completely and go back to your courtship days with plenty of kissing, hugging, massage and closeness. It may help for your partner to share her fantasies so that you learn to appreciate how much she can enjoy sex. Masturbation may also help to prove to yourself that you still can get an erection.

If none of these steps work – or if they only partly work – you should see your doctor or a marriage guidance counsellor about sex counselling. Usually about ten therapy sessions and suitable sex exercises restore you to full potency.

- Stress and tiredness at home and at work can cause impotence. Learn to avoid it, or to cope with it better (see chapter on Stress and Mental Health).

- Forget about work while you are at home. Relax, play music and eat food you enjoy. Share an activity or sport with your partner that you both enjoy. Take the pressure off yourself and your partner, and don't feel obliged to perform.

INCONTINENCE, FAECES

Faecal incontinence is the inability to control the contents of the bowel and to expel them at an appropriate time and place. It is less common than urinary incontinence. It occurs more frequently in elderly people but must never be thought of as an inevitable consequence of getting old.

The most common symptom is the uncontrollable leakage of runny faeces (like diarrhoea in appearance) from the anus due to faecal impaction. What happens is that in very constipated people (usually elderly, immobile, and on a low-fibre diet) there is a build-up of hard faeces in the rectum which ruins the normal emptying mechanism of the bowel. As a result the bowel cannot empty normally and all that happens is that a little faecal fluid trickles round the hard mass and out through the anus.

Leakage of fully formed faeces is much less common and is more serious and difficult to treat.

Self-health

- Since the most common cause of faecal incontinence is impaction it is vital to eat a high-fibre diet to prevent constipation (see separate entry), particularly for the elderly and immobile.

- Another common preventable cause of incontinence is depression (see separate entry). Depressed people may become so miserable that they no longer even bother about bodily functions; indeed they may use this lack of concern as an outward sign to everybody of their misery. As soon as the depression is treated and the mood lightens, the incontinence stops.

- See **Incontinence, Urine** for advice about clothing, bedding and household goods.

INCONTINENCE, URINE

Incontinence results when you lose control of your bladder and accidentally leak urine. Under the age of sixty-five it affects about one woman in twelve and one man in seventy-five. In people over sixty-five, one woman in nine and one man in sixteen is incontinent. This means about two to three million people in the UK suffer from incontinence. There are three types:

1. **Stress incontinence.**   Urine leaks when you run, play sport or cough. Later in life, any physical effort will cause it. It is due to weakness of the bladder outlet mechanism and the pelvic muscles round it. During pregnancy and childbirth these muscles are stretched and may never quite recover. After the menopause too, the bladder outlet becomes less watertight.
2. **Urge incontinence.**   You may find that you have to pass urine more often than before and that you get far less warning. Unless you get to a lavatory quickly, urine leaks uncontrollably. This may be caused by a problem of the nervous system (e.g. a stroke or multiple sclerosis) but in most people the cause is not known. Occasionally an infection may cause it.
3. **Dribbling incontinence.**   If the bladder fails to empty

properly it quickly fills again and 'overflows' uncontrollably. Older men with enlarged prostate glands are prone to this type of incontinence. People who have damaged their spine may also suffer from it.

Self-health

- Incontinence is not inevitable, and it is certainly worth taking action to try to prevent it.

- Good general health care does much to help. Stay as fit and active as possible; eat a good diet (high in fibre to prevent constipation, low in calories to prevent weight gain); don't smoke (a frequent cough puts strain on the bladder muscles); drink plenty of fluids.

- Many health problems can lead to incontinence, so always discuss any new symptoms or illnesses with your doctor and get treatment as soon as possible.

- For women, daily exercises after childbirth are important for strengthening the pelvic floor muscles. Indeed, all women can benefit from pelvic floor exercises (see separate entry).

- Some women find hormone replacement therapy (see separate entry) after the menopause helpful.

- Good bladder habits will help. For example, it is not good to hang on all day and ignore the need to go, but neither is going too often 'just in case' a good idea. Try to achieve a happy medium. Some people find using a timer to make sure they pass water regularly often works well.

- Do not cut down on fluids. This can make incontinence worse. Drink about six to eight cups of fluid a day but drink less before you go to bed. Choose water or fruit juices. Tea, coffee (except decaffeinated), cola and alcohol can make you produce extra urine, so if one of them causes you a problem, cut down or avoid it altogether.

- Make sure your diet includes plenty of fresh fruit, vegetables, cereals and bran-based biscuits. This will keep you healthy and active and prevent constipation.

- Go to the toilet regularly, using a clock or alarm if necessary to remind you. Make sure your bathroom is warm and well lit, with rails by the toilet to help you up or down if needed. Sit correctly with your bottom and back well supported and your feet firmly on the ground.

- Sleep in a firm, comfortable bed which supports you well and is easy to get out of. If necessary use a fitted waterproof mattress cover or waterproof bedding protection. Both disposable and reusable absorbent sheets are available. There are even sleeping bag liners if you are feeling adventurous.

- Try to have your bed near your toilet. An alternative is to have a commode or urinal nearby.

- Choose clothing which is easily removable, especially if you have arthritis or are paralysed. Full skirts are best for women. Trousers which open widely and use velcro fastenings are best for men.

- Disabled people may find raised lavatory seats, grab rails and clothes that allow quick undressing useful. If getting on to a lavatory proves impossible, a commode or hand-held urinal may help.

- If your own efforts fail to control the incontinence see a doctor. It may be that further exercises, bladder retraining, medicines or surgery (e.g. an operation to remove the prostate gland for men or to repair weak muscles for women) may prevent your incontinence.

- In a few people it is not possible to prevent incontinence. But these days it is possible to prevent anyone knowing you have a problem because there is such an excellent range of protective pads and clothing. Ask your doctor, continence adviser, district nurse or health visitor for advice. They will be able to suggest something suitable and give you advice on skin care. Whatever you choose should be comfortable to wear and easy to fit. You will feel better because your skin will be drier and you will have less leakage and smell.

- Other important points to consider are the absorbency and style of product to match your need:

  1. **Light incontinence**. Reusable pants or slim disposable pads may suit you.

2. **Moderate incontinence**. Shaped pads with a waterproof backing and pants may be what you need. Alternatively an all-in-one brief may be suitable for heavier degrees of incontinence if leakage is a problem.
3. **Heavy incontinence**. All-in-one disposable briefs or shaped pads with snug-fitting pants will be helpful for heavier urinary or faecal incontinence and can be used day and night.

- There is also a wide range of chair and bed pads available which can minimize soiling of bedding and furniture.

- Men with urinary incontinence can use a collection appliance. Many types are available on prescription, so ask your doctor.

- *Disposal*. You can dispose of soiled pads by wrapping them in a sealed plastic bag and placing them with your normal domestic waste. **Never flush pads down the toilet**.

- *Cost and availability*. Unfortunately there are no special DSS cash benefits available for people with incontinence apart from Attendance Allowance (leaflet NI.205 available at a DSS office or post office). However, some health authorities may provide incontinence products to help you and may also provide a laundry collection service. You can also purchase products from chemists, specialist wholesalers, home delivery services or from mail order firms, some of whom operate a discreet twenty-four or forty-eight hour delivery service to your door.

INFERTILITY

An infertile couple is usually defined as one which has not conceived a baby after a year of unprotected, unlimited intercourse. It is a common problem. In Europe about ten per cent of couples have a period of infertility and eight per cent of marriages are childless after ten years.

Self-health

- If possible, don't leave it too long to have children. All your ova (eggs) are present when you are born, and the longer they are in your body the poorer quality they become. Over one third of women aged forty to forty-five are infertile for this reason, and even by the age of thirty your fertility is reduced.

- Avoid sexually transmitted diseases such as gonorrhoea (see separate entry) which damages the Fallopian tubes, preventing your eggs from reaching your womb. If you do develop symptoms the earlier treatment starts the less likely you are to have infertility problems.

- If you are hoping for a family do not use an intra-uterine device (IUD) for contraception without first discussing it with your doctor. IUDs are associated with pelvic infections which can cause infertility.

- Make sure you use an effective method of contraception so you do not need an abortion. Abortions sometimes cause pelvic infections and infertility.

- A few women (about two per cent) find they do not produce eggs (ovulate) once they stop taking the Pill. This usually rights itself after a few months, but see your doctor if it does not.

- Both partners should eat a healthy, balanced diet. Avoid becoming too thin because this can affect ovulation. Both partners should not drink too much alcohol (see **Alcoholism**), because alcohol reduces fertility in both and may damage the precious new fetus.

- Both partners should avoid smoking since this may reduce fertility.

- Some medicines reduce fertility (e.g. certain anti-malarials, sex hormones, cancer drugs). Consult your doctor if you are taking any of these regularly.

- Exercise is good for both partners but very hard exercise (e.g. marathon running) may stop you ovulating.

- Sex should be enjoyable for both partners. If it is not there will be tension and stress which will reduce the chances of starting a baby. In fact all forms of stress (e.g. at work) inhibit ovulation in women and sperm formation in men. Consult a professional if you continue to have problems with sex after talking it over between yourselves.

- For sexual intercourse to be most effective the sperm should be placed near the neck of the womb, ready to race up through the womb and Fallopian tubes to fertilize the egg released by the ovary. Impotence may prevent this (see separate entry) but treatments are available. Premature ejaculation (see **Ejaculation, Premature**) may also prevent the sperm being placed high enough in the vagina.

- Some doctors suggest the woman should lie on her back with hips slightly raised on pillows after intercourse so that the sperm have the best chance of reaching the womb. This probably helps most women with normally positioned wombs, but a few have retroverted wombs (i.e. tilted backwards), which make this position unhelpful. Your doctor will be able to tell you whether your womb is retroverted by examining you internally.

- A woman does not need to have an orgasm for conception to take place. Orgasm shows she has enjoyed the sexual experience but it is not necessary.

- You must make love around ovulation for the sperm to meet the egg at the right time and place. Most women produce their ovum at about the twelfth to fourteenth day of their cycle. So count the first day of proper bleeding of your period as day one, have sex on day ten, and maybe again on day twelve and days fourteen or fifteen. In order to build up plenty of sperm men should not have sex or masturbate two to three days before lovemaking. The gap between days ten and twelve, and days twelve and fourteen is designed to allow sperm to accumulate again. These dates are guidelines only, so do not feel obliged to stick to them rigidly, particularly if it feels unnatural for you. Besides, many women have such irregular cycles that they will need to do the following special tests to know when they are ovulating:

  1. Keeping temperature charts will help you pinpoint ovulation. Just before ovulation there may be a small drop in temperature followed by a 0.5°C rise which continues until your period begins.
  2. Some women also notice a difference in their cervical mucus (noticed as a slight discharge from the vagina) at the time of ovulation and are able to time intercourse this way.

3. Just before ovulation the level of one of the hormones, luteinizing hormone, rises. A test to monitor this rise in the urine can now be bought from the chemist and is an accurate way of pinpointing ovulation.

- There is not a great deal a man can do to improve his fertility. Tight underpants and trousers, though, reduce your sperm count so avoid them.

- If, after twelve to eighteen months of unprotected, enjoyable sex, you still have not conceived you should see your doctor, who may be able to help you or may refer you to a specialist. Nowadays there are many remarkable procedures (of which in-vitro fertilization is only one) which can help you.

- Do not think of adoption as a last resort. For many couples it is a very rewarding experience.

INFLUENZA

Influenza, better known as flu, is caused by a virus and spreads from person to person in the air by droplets, from coughs or sneezes, or by contact (e.g. touching hands). Symptoms include feeling unwell, headache, high temperature, muscle and joint aches and pains, coughing and a runny nose. After two or three days you should start to feel better. The only serious complication that may occur is pneumonia (see separate entry).

Self-health

- You are infectious while you have flu, so keep away from public places to avoid infecting others. The problem is that you don't develop symptoms until one to three days after catching the virus and so you can be infectious before symptoms appear without knowing it. Once your symptoms disappear you can safely assume that you are no longer infectious.

- Keep away from other people with coughs, sneezes and runny noses. You are most likely to catch flu in crowded places in winter.

- Older people over sixty-five are most at risk from flu and should take special precautions, including asking their doctor about vaccination.

- The only way of preventing flu is by vaccination. This is about eighty per cent effective against known viruses. The difficulty is that it does not work against new strains of flu, which may sweep through a country every two or three years. The risks from vaccination are low, so anyone at risk (e.g. people over sixty-five, health workers), should seek advice from their doctor.

- Once you have the symptoms you can prevent them getting worse by going to bed, taking paracetamol or aspirin (don't give aspirin to children), and, if you are sweating a lot, drinking plenty of fluids, such as fruit drinks or hot lemon and honey.

- If your fever lasts more than three or four days or you develop chest pain or shortness of breath you should call your doctor.

- Do not be surprised if you feel depressed for two or three weeks after your illness. This is common. It will get better and you will not need to see a psychiatrist!

INGROWING TOENAIL

A nail is ingrowing if it cuts through the skin near it, causing a wound. The wound may not be infected, in which case it weeps clear fluid, or it may be infected and pussy. If the flesh is piled up round the nail, which may have an exaggerated U-shaped curve, and there is no wound, the condition is known as an involuted nail.

Self-health

- Look after your toenails regularly and carefully. Do not cut them too short or with too much of a curve because this will make an ingrowing or involuted toenail more likely.

- Generally use clippers rather than scissors because they are safer. If you do cause an accidental cut, wash it with an

antiseptic lotion, apply some cream and cover with gauze.
Change the dressing each day and see your doctor or
chiropodist immediately if there is any sign of infection.

- Ask someone else to cut your toenails if you cannot reach
  them, have shaky hands or cannot see well. Filing is safer than
  cutting; file along the length of the nail rather than across it.

- Cutting a 'V' in the free edge of the nail does not prevent
  ingrowing nails; instead it may catch in socks or stockings and
  even cause the nail to be pulled off.

- If you do get an ingrowing toenail, it can be prevented from
  getting worse. Bathe it daily in boiled salted water or a gentle
  antiseptic and dress it with sterile gauze. Wear large, roomy
  shoes or slippers. Sometimes a small wad of cotton placed
  between the nail and wound helps, but place it carefully and
  change it every day. Beware of cutting the nail at this stage as
  your efforts may damage the skin and cause infection.

  Do not continue with the treatment for longer than three or
  four days if the toe is not getting better. Your doctor or
  chiropodist will prefer to treat the condition early rather than
  late.

INSOMNIA

You are suffering from insomnia (sleeplessness) if you are
sleeping so badly that you are tired and sleepy during the day.
How much sleep you need varies from person to person; some
people need eight or nine hours, others three to four. What
matters is that you get the correct amount to suit you.

Self-health

- Develop a regular routine before going to bed so that you can
  wind down and feel peaceful and relaxed. It doesn't matter
  much what you do provided it's roughly the same each night.
  In other words, make yourself a hot drink (not coffee, tea or
  cocoa), play music, watch TV, have a bath, read a book or
  whatever, in the same order each night so that sleep comes
  naturally as the last thing you do.

- You won't sleep well if you are in pain. Discuss any pain you have with your doctor, who may suggest painkilling tablets. These are best taken just before you go to sleep so that the pain (see separate entry) is prevented, otherwise you may wake in pain and have to wait half an hour or so before the tablets start working again. A good sleep will also help you to cope better with pain during the day.

- Try not to eat within three hours of going to bed. A full stomach makes sleeping difficult. If you are regularly woken by indigestion (see **Heartburn**) see your doctor, who may be able to treat this problem.

- A small amount of alcohol (e.g. a tot of whisky) helps sleep; much more will make it disturbed.

- You may find that certain foods (e.g. cheese or other fatty foods) make it difficult for you to sleep, or wake you in the night. You can only pinpoint them by trial and error because they vary between people so greatly.

- Exercise during the day will improve your sleep. Some people find a gentle stroll before going to bed useful. Others use yoga or deep breathing exercises (see **Breathlessness**).

- Sex can help you sleep but bad sex can make sleeping more difficult. If you or your partner are not being satisfied discuss it frankly and try the suggestions in **Sex, Boredom**. If you are still having problems, see your doctor or a sex therapist.

- Shift work makes sleep difficult because the body cannot get into a routine. Some people find they have to insist on one regular shift or change their jobs. See **Jetlag** for advice on a related problem.

- Make sure your bed is comfortable. Many are too soft and don't give enough support. Many are also too small. For example, since the 1920s men have grown 5 cm taller on average, and the percentage of men 1.9 m tall or more has increased from one in 250 to one in forty. But beds have stayed the same size. Your bed should be at least 15 cm longer than you are. It is too narrow if when you lie with your hands behind your head you find that your elbows are overlapping the sides.

Sharing a double bed with someone you love usually helps sleep, but it can have the opposite effect, especially if one partner is much heavier, creating a 'valley' so that the other partner either rolls into it or spends the night clinging sleeplessly to the sides. The modern solution is two mattresses independently sprung but zipped together for closeness.

- Your partner may be temporarily unwell. Do not hesitate to sleep in another bed so that you both get a good night's sleep. Snoring is another problem for some couples and can usually be overcome (see **Snoring**).

- Some couples, especially when they get older, find they cannot sleep unless they have separate beds, or even separate rooms. Do not hesitate to take this step if it is necessary; it does not mean you love each other any the less. It is probably worth one of the partners keeping a double bed to encourage regular lovemaking and closeness.

- You will sleep best if your room is about 16–18°C and well ventilated. Old blankets work badly because they become thick and matted instead of light and fluffy, so buy new ones rather than piling more on.

- Earplugs may help you sleep if your room is noisy at night. Some people find that eyeshades or fitting thicker curtains to cut out light help them sleep better.

- If, despite your efforts, you are still having difficulty sleeping, see your doctor. He or she may prescribe sleeping tablets for a short time to break the cycle. Be wary of taking them for more than two or three months because some can become addictive.

- Depression (see separate entry) commonly disrupts sleep, but treatment will prevent this problem.

CHILDREN

- Most children have problems with sleep at one time or another so don't despair if your child does. Remember that even if you can't prevent it in the short term your child will probably grow out of it within two or three months.

- Most problems are related to anxieties and a need to be

reassured. So try to maintain a calm and loving atmosphere in the home and develop a regular routine which reassures the child that all is well. Singing, patting the back, rocking the cot or playing a musical box are often helpful.

- Try to persuade your baby to fall asleep in his or her cot from the earliest days. If your child gets used to falling asleep at your breast, in your arms or in your bed, you may have difficulty getting him or her to sleep independently.

- Some parents give rewards or a star for every trouble-free night but the important point is to be generous with your praise.

- School may cause your child problems which are expressed as sleep problems. Only when the difficulties at school are resolved will you all get a good night's sleep.

- Many children suffer from nightmares, especially when they are aged three or four. Often there is no obvious cause but sometimes they can be prevented by cutting out unsuitable TV, bedtime stories or certain foods (e.g. cheese or other fatty foods).

- Be cautious about sending a child to bed as punishment because sleeping will then become associated with punishment and you will have an even more difficult problem.

- Never give a baby or child a sleeping pill prescribed for an adult.

IRIDOLOGY

Iridology is a system of diagnosis in which the practitioner examines the coloured part of the eye, the iris, from which he or she then draws conclusions about the person's mental and physical health. For centuries the Chinese have used the eye for diagnostic purposes, and orthodox doctors are able to diagnose certain conditions from it (e.g. diabetes and raised blood pressure), but it is only since the nineteenth century, following work by the Hungarian Ignatz von Pezely, that the iris alone has been used by practitioners of this form of diagnosis.

According to iridology the right eye reflects the right side of the body and vice versa. Brightness, lines, flecks and pigment changes are all significant, and particularly the texture of the iris, which can vary from very fine to very coarse.

The advantage of iridology is that it is painless, quick and harmless. However, there is little research to suggest it works and it should not be relied upon by anyone as the only form of diagnosis of serious conditions.

IRRITABLE BOWEL SYNDROME (IBS)

Some people have very active bowels which cause a variety of bowel symptoms known as irritable bowel syndrome (or spastic colon). Women aged between twenty and forty are most commonly affected.

The most common symptom is lower abdominal pain (almost in the pelvis), either at one side or flitting from side to side. Sometimes the pain is brought on by certain foods (see below), sometimes it is helped by opening your bowels. Most people notice pellet-like stools, often with mucus, at some stage but constipation and diarrhoea (often alternating) are common.

Other symptoms include a bloated feeling, often with a lot of wind and stomach rumbles, a feeling that you have not opened your bowels completely, and generally feeling sick, tired and headachy.

The diagnosis of IBS is often difficult to make and may cover a variety of different problems. But there are several measures you can take.

Self-health

- Research has shown that food allergies can cause IBS. Common culprits include wheat, maize, milk products, coffee, tea, alcohol and citrus fruits. It is probably worth going on an elimination diet (see **Allergy, Food**) to discover if any of these foods affect you.

- Many studies have shown that stress and anxiety make the symptoms worse, although it seems unlikely that they cause them. People with IBS are also often depressed but again this probably results from symptoms rather than causes them.
  Learning to cope with stress (see chapter on Stress and

Mental Health), relaxation techniques, plenty of exercise, yoga, hypnosis or psychotherapy may also help and are all worth considering. Sometimes anti-depressive medicines prescribed by your doctor can alleviate symptoms.

- If constipation and pain are your worst problems increase your fibre intake and stop taking laxatives, which tend to make your bowel habits unpredictable.

- Painless diarrhoea is often caused by specific foods such as fruit and salads, so consider eliminating these from your diet. If you also get pain you may need an anti-spasmodic medicine from your doctor.

  If your diarrhoea is difficult to control, carry the medicines codeine phosphate or loperamide (Imodium) with you at all times. They work quickly so they can be taken in an emergency or, better still, taken at a time when you have learned to expect diarrhoea. Loperamide is available from your chemist, codeine on prescription.

- Some experts believe IBS may be caused by candida or chlamydia (see **Thrush, Vaginal**), which explains why antibiotics (which change the bowel's normal bacteria and yeast populations greatly) make symptoms worse. You may wish to discuss this possibility with your doctor.

Screening

- Many people with unusual bowel symptoms understandably worry they may have cancer or some other severe illness. If you have such worries see your family doctor immediately so you can be thoroughly examined and your worst fears settled. You should then notice an improvement in your symptoms.

J

JETLAG

The symptoms you experience when you fly across time zones, especially from west to east, are known as jetlag. They include mental and physical tiredness, difficulty concentrating, difficulty sleeping, headache and nausea.

Self-health

- Before flying, prepare yourself in advance by changing your eating and sleeping habits to match the country you are visiting. So, if you are travelling from west to east you will need to eat and sleep earlier and later if travelling from east to west.

- As soon as you get on the plane adjust your watch to the time in the country you are visiting. This encourages the process of adjustment to the new time zone.

- Drink plenty of fluids to combat the dehydration every plane traveller experiences. Avoid alcohol because it dehydrates the body (for example, you will notice you pass water in larger quantities and more often after drinking alcohol).

- Avoid large amounts of indigestible, fatty foods. Instead select salads and fruit (although you may have to bear in mind where this food comes from and its chances of being contaminated).

- Get as much sleep as you can. You can now buy neck supports which make sleeping in aircraft seats more comfortable, and you can discuss with your doctor whether to take sleeping pills. There is one, Temazepam, which claims to be particularly useful for jetlag.

JOINTS, STIFF AND PAINFUL

There are two main causes of painful, stiff joints. One is arthritis (see separate entry) and the other is injury. In both cases you may need to see a doctor for specific treatment but there are some ways you can help yourself.

Self-health

- See **Sports Injuries** for tips on how to prevent them. It is a good general rule that the fitter you are the less likely you are to damage your joints and cause pain and stiffness.

- Immediately after an injury a stiff, painful joint needs rest. There is nothing to be gained by ignoring the symptoms – you will simply delay recovery. It is also important to rule out the possibility of a fracture so go to Casualty for an X-ray if you are at all worried.

  Do not be surprised by how long some injuries take to heal. A sprained ankle may take a few weeks to a few months. A whiplash injury of the neck may take up to two years.

  If the joints of your legs are affected you should rest them by taking the weight off them. If your arms are affected you must not carry or lift heavy objects. If your neck or back are affected you need to lie down.

- Stiff, painful joints need to be moved through their full range of movements or they will stiffen further. This should be done several times a day and you should concentrate on all the movements the joint is capable of. Try and exercise the muscles around the affected joint to prevent them becoming thin and wasted. Your doctor or a physiotherapist will advise you.

- Never leave a joint in one position all day (e.g. with a pillow under a bent knee) however comfortable it might seem, or you will lose the ability to bend and straighten it fully.

- Painkillers are important when coping with a stiff, painful joint. You may need to discuss which ones to take with your doctor but the principle is that you should take fewer more often rather than many infrequently. The idea is to prevent pain coming rather than treating it once it is there.

- Applying heat (e.g. from a heat lamp or a covered hot-water bottle) or cold (e.g. from a covered ice-pack or packet of frozen peas) to the area may relieve pain and stiffness and allows you to exercise the joint more.

K

KIDNEY STONES

Kidney stones are made of salts (e.g. calcium) and vary in size from a pinhead to several centimetres in diameter. Many cause no symptoms, but if one passes into the ureter (the tube leading from the kidney to the bladder) it may cause what has often been described as the worst pain suffered by people.

Self-health

- It seems people fall into one of two categories – stone-formers or non-stone-formers. If close relatives suffer from kidney stones it is likely you are the former, in which case you should take precautions more seriously. Unfortunately there are no tests that will accurately predict whether you are a stone-former.

- Drink plenty of fluids, but avoid alcohol, which increases the concentration of calcium, uric acid and phosphate in the urine, making stones more probable. If you go to a hot, dry place where you sweat a lot, be sure to drink even more so there is plenty of urine to flush the ureter and prevent stones forming. During the Second World War soldiers fighting in the desert were far more prone to stones than those in cooler places.

- Some experts believe that diet can affect your likelihood of developing kidney stones. They claim that a diet rich in fibre and low in animal protein and sugar will increase the rate of absorption of calcium from the gut and thus make calcium stones more likely. By the same token a diet rich in calcium (e.g. dairy products) has the same effect. The problem is that these constituents are important for health in other respects (see **Osteoporosis**). So the wise course for most people is to eat

KIDNEY STONES

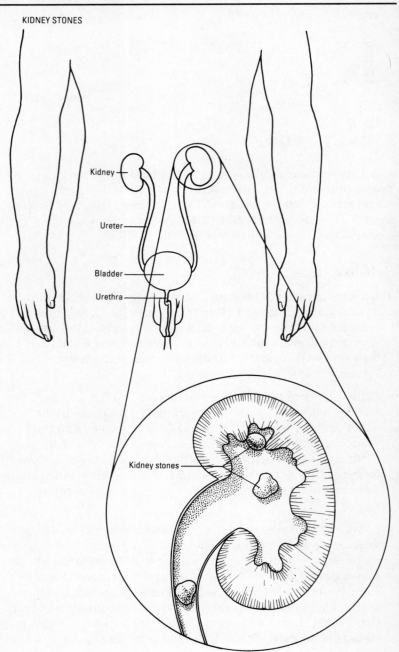

a balanced diet and consider a special diet only once stones have been diagnosed.

- Another problem caused by stones is that they block the free flow of urine, making infection more likely. It is important that infections are treated quickly by your doctor to prevent the development of kidney failure. Symptoms include back and loin pain, fever, chills and hot flushes (rigors), and a change in the colour, smell and consistency of your urine.

KYPHOSIS (CURVATURE OF THE SPINE)

If the spine is too curved in its upper part it is called kyphosis. Hunchbacks have a very severe form of kyphosis, people with round or humped backs a milder form. A baby may be born with it, or it may develop over the years due perhaps to the bone disease, osteoporosis (see separate entry). The roadsign for 'elderly people crossing' shows someone with kyphosis.

Self-health

- The congenital form cannot be prevented, and a baby born with kyphosis must be seen regularly by a doctor to limit the complications, of which chest infections are the most serious. Physiotherapy, bracing or even surgery may be necessary.

- The kyphosis caused by osteoporosis can be partially prevented (see **Osteoporosis**).

L

LAXATIVES

Laxatives are medicines to prevent or treat constipation (see separate entry). They should be needed only in special circumstances (e.g. after an operation), or if a high-fibre diet has failed. There are three main types:

1. Bulking agents (e.g. methylcellulose or ispaghula husk). These are dietary supplements and are prescribed only if you find you cannot manage 30 g of fibre a day.
2. Osmotic laxatives (e.g. lactulose or magnesium hydroxide). These contain sugar and/or salts which are not absorbed by the body and which draw water into the stool, making it larger and softer.
3. Stimulant laxatives (e.g. bisacodyl). These act on the bowel wall, stimulating it to propel the stool forward. They are often used after an operation.

LEAD

Lead is found in car exhaust fumes, old piping, some paints, some crayons and pencils, and cigarette smoke. High levels of lead in the body, especially in children, have been linked with hyperactivity, emotional problems, and difficulty concentrating or learning. Research has found a link, too, between high levels of lead and low IQ (1981 Medical Research Council study of London schoolchildren). Children seem to be more at risk than adults, since they absorb more of the lead because they are growing.

Self-health

- If you have a car use unleaded petrol.

- If you have children consider moving from an area of high traffic and traffic jams.

- Wash fruit and vegetables thoroughly to remove traces of lead dust – this will also help to cut down your intake of pesticides, which are sprayed on to fruit and vegetables by farmers.

- Peel fruit and remove outer leaves from vegetables.

- Investigate whether you have old lead water pipes in your house. If so, consider renewing them. At least let the tap run a minute or so first thing in the morning to drain away contaminated water. You may be eligible for a council grant to replace them in some parts of the UK. Soft-water areas are most dangerous because the lead is more easily dissolved.

- Make sure your children use lead-free paints only.

- Avoid damaged or dented cans of food. The seams of many cans are made of lead and covered with lacquer for protection. Damage may break this seal and allow lead to contaminate the food within. For the same reason never store food in a can, it should always be transferred to a plastic container for storage in the refrigerator.

LEGIONNAIRES' DISEASE

Legionnaires' disease is an infection caused by the bacterium *legionella pneumophilia*, caught by breathing in a fine spray of airborne water which carries the bug. You cannot catch it directly from someone who has already been infected or from drinking water.

The first symptoms are a high fever, chills, and headache or muscle pain. Later a dry cough and pneumonia may develop. Most people recover without permanent damage but a few (generally older) people die. There are about 100–200 reported cases each year in the UK but this figure is probably an underestimate because it is a difficult condition to recognize and diagnose.

Self-health

- The *legionella* bacterium is found in soil, natural water supplies and many recirculating and hot water systems. Outbreaks occur in or near large buildings such as hotels, hospitals and office blocks. So far it seems that water systems in domestic homes are not a risk.

- Special precautions have to be taken to prevent the bacterium breeding rapidly in water systems:

  1. The presence of rust, sludge, scale, algae and organic matter encourage growth. So tanks, pipework and cooling towers should be designed to prevent water lying undisturbed for long periods and should be well covered to prevent dirt and debris getting into them. They should also be regularly inspected (e.g. six-monthly), cleaned and disinfected.
  2. The bacterium breeds in water temperatures 20–40°C so water in water systems should be stored at 60°C and circulated at 50°C (i.e. scalding hot).
  3. In cooling towers, drift eliminators should be fitted to reduce the escape of spray, which is the only way the bacterium can infect people. Water should be treated to prevent corrosion and the growth of bacteria. It may also be possible to replace cooling towers with dry cooling systems.

- If you think these precautions are not being taken by your employer at work you should contact your health and safety officer because the Health and Safety at Work Act (1974) places a legal obligation on employers and those who control buildings to take such precautions.

- If you work in an environment that might favour legionella or if you have been abroad recently and you develop the symptoms above you should see your doctor immediately and mention your fears. The quicker you receive treatment (usually antibiotics) the quicker you will recover. Also, if you report your symptoms it will help doctors to find the source of the bacterium, to identify other people likely to be affected, and to make sure the offending water system is dealt with to eradicate the source of infection.

LEPTOSPIROSIS

Leptospirosis (also known as Weil's disease) is a disease caused by bacteria called *leptospira*, which infect rats. If the rats' urine gets into water (e.g. ponds, canals or rivers) it can contaminate it with bacteria. These bacteria can then infect humans either through cuts, grazes or small wounds or through thin surfaces like the lining of the mouth. Three to fifteen days later a flu-like illness develops (aches and pains, headache and fever) which may get better or may deteriorate, with the development of kidney, liver or heart disease. Untreated it may be fatal; treated, you can expect to make a good recovery.

Self-health

- Anyone who works in rat-infested places is at risk especially abattoir and farm workers, or vets. If you do, take special precautions.

- Rubber boots and gloves should be worn anywhere there is a risk.

- Do not swim anywhere you suspect rats might live.

- If you think you may have swum in a dangerous place and are developing suspicious symptoms see your family doctor immediately. Precautionary antibiotics (e.g. penicillin) will prevent the disease if taken in time, and if you have already caught the disease they will certainly minimize symptoms the earlier you take them.

LEUKAEMIA

Leukaemia is an uncommon cancer affecting the white cells of the blood. The function of these cells is to recognize anything which is foreign in the bloodstream (e.g. bacteria) and either kill or immobilize it.

Leukaemia affects both children and adults. The symptoms include paleness, tiredness, shortness of breath, a tendency to bruising and bleeding, poor resistance to infection (especially infections of the mouth), loss of appetite and weight, fever and sweating at night.

Self-health

- There is controversy about whether children living near nuclear power stations may be at risk. Certainly in Britain more children living near these stations seem to have developed leukaemia than would be expected. Some experts, though, say this is due to chance clustering. However, if you have children, it would seem a sensible precaution to live as far from these stations as you can.

- Excessive radiotherapy or X-rays have been linked with leukaemia. There are strict regulations for anyone working with any type of radiation, and you should avoid having too many X-rays in one year – consult your doctor if you are worried.

- If you or your children develop any of the symptoms described above you should consult your doctor. Leukaemia is not a condition you can treat yourself and it needs careful medical supervision. However, modern treatment can cure many types of leukaemia, and greatly prolong the lives of people affected by other types.

LICE

A head louse is a small parasite no bigger than the head of a matchstick. It lives only on human beings and survives by sucking blood from the scalp.

Self-health

- The louse likes the warmth and moisture of the scalp, preferably covered with clean, healthy hair (dirty, greasy hair creates problems for it). It is not adapted to living on pets, clothing, furniture, hats or combs so you do not need to worry about these causing infection.

- What you do have to worry about is direct head-to-head contact because this is the only way lice spread; they cannot fly or jump. The problem is that someone can be infected – and so able to infect other people – for as long as two months before starting to itch. So if you or your child is at risk (especially during term time) the hair must be checked about once a week even if there are no symptoms.

- The louse is a difficult creature to spot because it is sly, flesh-coloured, avoids direct light and can move quickly. The fact that you cannot see any lice does not mean the hair is uninfected.

- Easier to see are the 'nits' or empty egg shells. These are firmly attached to hairs close to their base, quite different from dandruff, which is part of the scalp.

- To inspect a head, dampen the hair a little and then place it over a sheet of white paper so you can see what falls out when you comb the hair.

  Use a fine-toothed comb or nit comb (these are often included with family treatment packs) to comb the hair thoroughly. After combing, check to see if any damaged lice or nits have fallen out on to the paper.

  Next, part the layers of hair quickly, looking for moving lice or nits. Work methodically across the whole head, paying special attention to the nape of the neck, the ears and under a fringe.

- If you find that your children (or you) have lice you should inform the school and anyone who may have been in close contact with them. In the past people may have been disapproving but this attitude has changed now that we understand more about how lice behave. Reporting the existence of lice will help to prevent an epidemic.

- Keep your children off school and away from other children while they are infested. This will probably only be for one day because modern one-application treatment is so effective.

- The whole family will need treatment to make sure the infestation is killed. There are two main insecticides, malathion and carbryl, available as lotions or shampoos.

LISTERIOSIS

Listeriosis is a kind of food poisoning caused by the bacterium *listeria monocytogenes*. This bacterium lies in soil and can enter the human food chain by several routes. It can be found on unwashed vegetables, it can contaminate meat in the slaughterhouse, or it can infect milk by faecal contamination or cow udder infections.

Listeriosis is relatively rare. In the UK in 1988 there were 287 reported cases (compared to 24,000 cases of salmonella poisoning). Although as many as one in twenty of us have the bug in our bowels at any one time, it does not usually cause more than a mild, flu-like illness, which a healthy adult would hardly notice. Only young children, elderly people, pregnant women and people with weakened resistance to infection (e.g. with cancer or after transplants) are at risk of serious illness and should take special precautions.

Self-health

- Listeria is a great survivor and can exist in refrigerators at temperatures that would kill other bacteria. So make sure your fridge is kept at 5°C or below.

- Listeria can cross-contaminate food in a fridge so it is safer to cover all foods. Separate cooked foods from raw vegetables and cheeses.

- Listeria can also survive quite high temperatures so make sure foods are well cooked. It will be killed by constant temperatures over 70°C. Microwaving may present a problem because it heats food unevenly, so make sure you follow the times recommended by the manufacturer.

- Keep foods for as short a time as possible, follow storage instructions carefully and observe the 'best before' and 'eat-by' dates on the label.

- Do not eat undercooked poultry or meat products. Make sure you reheat cooked chilled meals thoroughly.

- When reheating food make sure it is heated until piping hot all the way through and do not reheat more than once.

- Cooked food which is not eaten straightaway should be cooled as quickly as possible and then stored in the fridge.

- People who are at special risk of listeriosis (see above) should avoid the following foods:

1. Soft cheeses, which are less acid than hard cheeses and so are more welcoming to listeria, which does not thrive in acid conditions.
2. Food prepared by the cook-chill method.
3. Pre-packaged salads with dressings.
4. Unpasteurized milk or any unpasteurized milk product (e.g. unpasteurized yogurt).
5. Pâtés – in the summer of 1989 unacceptably high levels of listeria were found in some Belgian pâtés.

LONELINESS

Loneliness is the unhappy feeling of being alone in the world. Unlike solitude, which you may have chosen, loneliness is a negative emotion since it suggests you would prefer not to be alone. Loneliness is often felt most when you are surrounded by other, apparently happy people.

Self-health

- Prevention starts from the earliest days when you teach your baby, firstly by example, the social skills that will help him or her to discover how interesting life is. Babies should not be left alone for long hours. Carry your baby around with you in a sling or put him or her in the kitchen while you are working there. Later, as your baby grows older, teach him or her that you cannot always be around and that he or she must learn to be alone sometimes.

- If you have no alternative to living alone make a virtue of it. Enjoy the freedom it brings, and take part in your favourite hobbies and activities.

- Get to know yourself better. There are plenty of good books about self-discovery, and social-skills training courses are widely available.

- Some experts believe that talking to yourself is helpful because it releases tension. Others recommend keeping a diary in which you write down your fantasies and wildest hopes.

- Try to meet other people in a social or community-based

setting (e.g. helping with a toddler group or going to church).

- If you would like to (re)marry or have a close relationship join a marriage bureau (you will be pleasantly surprised by how many like-minded people there are in the good ones).

LUNG CANCER

Lung cancer is a tumour of one or both lungs. Before smoking became popular it was practically unknown. Now it kills about 40,000 people in the UK alone each year and is the most common cause of death.

In the past more men died of lung cancer than women because they smoked more. However, since the Second World War smoking has become more popular with women and already many more are dying from lung cancer. In fact in one year in Scotland lung cancer overtook breast cancer as the most common cancer killing women and this trend can be expected to continue in the future, particularly as more young girls are taking up the habit (see **Smoking**).

Symptoms vary greatly. Some people have no chest symptoms until they start feeling unwell, losing appetite and weight or have unexplained fevers. Others get a cough which is worse than usual and may have blood streaks in the sputum. Shortness of breath, chest pains (worse when breathing in) and wheezing are also common.

Self-health

- If you smoke, stop immediately (see **Smoking**). The risk of cancer is in direct proportion to the number of cigarettes you smoke a day, so if you smoke forty cigarettes a day you are forty times more likely to get cancer than someone who smokes none. Some experts have suggested that after five years as a non-smoker your chances of getting cancer are similar to those of someone who has never smoked. However, recent research contradicts this viewpoint and suggests that you never return to the low risks of a lifelong non-smoker. Nevertheless your chances will still be a lot better than if you had continued smoking.

- If you have not succeeded in giving up smoking you should watch your health carefully, particularly for any of the symptoms described above. If you have any cause for concern, consult your family doctor immediately. The outlook for lung cancer is generally poor but it is still true that the smaller the tumour is at diagnosis, the better your chances are.

- If you work with asbestos you are at risk of developing a tumour called a mesothelioma. There are now very strict regulations designed to protect you at work, but if you are worried that these may have been ignored at your workplace you should consult your health and safety officer or local Government Health and Safety Office.

- Experts are now becoming ever more conscious of the dangers of 'passive' smoking – the inhalation of smoke from other people's cigarettes. Research in Japan and Greece has shown that non-smoking wives of smokers are at risk of lung cancer. In the Japanese study 91,500 women were studied and it was found that if a man smoked over twenty cigarettes a day his wife had twice the expected risk of cancer.

- Make use of non-smoking areas. These are available in all trains, planes and buses, and most public places such as theatres, cinemas and restaurants.
  Make sure you have non-smoking areas at work, and at home ask smokers to smoke outside the house or in one room which you and your family can avoid.

- Since ninety-five per cent of people who die from lung cancer are smokers many will blame themselves for causing their illness. Relatives and friends should beware that this added burden of guilt often has a devastating effect on the person's morale which it is difficult to shake. The best that can be said is that smoking does not cause cancer, it merely makes it very likely in those unfortunate people who are susceptible to it.

Screening

- The mass chest X-ray campaigns of the 1960s and early 1970s have now been abandoned because it was realized that for the time and money spent, only a few cancers were being found and many of them were so advanced that cure was impossible.

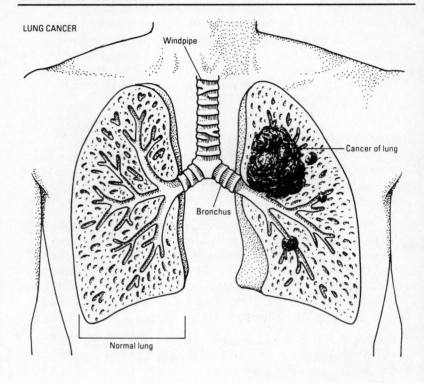

LUNG CANCER

Windpipe

Cancer of lung

Bronchus

Normal lung

- If you are a smoker you should see your doctor regularly for check-ups and especially if you develop any of the symptoms described above. You are at risk not only of lung cancer but also of heart, chest and artery disease.

LUNG, FARMER'S

People who suffer from farmer's lung are allergic to the fungus that grows on mouldy hay or grain. The allergy causes lung inflammation which narrows the air passages and causes shortness of breath and coughing, usually a few hours after exposure to the hay.

Self-health

- Avoid exposing yourself to hay or grains. Change your job if necessary.

- If possible wear a mask over your nose and mouth when you are exposed to the fungus.

M

MALARIA

Malaria is caused by a tiny parasite, plasmodium, which passes from infected people to others via the female anopheles mosquito. One bite is enough to give you the illness. Symptoms start from nine to thirty days after the bite (or sometimes even longer) and include headache, joint and muscle pains, tiredness, feeling sick, and sudden chills followed by sweating attacks. If the infection attacks the brain (cerebral malaria) the outlook is particularly poor without prompt treatment.

Self-health

- Malaria is a serious illness which can be fatal, especially in children, so precautions must be taken against it.

- See your doctor before travelling abroad to find out whether the country you are going to is affected by malaria and what tablets you should take if it is. Some forms of malaria have built a resistance to some anti-malaria tablets, so do not think every anti-malaria medicine will work for you. You need expert advice. In general take your tablets a week before leaving and for a month after returning home.

- Keep your arms and legs covered after sunset when the mosquitoes are active, and use insect repellents liberally.

- Use nets or screens for sleeping.

- Burn anti-malaria coils if you are sitting in one place.

- The more you move and thrash about the more you will be attacked by mosquitoes because they are attracted by hot, moist, turbulent air.

- If you become ill for no obvious reason while abroad tell the doctor if you think you may have missed taking all your anti-malaria tablets at the right time.

- If you become ill after returning home tell your doctor you have been abroad.

MASSAGE

The beauty of massage is that it is instantly calming, stimulating and healing, and you can do it all yourself! Most people are not instant expert masseurs, but with practice you can get pretty good. Try some of the following and see what suits you best.

Neck and shoulders

Your neck and shoulders are the most likely places to get stiff and sore from tension, so start massaging before that headache or migraine comes on.

- First turn your head to the right and put your left hand on the back of your neck. Pull your hand firmly to the left across your head while at the same time allowing your head to swing into the neutral position. Repeat ten times and then turn to the left, using your right hand to stroke your neck.

- With your left hand grip the flesh where your right shoulder meets your neck. Massage it firmly using your fingers in a circular motion. Next rock your head from side to side (as if you were looking for something under a table), all the time keeping a firm pressure on the flesh. Try nodding your head backwards and forwards several times and then swinging your head in as wide a circle as possible. Repeat using your right hand on the left side of the neck.

- If you find any particularly sore spots, you can work on them separately. Start with a gentle, circular, rhythmical massage round the sore spot and slowly increase the pressure as the muscles loosen up. You will be amazed how as little as five minutes' massage can take away pain and improve the range of movement in your neck and shoulders.

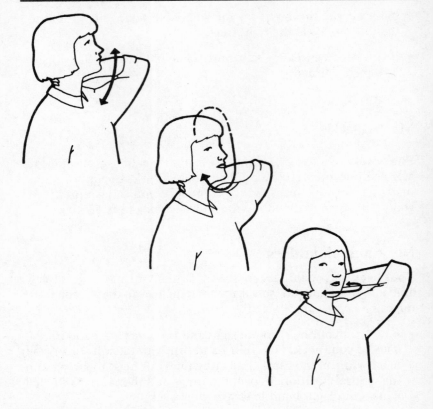

Back

Sadly you cannot massage your own back easily, though you can teach your partner and enjoy some mutual massage. On your own, though, the easiest and cheapest way is to use a rubber ball.

- Buy a rubber ball the size of a tennis ball.

- Stand about 20 cm away from a wall with your back to the wall, your feet apart and your knees bent.

- Hold the ball halfway down your back, then lean against the wall. Keeping some pressure on the wall gently roll the ball all over your back by bending and straightening your knees and swinging your hips, finding the sore spots and massaging them away. You'll love it and after a few sessions you will have helped firm up your thighs too.

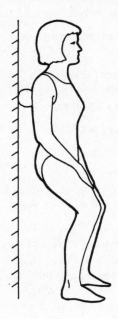

Hands

Don't neglect your hands. A good, firm massage will make them feel like a new pair.

- Start by stroking each finger in turn, followed by a gentle massage.

- Next stroke and massage the palm of each hand using the thumb of the other. Don't forget the pad of muscle at the base of the thumb; you will be amazed how much better you and your hands feel after a good massage there. It's no coincidence that it's a popular area for acupuncturists to use for all sorts of problems.

Feet

Aching feet are so common. But a good massage can make all the difference, especially in the evening.

- While sitting, put one foot across the opposite thigh and give it a good massage, particularly the sole.

- Pull your toes in turn, spreading and curling them.

- Straighten your leg out and then exercise the ankle by trying to make as big a circle with your toes as you can.

- Finally put a ball (smaller than for the back – a squash ball is perfect) under the sole and then roll it round under your foot so that every part gets a massage.

- Repeat with the other foot.

Face

You may not think of the face as a place to massage but you will be amazed what a difference it can make, especially after a tiring, frustrating day.

- Start with the fingertips of both hands placed on your forehead. Slowly stroke the skin in a circular motion, first across the forehead, round the eyes and ears and down the jaw to round the mouth, finishing with the nose. Start gently, then slowly increase the pressure of your fingertips until you can feel the tension melting away.

- Some people find gently pinching the skin helpful. The best places are the eyebrows – start at the inner edge and work

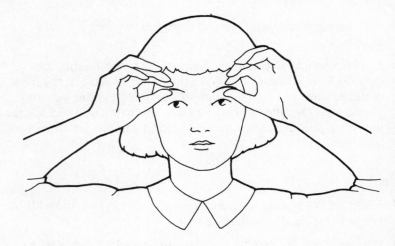

outwards pinching and releasing the skin – and just below the nose.

- Finish with a scalp massage. Start with a gentle stroke of your fingertips and gradually increase the pressure so you get the circulation humming (in your hands too!). Often you will find sore spots which you can massage away.

MEASLES

Measles is a contagious illness caused by a virus. It passes from person to person by droplet infection, usually sneezing or coughing. It causes fever, runny nose, watering eyes, cough and a rash, which often starts on the face and spreads to the rest of the head and body (but not usually the arms or legs). There may also be tiny, white spots inside the mouth. Symptoms start about ten days after you are infected and last for six or seven days. Rare complications include bronchitis, pneumonia and ear infections. Encephalitis develops in one in 5,000 cases. You are most infectious when your symptoms first begin and until about four days after the rash appears.

Self-health

- The key to prevention is the very successful measles vaccine. Using this vaccine the World Health Organization has set a goal of eliminating measles worldwide by the year 2000.

- Children should be vaccinated shortly after their first birthday. There is no point having it done sooner because there will still be anti-measles antibodies from the mother circulating in the child's blood, which will inactivate the vaccine.

- The best method is to combine vaccination against measles, mumps and rubella in one injection, MMR (see separate entry). In future, health authorities will make sure every child has received this vaccine by the time he or she starts school unless there is a specific contra-indication, the parents have refused permission, or the child has already had measles.

- If your child gets measles the illness will last for about one week.

- Painful, red eyes are common, so keep bright lights away and bathe the eyes often, using cottonwool dipped in boiled and cooled water.

- A high temperature will need to be controlled (see **Temperature**), especially if your child has had fits in the past.

- Offer plenty of nourishing drinks; your child may not feel like eating.

- Consult your doctor immediately if you notice your child's breathing becoming fast or difficult or if he or she starts coughing up thick sputum. These may be signs that bronchitis or pneumonia is developing which will need urgent treatment.

MEMORY LOSS

The ability to remember things easily varies greatly from person to person, but in most people it begins to deteriorate after the age of fifty or sixty. Memory for recent names, faces or facts usually gets noticeably worse before we start to forget things from the distant past. The reason is probably that concentration also gets worse as we grow older, and concentration is important for memory. It may also be that older facts have been recalled, both consciously and unconsciously, so often that they cannot fail to be well lodged in the brain.

Self-health

- Keep healthy because this will keep your mind lively.

- Avoid drinking much alcohol (see **Alcoholism**) because alcohol worsens your memory.

- Learn to improve your level of concentration. Repeat facts you need to remember and make a conscious effort to remember them.

- Link something new with another fact you already know, or with a picture or word that will trigger your memory immediately.

- Make lists and write notes for yourself.

- Use modern technology, such as telephones with the numbers you use frequently preprogrammed into them.

- Avoid tiredness because this will affect your memory.

- Research has shown that you are more likely to remember things if you are feeling happy rather than sad.

MENINGITIS

Meningitis is infection or inflammation of the outer layer or lining of the brain and spinal cord (the meninges). It is most commonly due to a virus (e.g. mumps or polio), but may also be caused by the bacterium *neisseria meningococcus*, particularly in epidemics, and by the tuberculosis organism.

The first symptom in an adult are cough, sore throat, feeling unwell, and fever, followed by a very severe headache. The person may begin to vomit, avoid bright lights (photophobia), become delirious or even have a fit. As the condition worsens the patient develops a stiff neck, a spotty rash over the body, and may become unconscious or even die. Occasionally the illness is very sudden and severe with no warning symptoms and a quick deterioration within hours into unconsciousness and death.

Children or babies with meningitis usually have a high temperature, are miserable and irritable and, if old enough, complain of headache. They may shield their eyes from bright lights and hold their necks stiffly. They may vomit or even have a fit. In very small babies the soft spot on top of the skull (the fontanelle) may feel taut and bulging instead of soft, because of the inflammation causing increased pressure on the cerebrospinal fluid within.

Self-health

- The risks of meningitis are greater in small babies and children than in adults, but it is a dangerous illness for everyone.

- The secret of success in preventing death and limiting complications (such as mental handicap or cerebral palsy) is early diagnosis. A doctor should be called immediately if anyone shows the symptoms above, and particularly if they become drowsy or delirious.

- Once the diagnosis has been made the sufferer will be put under close medical supervision. Antibiotics will be given if the cause is bacterial or tuberculosis. No specific treatment is available for viral meningitis but fortunately it is usually the least serious type of meningitis.

- The most serious form of meningitis is meningococcal meningitis which often occurs in epidemics, particularly within closed communities such as schools. No one fully understands why such epidemics occur, and this of course makes prevention difficult. The action of some people in taking their children away from affected schools is quite understandable, therefore. Some doctors also recommend antibiotic treatment for anyone at risk in an effort to kill the bacteria, which live mostly in noses and throats.

- The most effective means of prevention in an area where there is known to be a lot of meningitis is vaccination. This is a single injection of a dead vaccine which causes few side effects. It can safely be taken with other vaccinations and becomes effective seven to ten days later. Ask your doctor for details if you think you may be at risk.

THE MENOPAUSE

Strictly speaking the menopause is a woman's last menstrual period, but the term is more commonly used to describe the two to three years around the last period.

It happens to every woman, usually between the ages of forty and fifty-five although it can happen as early as thirty-five and as late as sixty-five. The average age is fifty and slowly getting older, perhaps because of better nutrition and general health.

The menopause is mainly due to a fall in activity of the female glands, the ovaries, causing a reduction in the amount of hormones (especially oestrogen) they produce. This fall causes the symptoms described below.

Self-health

- Hot flushes (see separate entry) and night sweats affect about two-thirds of menopausal women. The exact cause is unknown but is probably linked to the release of chemicals into the bloodstream at this time. They will disappear, usually within two years. Here are some practical tips:

  1. Wear several layers of light clothing so you can take them off and put them on easily to suit your temperature.
  2. Wear cotton clothes and use cotton sheets. Keep a spare nightdress by your bed in case you need a change.
  3. Avoid alcohol and coffee as far as possible because these tend to cause flushes.
  4. Take a tepid shower when you are feeling uncomfortable. It will cool you down better than a bath.
  5. Keep a solid cologne stick ready at all times, especially if you expect to meet people.
  6. If you are taking medicines for high blood pressure, find out from your doctor whether they may cause hot flushes (as some do). An alternative medicine might make all the difference.
  7. Check in the mirror when you are having a hot flush. It may not be nearly as noticeable to other people as you had imagined.

- One of the effects of the fall in oestrogen levels is to make the lining of the vagina thin and dry, which can result in painful intercourse. Here are some tips:

  1. Continue to make love with your partner. Research has shown that women who do continue to have sex also continue to lubricate their vagina, though they may need help from a lubricant as well.
  2. Use a lubricant like KY jelly which can be bought from the chemist.
  3. Oestrogen cream or hormone replacement therapy (see separate entry) from your doctor help many women. Remember not to use the cream just before sex because it will be absorbed by your partner!
  4. Avoid tight, synthetic clothes which make the vagina prone to infection.

- During the menopause you may find you are prone to urine infections. Take the same precautions as those for cystitis (see separate entry), and you may also find that oestrogen creams or hormone replacement therapy help.

- Osteoporosis (thinning of the bones) may start with the menopause. See **Osteoporosis** and **Hormone Replacement Therapy**.

- Some women put on weight during the menopause. But it is not inevitable and many women only imagine they have put on weight because they feel bloated. However, if you have put on weight see the chapter on Understanding Weight Loss for advice. Bloating is difficult to prevent but avoid large amounts of pulses such as beans and lentils which tend to cause wind.

- Palpitations are common during the menopause, often at the same time as hot flushes. They will disappear within two years in most cases; some women are helped by hormone replacement therapy.

- Depression and anxiety are also common during the menopause. The causes are not fully understood but are probably a combination of chemical changes in the body and because you are going through a difficult time in your life. Not only are your reproductive years coming to an end but changes may be happening at home, for example children leaving. Drugs such as anti-depressants and anxiety medicines are not often helpful at this time. But you will find that as you learn to cope with physical symptoms better and come to realize that there are advantages to the menopause (for example you no longer need to use contraception), the depression and anxiety will lift. Some doctors claim that hormone replacement therapy helps these symptoms.

- Some women experience an unpleasant sensation like ants running all over their body. Again the cause is not fully understood but is probably chemical. Most women do not need treatment and the sensation usually passes within months. Occasionally tranquillizers or hormone replacement therapy are needed.

Screening

- Bleeding after the menopause may be a sign of serious illness and so should never be ignored. The difficulty is knowing when your last period is and so being able to decide that the bleeding is abnormal. However, if you have not bled for six months or more and then have a bleed you should see your doctor immediately.

MIGRAINE

Migraine is a type of headache accompanied usually, but not always, by a regular pattern of other symptoms such as lightheadedness, visual problems like flashing lights, finding bright lights unbearable, seeing zigzags, temporary blindness, nausea or vomiting. The headache usually starts on one side but often spreads to the whole head. The whole episode may last from a few minutes to two or three days.

Migraine affects about one in ten people and affects three times more women than men. It can affect children, so parents should be aware of this possibility. It very rarely starts after the age of forty and often gets better, even disappears, by middle age.

Self-health

- Consider your lifestyle carefully because stress may bring on migraine, often during the relaxation period afterwards (e.g. at weekends or holidays). Learn to avoid or cope with stress (see chapter on Stress and Mental Health). Some people find meditation or relaxation exercises help.

- Certain foods – cheese, chocolate and red wine particularly – bring on migraine. By a process of elimination you should be able to pinpoint whether a food is causing the problem. Some experts believe the Pill may cause migraine. If you are on the Pill discuss with your doctor whether you should use an alternative contraceptive method.

- Even if you cannot identify the cause of your migraines, you can often prevent the attack becoming unbearable. As soon as your warning symptoms start take two painkillers (e.g. aspirin, paracetamol, codeine or specific anti-migraine tablets) and go to bed in a darkened, quiet room. Every minute counts so do not waste time hoping the attack will go of its own accord.

- If your attacks are frequent and severe, or if you cannot prevent them yourself, see your doctor. There are anti-migraine medicines which, if taken regularly regardless of whether you have an attack, can prevent attacks happening.

MISCARRIAGE

A miscarriage is the natural loss of a fetus before it is old enough to survive outside the womb – twenty-eight weeks is the legal age at the moment (after twenty-eight weeks it is a stillbirth). Doctors call it a spontaneous abortion.

As many as eight out of ten conceptions are lost spontaneously shortly after conception, though no one knows why this happens to humans more than any other species. It may be that the mother's body is better equipped than other species to detect abnormalities and imperfections at an early stage. As many as one out of five confirmed pregnancies are also lost, some women being more prone than others.

Self-health

- When you are trying to become pregnant eat a healthy diet, get plenty of sleep and avoid stress, too much alcohol and smoking. There is no absolute proof that this will lessen your chance of a miscarriage but it is common sense to stay as healthy as possible.

- Avoid genital infections, especially herpes and gonorrhoea (see separate entries) because they may make you more prone to miscarriage.

- There is no evidence that strenuous exercise, jumping, falling or intercourse increases your chances of a miscarriage. However, it makes sense not to take anything to extremes, especially if you have had a miscarriage previously.

- A nasty shock or fright may be linked with miscarriage but there is usually little you can do to prevent these unexpected emotions.

- One in five miscarriages is due to cervical problems. The most common cause is known as cervical incompetence, when the cervix is too loose to hold the fetus in the womb. Most cases happen for no known reason but occasionally an abortion may cause cervical incompetence. The best way to prevent it is by closing the cervix with surgical stitches. Your gynaecologist will usually do this in about the fourteenth week of your pregnancy, or earlier if you have previously miscarried before this time. The stitches are removed at about thirty-eight weeks or earlier if labour begins.

- If you start bleeding from the vagina during early pregnancy with or without cramps (threatened miscarriage) you should go to bed immediately and call your doctor, who will probably examine you to decide whether the mouth of your cervix is opened or closed. If it is open you will usually be sent directly to hospital, because miscarriage is then probably inevitable. Try not to be too sad because this may be nature's way of preventing you having a very abnormal baby.

  If your cervix is closed you will be advised to stay in bed until twenty-four hours after the bleeding has stopped and to avoid sex for a few days.

- If you experience pain and contractions later in your pregnancy when your baby could survive it is called premature labour and occurs for a different reason. Rather than ridding itself of an abnormal baby, the body has mistimed delivery. In addition to bed-rest there are medicines which can reduce the premature contractions and help prevent an early delivery.

- If you are young and have had one miscarriage it is probably not worth investigating the cause. If you have three consecutive miscarriages this is known as habitual miscarriage and your doctor will wish to investigate you to discover whether there is anything that can be done to prevent you miscarrying. These tests might include:

1. Genetic studies of you and your partner's family to see whether there is a genetic problem.

2. Hormone studies to decide whether a lack of hormones may be the cause. Appropriate hormones could then be given during your next pregnancy.
3. A tiny piece of the lining of the womb may be taken for examination under a microscope to make sure it is reacting correctly.
4. A special X-ray of the womb and tubes (hystero-salpingogram) may show anatomical problems which could be corrected surgically.

- Do not worry excessively, even if you tend to miscarry easily. Research has shown that you still have a seventy to eighty per cent chance of a successful pregnancy even if you have had three consecutive miscarriages. It seems the body gradually learns how to control all the different stages of pregnancy.

- If you are over thirty-five, have never had a baby, and have a miscarriage it may be worth starting investigations earlier. Stories about the reduced fertility of older women have been greatly exaggerated but the fact is you have less time to get things right.

MITES

Some people are allergic to tiny insects called mites living in house dust. This allergy may cause a runny nose and streaming eyes (see **Allergic Rhinitis**), or even asthma. Symptoms can be made less severe by reducing the number of mites you have in your house.

Self-health

- Keep your house dust-free. Hoover frequently, and try not to have objects on floors round which dust can collect.

- Replace natural-fibre carpets with synthetic carpets.

- Foam mattresses are less likely to encourage mites. If you want to keep a mattress made of materials other than foam, iron it (to kill the mites) and cover with a plastic mattress cover.

- Use duvets and pillows made from synthetic materials.

- Dry dusting may simply spread the mites around, so use a damp mop.

MMR VACCINE

MMR vaccine is a combined measles/mumps/rubella vaccine. It should be given to all children (with a few exceptions, see below) preferably shortly after their first birthday and certainly by the age of five.

Nasty reactions to the vaccine can occur but are minimal when compared with the seriousness of the diseases themselves:

1. The most common reaction is feeling unwell for one or two days, with or without fever, five to ten days after vaccination. Treat with paracetamol.
2. Very occasionally, fits may occur, especially if your child has another infection which was not noticed before vaccination. If, however, your child (aged one to two) did not have the vaccine and caught measles he or she would have an eight to ten times greater chance of having a fit in the course of the illness. Prevent fits by keeping your child's temperature down (see **Fits**).
3. Encephalitis can, very rarely, follow vaccination, but, like fits, your child is much more likely to get encephalitis if he or she catches measles.

A few people should not have the vaccine:

1. Any child with a fever – the vaccination can be given a few days later.
2. Pregnant women.
3. Anyone receiving anti-cancer treatment such as steroids, drugs or irradiation.
4. Anyone allergic to the antibiotics neomycin or polymyxin. Allergy to eggs is no longer a reason for not having the vaccine unless you have a very serious reaction (anaphylaxis) to them. Dislike of eggs or allergy to chicken feathers is not a contra-indication.
5. Anyone who has had another live vaccine less than three weeks previously.

MULTIPLE SCLEROSIS

Multiple sclerosis (MS) affects the nerves of the brain and spinal cord. The disease attacks a sheath called myelin, which surrounds the nerves like insulation round an electric wire. The resulting damage prevents the nerves conveying messages as they should.

MS affects about one in 1,600 of the population, usually those aged twenty to forty, and more women than men. Symptoms vary enormously as does their severity. Some last just a few seconds, others get steadily worse and worse. Some people have just a single attack, others have a few over the years, others may suffer a new attack every month. The most common symptoms are tingling and numbness of the fingers or feet, weakness, unsteadiness, blurred vision, difficulty speaking, difficulty passing water or incontinence.

Self-health

- The cause is still unknown so specific prevention (e.g. a vaccine) is impossible. The illness does run in families but to such a limited extent that there is no value in isolating or avoiding people with MS.

- It seems there is no genetic risk. Certainly an identical twin of someone with MS is no more likely to get it than anyone else.

- Once the diagnosis has been made there are positive steps you can take to help yourself and slow the development of the condition.

  1. Come to terms with the illness and accept that MS is something you may have to live with for the rest of your life.
  2. Involve your family and enlist their support. MS may put a strain on you all but early understanding and explanation will help.
  3. Get all the professional help that is available. This may include your family doctor, practice nurse, incontinence adviser, occupational therapist, hospital physiotherapy department, social services department, home help service, meals-on-wheels, day centres, luncheon clubs, and social

clubs. Your house, lavatory, bathroom, kitchen, telephone, television, radio may all need adaption to suit you, depending on the severity of your symptoms. Parking discs will help convenient parking.

- Some people claim to have benefited from special diets (e.g. evening primrose oil or sunflower seed oil) but there is no scientific proof that they either prevent MS or improve symptoms. Equally, though, they appear harmless. Steroid medicines and high-concentration (hyperbaric) oxygen have also been tried but there is no scientific proof that they work and they can have unpleasant side effects.

MUMPS

Mumps is caused by a virus and is caught by contact with an infected person. Symptoms develop fifteen to twenty-one days later and include swelling of the salivary glands just in front of the ear and round the angle of the jaw, fever, feeling unwell, earache, and pain on swallowing.

Mumps is generally a mild illness lasting about a week but occasionally it can be more serious (causing about 1,200 hospital admissions each year in England and Wales). It is the most common cause of viral meningitis (see separate entry) under the age of fifteen. It can cause permanent deafness, and occasionally it can cause pancreatitis (see separate entry). If you are male you may notice pain and/or swelling of one or both testes; this usually disappears within about a week without further problems. Very rarely mumps may reduce the number of sperm you produce and therefore your fertility.

Self-health

- The MMR vaccine (see separate entry) is the best protection you or your children can have. In the USA it has been routinely used for over twenty years and has caused a dramatic fall in the number of people getting mumps and associated serious complications.

- Keep away from crowded places (e.g. buses and swimming pools) if you know there is a local epidemic of mumps.

- Mumps is infectious from about six days before the glands swell until about two weeks afterwards. Limiting the spread of infection before symptoms appear is clearly impossible but afterwards you should keep your child at home. Mumps is so infectious, though, that there is little advantage in confining your child to one room and you must expect anyone within the household who has not already had mumps or the vaccination to get it.

- Treat mumps with paracetamol to prevent a rise in temperature and to ease symptoms. If any of the more serious problems described above develop see your doctor.

MUSCULAR DYSTROPHY

Muscular dystrophy is a gradual wasting disease of muscle, which affects children. There are many different types but the outcome for most sufferers is poor, most dying by the age of twenty to twenty-five. The most common form is Duchenne muscular dystrophy, which affects about one in 4,000 boys — usually, but not always, from affected families.

Self-health

- If anyone in your family has had muscular dystrophy you should seek genetic counselling from a doctor before starting a family. Research has found the exact spot where diseased muscle cells differ from healthy cells but it is still not possible to change affected people's genes so they do not pass the disease on to their children.

- If a woman 'carrier' of the disease decides to have a baby and it is male it will have a fifty per cent chance of being affected. However, she can have amniocentesis (in the seventeenth or eighteenth week of pregnancy), or chorionic villus biopsy in the ten to twelfth week, to find out the sex of the fetus and then, if it is male, she will be offered an abortion if she wishes it.

MYALGIC ENCEPHALOMYELITIS (ME)

Myalgic encephalomyelitis (ME) is a new illness which has gradually become recognized over the last five years. It is a mysterious illness with many names, including ME, post-viral fatigue syndrome and, in the USA, chronic fatigue syndrome. It is estimated that about one in 1,000 people are affected.

ME is not a single disease with a specific cause, nor is there an effective cure. It is a collection of symptoms which, put together, have a similar pattern.

Most people first have a flu-like illness which seems to last longer than usual and from which they never seem to recover fully. This is followed by a feeling of exhaustion totally out of proportion to any effort made, worse after exercise. Later, muscle weakness and pain may develop, as well as blurred vision, poor concentration and memory, depression, moodiness, strange sweats and poor circulation, palpitations, headaches, distended stomach and difficulty sleeping.

The course of the illness varies greatly from person to person. Some people recover completely, others cope with help from friends and relatives, a few are permanently confined to a wheelchair. Because there is no known cause there is no cure. Some experts think it may be due to viruses, others suggest changes in the immunity system, or the bacterium *candida* or food allergies (see **Allergy, Food**), or even psychiatric problems.

Self-health

- In the early days every sufferer has difficulty persuading themselves and their carers that they have a specific illness – ME. This is made worse because there is no single test that will diagnose it and many doctors still do not recognize it. However, accepting the disease is a vital part of learning to live with it particularly as so little can be done by professionals and so much by you and your carers.

- It is vital you learn what your limits are and how not to exhaust yourself. Avoid unnecessary exertion or exercise. Organize your time well. It may even be necessary to give up or change your job.

- Eat a healthy diet containing plenty of protein, vitamins, and minerals. Carbohydrates are useful for giving you energy but make sure you eat complex, unrefined ones so you avoid high peaks followed by low levels of sugar in your blood.

- The question of whether you should take nutritional supplements (e.g. essential fatty acids such as evening primrose oil) is controversial. You should consult a sympathetic doctor first.

- If you think food or chemical allergies may be a cause you should consult a dietary expert before making any radical changes to your diet.

- Get plenty of sleep and think positively of this sleep as useful treatment rather than wasted time. Some people need as much as twelve to fourteen hours of sleep a day.

- Conserve your energy at home:
  1. Have your bedroom and bathroom on the same floor.
  2. Sit while cooking or ironing.
  3. Use modern aids (see **Gadgets for Disabled and Elderly People**) in the kitchen and bathroom, and for gadgets such as the telephone and TV.
  4. Use bed-baths or 'all-over' washes in warm bedrooms or bathrooms instead of having baths or showers which may be tiring.

Tips for carers of people with ME

1. You must believe in ME as a specific illness like any other, which needs its own treatment and care.
2. You cannot catch ME like measles or chickenpox so do not worry about close contact. Be patient and compassionate with your relative or friend. The sufferer will experience great mood swings so you must learn not to take them to heart.
3. Be aware of the limitations on your patient's behaviour, and be prepared to step in if he or she is beginning to go beyond them.
4. Learn to live a life of your own while still providing the emotional and physical support the ME sufferer needs.
5. Be prepared to get the help of the family doctor, local hospital or social services if you are no longer able to cope.

- You may find sex exhausting. If so, try new positions or early in the day when you are less tired. Many people find just holding and caressing each other very satisfying.

- You cannot give your child ME so there is no reason why you should not have children, providing your doctor has no medical reasons against it.

- Some doctors have found the use of medicines called monoamine oxidase inhibitors helpful, so discuss the possibility of this treatment with the doctor who is looking after you.

MYXOEDEMA

Myxoedema is a disease caused by a shortage of thyroid hormones. Since these hormones are necessary for good health, their lack leads to loss of energy and intolerance to cold. Dry, thin hair is common, and a thickened, coarse skin, constipation, slow speech and thought. If neglected, myxoedema can lead to death (myxoedema coma).

Self-health

- Apart from recognizing the symptoms and seeing your doctor there is nothing you can do to prevent myxoedema.

- Your doctor will probably prescribe thyroxine tablets to replace your own absent hormones and prevent symptoms occurring. These will need to be taken regularly and usually for life.

- In case of an accident, always carry a card (or a piece of jewellery, such as a bracelet) stating your dose of thyroxine.

N

NAILS, BITING

Nail-biting in both adults and children is usually a sign of underlying anxiety, boredom, excitement or insecurity. It makes the hands look unattractive, and may damage the nails and make you more prone to infections (e.g. paronychia, see separate entry).

Self-health

- Try to discover whether there is an underlying problem and, if so, what it is.
- Keep hands occupied, e.g. sewing, knitting, playing sports or enjoying hobbies.
- Teach your children to look after their nails properly.
- As a last resort there are proprietory products available from chemists. These are painted on to the nails and, because of their nasty taste, discourage nail-biting.

NAILS, CARE OF

The main purpose of fingernails is to protect the sensitive tips of the fingers. This allows us to concentrate on the pad of the finger for maximum sense of touch. Nail is mostly made of keratin, which also makes up much of our hair and skin. Nails grow slowly – from base to tip takes about six months.

Self-health

- Look after your nails and they will stay healthy.

1. Use rubber gloves to prevent prolonged contact with water, especially soapy water. Dry thoroughly afterwards and use a moisturizer if necessary.
2. Trim nails regularly, preferably after a bath when they are soft.
3. Avoid damaging the cuticle by too frequent or careless manicuring. Use only a cuticle stick or your thumbnail to push the cuticle back, again preferably after a bath.

- **Brittle nails**. The cause is uncertain but you may be able to prevent them by:

1. Seeing your family doctor if you think you may have a blood circulation problem with your hands or if you have psoriasis (see separate entry).
2. Use nail-hardeners. But if your nails have a tendency to loosen quickly beware of hardeners containing formaldehyde.
3. Consider taking zinc supplements (up to 20 mg a day) and eating more iron-rich foods (see **Iron**).

- **Ridged nails**. These may be caused by illness, damage to the nail bed, or shortage of zinc, or they may simply be a family characteristic.

1. Consider taking zinc supplements (up to 20 mg a day).
2. Once or twice a week buff the surface of your nails to smooth it. Also try a three-strength sloughing and buffing file.
3. Use a commercial ridge filler before applying polish.

- **Flaking, splitting or chipping nails**. Dry nails, or incorrect filing or shaping may be the problem.

1. Wear gloves when washing up. Moisturize daily with hand cream or special cuticle cream (even when wearing polish).
2. Use nail-hardener.
3. Use oily-based polish remover rather than suffering the drying effect of acetone-based ones. Leave polish on for longer (e.g. one week), retouching when necessary.
4. Use a pencil to dial the telephone.
5. File nails in one direction only. Don't shape nails into a point because filing down the sides will weaken them. Cut long nails; don't try filing them down.

- **Yellow nails**. Orange or red nail polish may stain nails. Nicotine and chlorine from swimming pools are other causes.

  1. Nails can be whitened by soaking them in lemon juice for a few minutes.
  2. Use pale polishes rather than orange or red.
  3. Try a base coat under the polish to protect the nail.
  4. Use a slougher or buffer designed for ridge removal. Some salons have electric buffers for stain removal. Be cautious with both methods.

- **White marks**. These may be due to minor damage to the cuticle. Zinc deficiency has also been suggested.

  1. Consider taking zinc supplements (up to 20 mg daily).
  2. Don't worry, these harmless spots will grow out.

NAPPY RASH

Nappy rash is reddened skin in the baby's nappy area. Sometimes it gets worse and painful, pussy spots or raw, ulcerated skin develops. It is usually due to bacteria in the baby's stools breaking down urine collected by the nappy. The urine then releases ammonia, a strong skin irritant.

Self-health

- Change your baby's nappies often. Try not to leave your baby in a wet or soiled nappy for long.

- Wash your baby's bottom frequently – especially after a soiled nappy. Dry thoroughly and then apply a barrier cream (e.g. zinc oxide).

- If practical, leave your baby without a nappy for as long as possible.

- If possible use disposable nappies, since they are less likely to encourage nappy rash than towelling ones. If your baby still develops a rash, change to another brand.

- If your baby continues to suffer with nappy rash despite using disposable nappies, then change to towelling ones and use a one-way fabric nappy liner (avoid paper ones which often make the rash worse). After use, soak the towelling nappies in a sterilizing solution before washing and rinse thoroughly afterwards to remove soap and detergent. Try not to use plastic pants because they stop air circulating round your baby's bottom.

- If the rash starts at the anus and spreads outwards it may be caused by thrush (see separate entry). If your baby also has white patches inside the mouth which are difficult to rub away with a handkerchief or leave raw, ulcerated areas, this makes the diagnosis of thrush more likely. See your doctor immediately for treatment.

NAUSEA

Nausea is the sensation that you are just about to vomit. It is a symptom of many different types of illness so you normally need to treat the illness first before the nausea will disappear. See also **Vomiting, Pregnancy**

Self-health

- All of us feel sick from time to time and often we never discover the cause. At such times it is sensible to rest and to avoid food and alcohol. After a few hours the feeling passes and we can carry on as normal. However, if the sensation persists or recurs often, particularly if you also notice other symptoms such as weight loss, feeling unwell, pain, constipation or diarrhoea, you must see your doctor immediately.

- There are medicines (available from chemists and on prescription) which can prevent nausea. Generally they work best for specific causes of nausea (e.g. travel sickness). They should not be used often to prevent a feeling of nausea for which you have no explanation, since the nausea may be a warning that something is wrong with your body.

NECK PAIN

Neck pain affects old and young people alike. It may be caused
by several different structures – joints, muscles, and nerves.
Some people with arthritis in their joints suffer from neck pain
as part of their condition but most problems are not truly
arthritic.

In young people it is usually due to one or more of the joints of
the neck moving out of position, causing irritation of the nerves
and muscles nearby.

In older people it is usually due to soreness and inflammation
in worn joints of the neck, sometimes known as cervical
spondylosis.

Self-health

- A 'cricked' neck affects young people mostly and usually gets
  better of its own accord within a week or so. There are several
  things you can do to speed recovery and ease the pain.

  1. Warmth from a heat lamp or covered hot-water bottle helps.
  2. Take a painkiller such as aspirin or paracetamol.
  3. Wrap your neck during the daytime in a thick scarf or towel
     to rest it and limit movement.
  4. Stand and sit upright, looking straight ahead if possible.

- Cervical spondylosis tends to affect older people. Symptoms
  come and go but below are some ways of helping yourself.

  1. Sleep on a firm mattress with only one pillow. Try not to
     sleep on your stomach with your hands above your head.
  2. Make sure your car seat is the right height so you don't
     have to strain to see when driving. Also make sure the
     headrest on the back of your seat is correctly positioned
     and your seat belts can be easily reached without twisting
     violently.
  3. Don't make sharp neck or arm movements.
  4. Don't read or watch TV partly lying down with your head
     and neck bent forward. Avoid chairs without armrests.
  5. Try not to lift heavy weights, but, if you do have to, hold
     them equally balanced between each arm.
  6. Take regular exercise.

7. Try to avoid stress and tension (see chapter on Stress and Mental Health), which can tighten the muscles of your neck and shoulders, making you more prone to neck pains.

NIGHTMARES

A nightmare is an unpleasant dream from which you (or more commonly your child) awake feeling frightened and upset.

Self-health

- If your child has a temperature give him or her a medicine (e.g. paracetamol) before going to bed to bring the temperature down, because high temperatures are common causes of nightmares.

- Avoid letting your child get overtired because he or she may well wake having a nightmare after one or two hours of sleep.

- Beware of television programmes or bedtime stories that may frighten your child.

- Consider whether your child dislikes the dark or hates being alone in his or her room.

- Anxiety about going to school, the arrival of a new baby, or moving home may be the cause of nightmares. Take time to reassure your child about these events.

- Never allow a child to suffer a nightmare alone because this will make the problem worse and may cause the child to fear falling asleep. Hurry to your child, turn the lights on, cuddle and speak gently to him or her. Usually you should be able to persuade the child to go back to sleep. Don't try to discover the problem there and then, but next day you may wish to question your child gently to discover underlying anxieties.

- If nightmares become daily occurrences see your family doctor.

NOSEBLEED

Most nosebleeds happen for no apparent reason but some are caused by damage to the lining of the nose (colds), blowing your nose too hard, picking your nose, injuries to the nose or head, blood disorders, and raised blood pressure.

Self-health

- Avoid picking your nose or putting objects up it.

- Blow your nose gently. For advice see **Nose, Stuffy**.

- As soon as the bleeding starts sit down with your head forward so that the blood does not go down your throat. Pinch the soft part of the nose (not the bone) between your fingers. Breathe through the mouth. After about fifteen minutes release the nose and sit quietly for a few minutes. In most cases bleeding will have stopped. If not, squeeze the nose again for a further fifteen minutes. Sometimes applying an ice-pack (e.g. a small pack of frozen peas) also helps.

- If the bleeding is so bad it makes you feel dizzy and weak, or squeezing your nose for thirty minutes has not worked, see your doctor.

Screening

- If you are young and have more than two or three nosebleeds for no apparent reason you should see your family doctor, who may want to test you for blood disorders such as haemophilia or thrombocytopenia.

- If you are over thirty and have unexplained nosebleeds, see your family doctor, who may wish to check that your blood pressure is not raised.

NOSE, STUFFY

There are many causes of a stuffy nose. Infants and children up to the age of about eight suffer particularly from colds, and there are many irritants (such as pollen and animal fur) which can cause allergic rhinitis, or hayfever (see separate entries).

Self-health

- For preventive steps you can take against colds, allergic rhinitis and hayfever see separate entries.
- To unblock a stuffy nose and prevent it recurring there are several things you can do.

  1. Preparations (often containing menthol) can be bought at the chemist which, when dissolved in hot water and breathed up through the nose (steam inhalation) will help to unblock stuffy noses and prevent the symptoms returning.
  2. There are also other medicines (decongestants), available from the chemist as tablets, sprays or drops, which dry out the inflamed lining of the nose and help clear and prevent stuffy noses. Never take more than the recommended dose of these nasal decongestants and use them sparingly, because over-use can lead to a 'rebound effect' in which the lining of the nose reacts to the medicine by producing more, not less, mucus. Over-use can also damage and scar the lining of the nose permanently, making the problem worse.

- Beware of trying too hard to blow your nose if both nostrils are completely blocked. This may force air and germs, which cannot escape along the Eustachian tube, to the middle ear, causing an infection or, in bad cases, a ruptured eardrum. Instead try the medicines mentioned above or gently unblock one nostril at a time.

OBSESSIONS

An obsession is an activity or thought which grips you out of all proportion to its worth. It may be harmless (like always walking on one side of the street) but it may also become so strong that it interferes seriously with your lifestyle.

An obsession may start as an interest in something like religion, safety, personal cleanliness or politics. Gradually you may start to brood about it until eventually you can think of little else.

Self-health

- Do not worry about minor obsessions provided they do not interfere with the person's lifestyle.

- Occasionally the development of a serious obsession can be prevented by someone close noticing and patiently talking the person out of it.

- In most cases the development of an obsession is not rational and does not respond to good sense. A professional such as a family doctor or psychiatrist will need to be consulted and even they are often not successful.

ORGASM, LACK OF, FEMALE

Female orgasm is the feeling of intense pleasure due to the release of pelvic congestion and muscle tension which is usually the 'climax' of a sexual experience. In the past it was believed there were two types of orgasm – the 'vaginal' orgasm and the 'clitoral' orgasm but since the work of the Americans Masters and Johnson it seems there is probably just the one clitoral orgasm accompanied by the rhythmical contraction of the vagina, surrounding tissues and uterus. Though not everyone agrees with Masters and Johnson all are agreed that there is a huge range and variety of orgasm and that all are good whatever the method of achieving it.

For some women, orgasm may be an intense experience lasting just a few seconds. For others it may be a plateau of pleasure lasting minutes. Some find it so intense they do not want it repeated immediately, others enjoy continued stimulation and 'multiple orgasms' with just a few seconds or minutes in between. On average women take about fifteen minutes to reach orgasm – longer than men – and this time does not increase with age (unlike men).

Self-health

- Many women do not have an orgasm during every sexual experience. Statistics show that only one in three regularly reaches orgasm through sexual intercourse. The remainder need extra stimulation (e.g. of the clitoris) and as many as five to ten per cent never have an orgasm (even during masturbation). So, experienced women do not need to feel deprived if they do not have an orgasm after every sexual experience, provided the experience is happy and pleasurable. Problems and frustrations may arise, however, if orgasm is rare or non-existent.

- If you are dissatisfied with how often or how easily you have an orgasm, the first step is to have a frank talk with your partner. This may reveal all sorts of underlying anxieties, or that poor sexual technique or pain is making orgasm impossible (see **Sex, Painful, Female**).

- Anxieties can sometimes be resolved by the partners themselves but deep-seated prejudices (e.g. believing sex is shameful or dirty) will need professional help.

- Poor sexual technique may result from ignorance, inexperience or lack of care and consideration (see **Sex, Good**). Here are some tips:

  1. There are plenty of good sex manuals now which can help you overcome ignorance, but remember, just because a

book says a technique will be enjoyable does not always mean it will suit you both. One person's turn-on may be another's turn-off.

2. Books alone cannot make you a good lover so you will need to practise. You may even need to forget all you have practised in the past and start afresh. You may not be very successful to start with but gradually you will get better and in time you will have a mutually satisfying relationship.

3. Books cannot teach care and consideration within a sexual relationship, and nothing is more likely to prevent you having an orgasm than the knowledge that your partner has no interest in your pleasure, only his. So, pick your partner well and keep communicating.

- Do not worry if you are one of the women who does not have an orgasm despite skilful and loving intercourse. Instead experiment with alternatives like masturbation or vibrators, which may bring you satisfaction.

- Many couples try very hard to make sure both partners 'come' at the same moment. This is fine but do not worry if you cannot manage it. In fact many experienced couples believe they can double their pleasure by having their orgasms separately since each can enjoy their partner's orgasm to the full before or after their own. Remember, though, it will normally need to be the woman who climaxes first because most men cannot maintain an erection for long after ejaculation. Boys aged fifteen to twenty may be able to regain their erection within a minute or so but this ability gradually declines over the years so that, on average, men aged fifty and over take about twelve hours.

ORGASM, LACK OF, MALE

The male orgasm is a feeling of intense pleasure accompanied by the ejaculation of semen, which is usually the 'climax' of a sexual experience. Most men can reach orgasm within three minutes and failure to have an orgasm is very rare. Indeed, quite the reverse, the most common sexual difficulty is having an orgasm too quickly (see **Ejaculation, Premature**).

Self-health

- The main cause of failure to have an orgasm is failure of erection (see separate entry).

- Failure of orgasm does not mean you are infertile. In these special circumstances your semen can be harvested by specialist doctors for implantation (insemination) into your wife, and many babies have been successfully conceived in this way.

OSTEOARTHRITIS

Osteoarthritis is the medical term for wear and tear in the joint. Some people are more prone to it than others. There is nothing you can do to prevent it, but there are some measures you can take to slow the speed at which it develops.

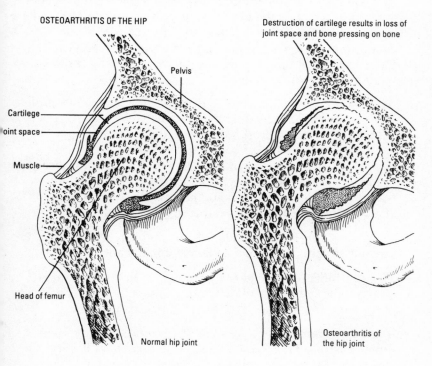

OSTEOARTHRITIS OF THE HIP

Destruction of cartilege results in loss of joint space and bone pressing on bone

Pelvis

Cartilege

oint space

Muscle

Head of femur

Normal hip joint

Osteoarthritis of the hip joint

OSTEOARTHRITIS OF THE HIP

Symptoms include pain, often at night, and stiffness, usually in the morning. Later the joint may become fixed in one position, often flexed forward a little.

OSTEOARTHRITIS OF THE KNEE

Symptoms include pain, swelling, and difficulty bending and straightening the knee.

Self-health

- Try not to become overweight because the more weight you put on the joint, the more you strain it.

- Keep as mobile as you can. Research has shown that gentle exercise slows the destruction of cartilage coating the ends of the bones (which is the main problem in osteoarthritis), and may even stimulate the cartilage to grow again. The best exercises are non-weight-bearing, e.g. swimming and cycling. If the arthritis becomes more serious hydrotherapy (exercise in warm water) is often helpful.

- Be certain to use the correct equipment for sport, for example well-padded running shoes. If you know you have arthritis in your hips or knees you should avoid distance running completely, especially on roads. Never put a great strain on your hips or knees (e.g. gymnastics) without training correctly, preferably under the supervision of a qualified coach. Always warm up before a vigorous sport and gently 'warm down' afterwards with stretching exercises.

- Sadly, avoiding certain foods has not yet been proven to prevent arthritis, despite the claims of many enthusiasts.

- The anti-inflammatory tablets your doctor may give you will help relieve symptoms of pain and stiffness but none have yet been found to have any effect on the arthritis itself.

- In the end your doctor may suggest you have a hip or knee replacement. Do not fear this operation because it is very successful for most people and is one of the great medical advances of the last twenty years. Take heed when the surgeon tells you how much you can do afterwards. Do not imagine you will have the same flexibility as when you were younger because the replacement is prone to work loose if you overuse it. But you will be pleasantly surprised with how much you can do and delighted by the relief from pain.

OSTEOPATHY

Osteopathy is a system of healing based upon manipulating the back. It was founded by the American Andrew Taylor Still (1828–1917), an orthodox doctor, who found that illnesses could often be traced to a defect or distortion of the spine. In this sense osteopathy is similar to chiropractic (see separate entry), although the techniques of manipulation are different.

There are two osteopathic schools of thought. One believes in the concept of holistic osteopathy, in which manipulation is just one of many adjustments necessary to restore good health. The other school takes a more limited view, using osteopathy as a valuable method of treating backs and joints that have been 'put out'.

Self-health

- Manipulation is an important part of treatment. See **Chiropractic** for advice about its uses and risks because they also apply to osteopathy.

- You should avoid untrained osteopaths. For further information about training and a register of osteopaths contact British School of Osteopathy, 1–4 Suffolk Place, London, SW1 4HG.

OSTEOPOROSIS

Bone is a living substance that is continually being removed and replaced. When the amount removed by bone breakdown cells is greater than the amount produced by bone repair cells, bones become more fragile and likely to break. The bone is still normal but there is less of it, so the skeleton is weaker. This condition is known as osteoporosis.

What happens is that the narrow cavity inside the long bones of the arms and legs becomes larger and the outer tube of tough, dense bone becomes thinner, so that these bones are more likely to break. In some people the spongy bone in the front part of the spine – the vertebrae – also gets weaker, and is more likely to be damaged. The spine then curves forwards. This is why very old people shrink and often have very curved spines and hunched backs.

Women are much more at risk than men and at an earlier age. This is because they lose the benefits of oestrogen after the menopause and they have lighter bones anyway. For the same reason small, thin, lighter women are more at risk than women with heavier frames.

White people are more likely to get osteoporosis than black people although no one knows why. One in every four white women has broken a wrist or hip bone or suffered a crush fracture of the spine by the age of sixty-five, and half of all women have had a fracture by the age of seventy-five.

The earlier the menopause occurs, the greater the risk. Young women whose ovaries have been removed surgically (usually at hysterectomy) and young women who have never had periods or who have had anorexia nervosa are at risk of osteoporosis.

Female athletes and dancers who exercise so strenuously that they stop having periods are at risk.

Women who have had children seem to have more protection against osteoporosis than those who have not.

The contraceptive pill, which contains oestrogen, may offer some protection against osteoporosis. Unfortunately, most people do not know they have the condition until they break a bone later in life. Osteoporosis is a silent disease, with few outward signs. You should suspect osteoporosis if you are losing height, and there are tests that your doctor can arrange if he or she suspects your bones are at risk.

Self-health

- The best protection against osteoporosis is having a strong, heavy skeleton. So it is important to make sure that children, especially girls, build good bones while they are growing. Calcium is very important for healthy bones. You should eat plenty throughout life, especially during childhood and

adolescence. If you are on a special slimming diet make sure
you are getting enough calcium. The best sources are dairy
products, because the body finds the calcium contained in
them easy to absorb, but it is possible to get adequate calcium
from other sources, including calcium supplements. If you
suspect you are not getting enough calcium ask your doctor for
advice.

- Take regular exercise. Exercise accelerates the flow of blood to
the bones, increasing the supply of essential substances
needed for bone-building.
    Remember, though, if your training is so hard that it stops
your periods, you will be at risk of getting osteoporosis.

- Drink alcohol only in moderation. Heavy drinkers have
abnormally light bones that break easily. Alcohol also prevents
calcium being absorbed into the body.

- Do not smoke. Smokers are more likely to be underweight than
non-smokers and pregnant mothers who smoke have smaller
babies. Oestrogen levels are lower in smokers too, and they
have the menopause at an earlier age.

- For women who have already reached the menopause and
suspect that they may be at risk from osteoporosis it is not too
late to do something about it. You can of course start taking
regular, gentle exercise, and you should increase the amount
of calcium in your diet, perhaps checking with your doctor on
the question of calcium supplements. At this stage, however,
such measures may not be enough to prevent fractures later
on.
    The only treatment that has been shown conclusively to
prevent bone loss after the menopause is hormone
replacement therapy (see separate entry). Doctors are finding
sixty per cent fewer fractures of the hip and wrist among older
women who started low-dose HRT within a few years of the
menopause.

- Osteoporosis affects many people, particularly women after
the menopause. But with the help of a diet rich in calcium,
regular exercise, sensible precautions and HRT if necessary, it
can be prevented and you can live a long and healthy life.

P

PAIN

Pain is a sensation known to all of us. It is usually caused by injury to the body tissues. Its function is to act as a warning that something may be wrong and to encourage the sufferer to stop doing whatever it is that causes the pain.

The location and type of pain may help make it possible to diagnose the cause. However, there are three circumstances which can cause confusion:

1. Pain may spread from its source to a wider area. For example, people suffering from angina often feel pain down the left hand as far as the fingers, or a slipped disc may cause pain down the back of the leg as far as the foot.
2. Pain from an injured or diseased organ may appear in a quite different part of the body. For example, inflammation of the gallbladder or lung may cause pain at the shoulder tip. Or arthritis of the hip may cause pain in the knee. This type of pain is often called referred pain.
3. Everyone has different thresholds of pain, so some people find a pinprick very painful while others hardly notice it. These different levels of appreciating pain have nothing to do with the sensitivity of the skin, but are probably controlled by levels of a chemical called endorphin in the brain. Low levels result in a low threshold of appreciating pain; high levels cause the opposite. Most strong painkillers probably work by raising the levels of endorphin in the brain. Redhaired people are said to have low levels and therefore a low threshold of pain.

Self-health

- Once present, pain should never be ignored. Take notice of the warning. As a general rule pain should not be treated until the cause is known. Clearly this is not always practical (e.g. with a headache) but the same pain repeated three or four times within a few days should be investigated.

- Once the cause of pain has been found there are many different ways its return can be prevented or its effect reduced:

  1. Eat a healthy diet and exercise as best you can within your limitations. You will be in a better position to resist pain.
  2. Take a positive attitude to your pain, illness and life. Such an attitude probably raises the levels of endorphins in the brain and makes you less susceptible to pain. Enjoying a happy home life, hobbies and friends has a similar effect.
  3. Painkillers or anti-inflammatory medicines may be necessary. There are a few good rules:

     a. Take as few painkillers as you need to keep yourself comfortable. They all have side effects to a greater or lesser degree.
     b. Do not worry about becoming addicted to the minor painkillers such as paracetamol or aspirin. So long as you are taking them for a good reason addiction will not happen. Of course, strong painkillers such as codeine, heroin and morphine present a quite different problem.
     c. Small doses of painkillers taken often work much better than large doses taken infrequently.
     d. Research has shown that it takes much smaller doses of painkillers to prevent the onset of pain than to treat it once it has started. So if you know you are going to suffer pain in the middle of the night for example, take a painkiller before going to sleep.

- Placing a hot poultice (or even a hot-water bottle or a flannel dipped in hot water) or a cold poultice (or a bag of frozen peas) over a painful part of the body may help. If possible raising an affected part (e.g. a hand or foot) to encourage swelling to drain away is also worthwhile.

- In some cases acupuncture, nerve blocks or electrical stimulators are helpful. Consult your doctor about their value for you.

- Severe, uncontrolled pain is often what people fear most about dying. However, these days there is no need for such fears because painkillers are so effective. Everyone dying can be reassured they will not die in pain, and if anyone does die in pain it is usually because they are being badly treated. The amounts of strong painkillers (such as morphine) needed to keep the pain at bay may mean the dying person becomes addicted but this is a small price to pay for the relief they give.

PALPITATIONS

Most people are not aware of their heart beating. If you notice yours beating faster or more powerfully than normal and there is no obvious cause (like exercise), these heartbeats are called palpitations. Preventing them is important for two main reasons:

1. They may make your heart work inefficiently as a pump, causing heart failure (see **Heart Disease**).
2. They may cause a clot of blood to fly off from the lining of your heart and lodge either in an artery of the brain, causing a stroke (see separate entry), or in one of the arteries supplying the heart itself (coronary arteries), causing a heart attack (see **Heart Disease**).

Self-health

- If you notice palpitations more than two or three times you should tell your doctor. For some people (as many as ten per cent of people over sixty-five) no cause is found. Possible causes include too much thyroid hormone (see **Thyroid, Overactivity**) or coronary artery disease which, if treated, will prevent further recurrences.

- There are medicines (e.g. beta-blockers) that can help keep the heart regular.

- Occasionally a pacemaker may be needed to prevent palpitations. This is a tiny electrical box, powered by a battery, which is linked to the heart by an electrical wire running through the veins of the chest. Usually a permanent pacemaker is needed, in which case the box is placed under the skin of the chest during a small operation under anaesthetic. This procedure is now quite common; in the USA as many as one in every 4,000 people has one.

PANCREATITIS

Pancreatitis is inflammation of the pancreas gland. This gland lies behind the bowel in the abdomen and is responsible for producing insulin and digestive enzymes. Why it should become inflamed is not fully understood, although many sufferers have gall bladder disease or drink too much alcohol.

The symptoms are pain in the upper abdomen, vomiting, indigestion, and weight loss. Sometimes there is such a severe attack (acute pancreatitis) that the person needs to be taken to hospital urgently.

Self-health

- Apart from avoiding alcohol and sticking to a low-fat diet, as recommended by your doctor, pancreatitis is not a condition that can be prevented. In almost all cases it needs close medical supervision to prevent possible serious consequences.

PARKINSON'S DISEASE

Parkinson's disease affects the brain, particularly those parts of the brain that control movement. The cause in most people is unknown.

People over sixty, men more than women, are affected. Symptoms usually develop gradually over two or three years and include trembling of the hands, an uncontrollable shaking of the head, followed by a stiffness of the muscles which affects walking, speech, eating, writing. Because the mind stays clear until near the end, many people describe themselves as being encased in a stiff body which they cannot understand or control.

Self-health

- There is nothing you can do to prevent yourself getting Parkinson's disease. However, it is not inherited or infectious.

- You should see your doctor as soon as you notice the unusual symptoms described above. Effective medicines will help relieve the symptoms, although there is no cure as yet.

- An occupational therapist, physiotherapist and general practice nurse will help to make your home safer and more suitable for you. For example, bath rail supports, banisters, chairs with high arms and non-slip rugs will all help.

- Friends and family have an important role in supporting someone with Parkinson's disease. In particular they can help keep morale up, prepare nourishing, tasty food, and encourage the sufferer to take as much exercise as he or she can safely manage.

PARONYCHIA

A paronychia is an infection of the skin around the nail of the finger or toe. It is different from a whitlow (see separate entry). It is not always obvious what causes a paronychia but it may be because you are not looking after your hands or nails properly.

Self-health

- Keep hands dry by wearing gloves.

- Avoid cutting nails too short.

- A magnesium sulphate poultice and bathing in hot water may prevent the infection spreading. If not, antibiotic medicines, prescribed by your family doctor, will be necessary.

PELVIC FLOOR EXERCISES

Pelvic floor exercises are designed to build up the muscles of your pelvic floor. The main purpose is to improve bladder control for people with stress incontinence. An added bonus is that it may improve your and your partner's enjoyment of sex.

In women the pelvic muscles sweep down rather like a hammock, suspended from the bony pelvis to surround the anus, urethra and vagina. In men they surround the anus and the base of the penis. Men rarely have problems with the pelvic floor because their pelvis is narrowed and they do not undergo the traumas of childbirth. So the advice in this section is aimed at women.

First, discover your pelvic muscles. Imagine yourself trying to stop wind coming from your back passage. The muscles you contract are your pelvic floor muscles. Similarly pretend to control diarrhoea by pulling up the back passage muscles to a count of four. These are your pelvic floor muscles you are exercising.

Next try stopping your urine flow halfway through emptying your bladder. You will be exercising your pelvic floor muscles. At first you will not be successful but with time you may be able to stop the urine successfully. Do not repeat this exercise more than once a day at maximum.

Finally lubricate your fingers with a cream or jelly such as KY jelly and slip one or two into your vagina. This is perfectly safe. Then separate your fingers in a scissors action and try to squeeze the fingers together by contracting the muscles round your vagina. These are your pelvic floor muscles. Some women prefer to put a tampon into their vagina and pull gently on its string while contracting the vaginal muscles to stop it coming out. The stronger your muscles become the easier retaining the tampon will be. You can also do this exercise with your partner using his penis instead of a tampon – it can be fun and pleasurable for you both.

Once you are familiar with your pelvic floor muscles you should exercise them at least four times a day for two or three minutes. For many of the exercises no equipment is needed so you can do them at any time – while watching TV, standing in a queue, or cooking – no one needs to know.

PELVIC INFLAMMATORY DISEASE (SALPINGITIS)

Pelvic inflammatory disease (salpingitis) is inflammation of the Fallopian tubes. It may happen suddenly (known as acute) when you experience lower abdominal pain, a high temperature, a smelly discharge, pain having sex and changes in your periods

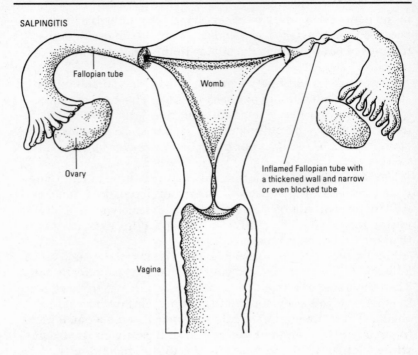

SALPINGITIS

Fallopian tube

Womb

Ovary

Inflamed Fallopian tube with
a thickened wall and narrow
or even blocked tube

Vagina

(e.g. very heavy or longer than usual). The causes include
sexually transmitted infections or infections caused by an
abortion, pregnancy or intra-uterine device (IUD).

Sometimes the symptoms are less severe, appearing
intermittently over a period of time, and this is known as chronic
pelvic inflammatory disease.

The main complication caused by pelvic inflammatory disease
is infertility. The inflammation blocks the tubes, preventing eggs
passing from the ovaries to the womb. This is most likely to
occur if a pelvic infection is treated late or inadequately. The
difficulty is that some women never have any symptoms, despite
the infection, so they never know they need treatment.

Self-health

- Take precautions to avoid catching sexually transmitted
  infections (see **AIDS, Gonorrhoea, Syphilis**).

- If you have any of the symptoms described above see your family doctor or go to a hospital special clinic immediately. If you are prescribed antibiotics make sure you complete the course, even if you have no further symptoms. If you continue to have symptoms after treatment, tell your doctor in case further treatment is necessary.

- Avoid an intra-uterine device (IUD) as a contraceptive because it makes you more likely to develop pelvic inflammatory disease.

- Avoid having an abortion, if possible, because infection may be introduced into your pelvis. Obviously 'back-street' abortions are the most dangerous.

- Tell your doctor if you have an unexplained high temperature after giving birth. You may have an infection which needs treatment.

Screening

- Special X-rays (hysterosalpingogram) or the use of a telescope to look inside your pelvis (laparoscopy) help diagnose whether pelvic inflammatory disease is the cause of infertility.

PERIODS, ABSENT

If you have not had a period by the age of sixteen, and certainly by eighteen, you have what is known as primary amenorrhoea and should see your doctor. Your doctor will examine you and organize tests to decide whether your sex organs are working properly, whether you have the correct balance of hormones, or whether you have a metabolic or genetic abnormality.

If you have had periods before but they stop for more than three months at a time when you would expect them to be happening (e.g. well before the menopause) you are suffering from secondary amenorrhoea. You may wish to consult your doctor but there is usually no pressing need to start investigations straightaway, unless you wish to become pregnant.

Self-health

PRIMARY AMENORRHOEA

- You cannot stimulate periods to start yourself. Some doctors believe periods will not start until you have reached a 'critical' weight but the difficulty is knowing what that weight is.

- Very hard training may prevent periods (athletic amenorrhoea).

- Many women with primary amenorrhoea are found to have nothing wrong, and periods eventually start normally.

SECONDARY AMENORRHOEA

- Consider whether you are pregnant or starting the menopause.

- Many women have very irregular periods so you may simply be more irregular than normal. Periods are most irregular when they first start, after coming off the Pill, and after pregnancy.

- Most women do not have periods while breast-feeding but they have usually re-started within six weeks of stopping breast-feeding.

- Failure to start periods within six months of stopping the Pill (post-Pill amenorrhoea) is worth consulting your doctor about. Some doctors believe stopping the Pill for two or three months every two or three years may prevent this amenorrhoea.

- Consider whether serious worries, stress or anxieties may be the cause.

- Very hard athletic training may prevent periods so you may need to reconsider your programme.

- Eating poorly and being very underweight may cause your periods to stop (see **Anorexia Nervosa**).

- If you continue not to have periods, see your family doctor, who may wish to investigate the cause.

PERIODS, HEAVY

Periods are heavy if they last longer than seven days, if you pass clots or if flooding occurs. About five to ten per cent of women are affected by heavy periods at some stage in their lives, usually as they near the menopause.

Self-health

- Women who persistently suffer from heavy periods are at risk of iron-deficiency anaemia because of the constant bleeding. So they should eat food containing plenty of iron (see separate entry).

- Women who start to experience heavy periods having never had them previously should consult their family doctor if they have more than three heavy periods. In most cases no cause will be found, but your doctor will wish to make sure you do not have fibroids, endometriosis, a pelvic infection, cancer of the womb or ovarian disease. An intra-uterine device (IUD) is another common cause. A diagnostic curettage (scraping of the lining of the womb) under anaesthetic may be necessary to exclude all possibilities.

- If your period was late and then is very heavy you may well be having a very early miscarriage. Consult your doctor because a dilatation and curettage operation on your womb may be necessary.

- If you have just one unusually heavy period and are convinced you cannot be pregnant go to bed with plenty of hot drinks and a painkiller such as paracetamol. If heavy bleeding lasts longer than twenty-four hours phone your doctor.

PERIODS, PAINFUL

Some women (especially girls and young women) suffer from pain in the lower abdomen or back just before or at the beginning of their periods. It may last for two or three days and varies in severity from mild to so severe that they have to go to bed. Menstrual cramp is particularly unpleasant and consists of spasmodic, colicky pain. The sufferer may also feel sick and faint.

Self-health

- Understanding about the pain, when, why and how it occurs, helps, particularly for young girls who may be experiencing it for the first time.

- Heat helps relieve the pain, especially spasmodic pain. Take a hot bath, place a hot-water bottle over your lower abdomen or try rubbing a deep-heating oil such as tiger balm into the affected area.

- Avoid standing for a long time.

- Some women find an alcoholic drink relaxes the womb muscles.

- Yoga or relaxation exercises (see chapter on Stress and Mental Health) may be helpful.

- Some women find orgasm temporarily relieves the pain.

- Exercise may help lessen the pain or it may make it worse. There is no anatomical reason why you should avoid exercise and some women find it helpful.

- Research has shown that painful periods may be due to affected women producing too much of the hormone prostaglandin, or having wombs which are very sensitive to it. Anti-prostaglandin medicines are now available from the chemist and may help you.

- If the pain interferes seriously with your daily life despite your own efforts, or if your periods become painful when previously they were not, you should consult your doctor.

PETS

The role pets can play in helping humans is starting to be recognized. The psychiatrist Freud used to have a dog in his consulting room because he thought it made conversation with patients easier. Studies have shown that blood pressure and stress levels are lowered when people hold or stroke their pet and that heart attack victims are more likely to survive if they have a dog. Pets ease the tension between people and make them laugh.

Having a pet at home teaches a child the first steps in being responsible and caring for others. Often the pet may act as a safety valve for pent-up emotions and it is a common experience to hear children pouring out their hearts to their pets when they cannot say a word to their parents.

For elderly people, too, pets are much-loved companions. Whereas health professionals have been called the 'hit-and-run brigade', pets are there twenty-four hours a day. At a time when older people are becoming increasingly isolated from friends and family and the suicide rate is rising dramatically, pets may seem to be the only reason for carrying on living.

All too often when their spouses, friends and family die older people are left feeling sad and lonely. Pets act as a comforting link with the past and a replacement in the bereaved person's affections. It seems more acceptable to talk to an animal than to oneself, so a pet may become a confidant with whom to talk over life's problems.

Pets can help to prevent apathy and confusion. During cold winters it's easy for old people to lose interest in themselves, but they will almost always make sure their pet is warm enough (and thereby keep themselves warm).

Even the warmth of a cat on the lap or a dog on the bed can help prevent the body temperature falling dangerously. The early-morning singing of a bird can remind the owner about the time of day, and a hungry cat will remind him or her to prepare food for both of them. The dog insisting on being taken for a walk establishes a regular pattern to the day and is a good excuse for exercise.

Pets can provide endless entertainment, from the gerbil digging tunnels in peat to the cheerful hamster dashing round the room, or the parrot shouting 'walkies' and 'dinner' at the dog. And in the evening, when elderly people fear intruders, dogs provide excellent protection.

There are all sorts of advantages in having pets but occasionally they can spread diseases. The ones to remember are toxocariasis, toxoplasmosis and cat scratch fever (see separate entries).

PHOBIAS

A phobia is an irrational, exaggerated fear of something which disturbs someone's life quite out of proportion to its cause.

Most of us have a minor form of phobia such as fear of snakes, spiders or heights. But the object of the fear can usually be avoided and panic attacks are rare.

However, many people (about 500,000 in the UK) suffer a more severe form and have repeated phobic attacks. These are basically panic attacks brought on by the fear of something specific. The two most common ones are agoraphobia and claustrophobia.

AGORAPHOBIA

Agoraphobia is fear of crowded public places (not open spaces as is often thought). It is the most common severe phobia affecting women more than men, usually in their early thirties. Most sufferers are able to continue working despite their phobia.

Symptoms include overwhelming anxiety and panic, dizziness, palpitations, clammy hands, tension cramps, and difficulty swallowing or breathing. Often these symptoms begin with a very bad panic attack shortly after an illness, shock, family tragedy or period of stress. Many agoraphobics describe the everyday fear of a return of this panic attack as their worst symptom.

CLAUSTROPHOBIA

Claustrophobia is fear of confined spaces. It often goes hand in hand with agoraphobia, but generally affects more men and is less common.

Self-health

- Minor phobias can often be prevented. As soon as you are aware of your dislike of something, try to overcome it by convincing yourself how irrational you are being, or getting your friends and family to do so. This is a simple form of behaviour therapy. By contrast, every time you express your fear or give in to it you are instilling it more deeply into your mind, thus making your problem worse.

- Severe forms of phobia cannot be prevented or treated by you alone. As soon as you recognize unusual symptoms see your family doctor, who will arrange appropriate treatment – the quicker you do this the less damage the phobia will do to your life (and to your family) and the easier it will be to treat. The good news is that many phobias.can be cured, usually by a combination of drugs and behaviour therapy, including desensitization therapy, and almost all can be prevented from getting worse.

- You may be able to prevent and cure your phobia if you come to realize that your major problems are a lack of confidence in yourself and a fear of fear. Confront this fear and the physical symptoms that go with it a little bit at a time, and you will find you grow in confidence each time you are successful until the fear is banished. Accept that you are human and there will be times you fail, but never accept defeat. In particular never compare yourself with others because this invites feelings of failure. Negative thoughts like 'if' or 'if only' should be avoided. Take up hobbies to distract the mind and encourage positive thinking. Even if you are housebound there is no reason why you shouldn't be adventurous with painting or reading, for example. Practise relaxation techniques (see chapter on Stress and Mental Health) to help cope with tension and stress.

- Many agoraphobics feel they can never have a holiday. But this is not so, provided you plan carefully. Select somewhere which will be as unthreatening as possible. You may surprise yourself how much you enjoy it.

- There is no reason why you should not have children if you suffer from agoraphobia or claustrophobia. In fact many women have found the joy of a new baby and the desire to show their child off to everyone has helped their problem. And phobias are not a genetic problem so you cannot pass them on.

PNEUMONIA

Pneumonia is inflammation of the lungs caused by infection either with bacteria (e.g. *staphylococcus* or *pneumococcus*) or a virus (e.g. measles or flu). It affects the lungs either in patches (bronchopneumonia) or in segments (lobar pneumonia).

The main symptoms of pneumonia are cough (which occasionally may be bloodstained), high fever, breathlessness, chest pain and feeling very unwell. In the past about one in three people with pneumonia used to die, often because it was the final complication of another illness that had reduced resistance and strength. Recently deaths have been fewer because better treatment is available. Old people and young babies and children are at special risk.

Self-health

- Do not smoke. Smokers are prone to pneumonia and get the illness more seriously than non-smokers.

- Try not to become overweight because you will be more prone to pneumonia.

- Avoid people with colds and flu, especially if you have long-standing lung diseases such as bronchitis or emphysema or are on medicines such as steroids, which reduce your resistance to infection.

- Keep as active as you can, especially after anaesthetics when the pain of the operation may discourage you from breathing deeply and coughing.

- Pneumonia is not an illness you can treat yourself. Get medical help as soon as you suspect the diagnosis. Modern antibiotics are very effective against bacterial forms of pneumonia, the most serious type.

- Some experts recommend that people who are prone to bacterial pneumonia should have a supply of antibiotics ready with them so they can start a course as soon as symptoms begin.

POLIO

Polio is a viral infection, often occurring in epidemics, which affects nerves and muscles. In over ninety per cent of cases patients suffer a flu-like illness and do not know they have had polio. But in a few cases it can be a serious disease which leaves the person with a permanently paralysed leg or arm. If the virus attacks the breathing or swallowing muscles it can even be fatal if intensive medical care is not available.

Polio has largely been eradicated from the Western world but this success depends on a high rate of immunization. It is still common in the Third World.

Self-health

- The virus is spread when it is excreted in the faeces of an infected person. Poor personal hygiene, particularly in overcrowded homes (and particularly as the person is often unaware he or she is infected), makes control of the illness difficult in some countries. However, with better sanitation, clean water, less crowding, and an understanding of how the infection spreads, the rate of cross-infection should come down.

- The best method of prevention is the live vaccine. This is given by mouth three times in the first year of life with the tetanus, diphtheria and whooping cough vaccine. It creates immunity in over ninety per cent of children. Booster doses are usually given before and after schooling.

- Anyone travelling to an area where polio may be common should consult their family doctor or local immunization centre to confirm their personal immunity.

PREMENSTRUAL TENSION

The group of unpleasant symptoms experienced by some women for up to two weeks before their periods is often described as premenstrual tension (PMT) or premenstrual syndrome (PMS). These symptoms include mood changes, depression and irritability, a bloated feeling and fluid retention (e.g. swollen feet or hands), tender breasts, headaches, difficulty concentrating, and a tendency to suffer recurring allergies. Only two or three per cent of women have symptoms so severe that they change their life, but many women experience some problems, especially in the few days before a period.

Self-health

- The causes of PMT are many and complicated so there is no single way of preventing it. Try a variety of remedies until you find the ones that suit you best.

- It is a good idea to start by keeping a record of your symptoms. They will form a regular and predictable pattern, and this reassuring discovery will help prevent you thinking you are going mad, as many women with PMT imagine.

- Changing your diet may help. Foods such as coffee, sugar and some processed foods, particularly those containing a lot of sugar, salt and spices, may make PMT worse. So try a low-salt, low-sugar diet taken in frequent, small meals.

- Research has shown that about half the women who suffer from depression as part of PMT may be short of vitamin B_6. Supplements can help, but discuss these first with your doctor as taking too many can cause unpleasant side effects.

- There is some scientific evidence that gamma-linolenic acid (GLA) from the seeds of the evening primrose plant may help relieve PMT symptoms.

- Take painkillers and long hot baths when symptoms are bad.

- If possible, try to avoid particularly stressful activities when you know your symptoms are going to be worst.

- If all these measures fail see your doctor, who may prescribe water (diuretic) tablets to prevent fluid retention, or hormones, particularly progestogen, in the form of tablets, vaginal or rectal suppositories or injections. Some women are helped simply by taking the contraceptive pill.

  Very occasionally your doctor may prescribe tranquillizers or anti-depressants.

PROLAPSE, UTERINE

A prolapse occurs when the uterus (womb) is no longer held in position by the muscles and ligaments of the pelvis so that it gradually falls into or through the vagina.

About one in 250 women consults her GP each year about a

prolapse. It affects all ages but most commonly women over sixty.

The symptoms include a feeling of heaviness and discomfort in the pelvis made worse by lifting, coughing or standing for a long time. Backache is quite common and occasionally the prolapse appears as a hard lump at the entrance of the vagina. If the prolapse affects the front wall of the vagina it may cause difficulty controlling the flow of urine (see **Incontinence, Urine**), or a desire to pass water often, or sometimes difficulty starting to pass water. If the prolapse affects the back wall of the vagina it may cause a lump which makes opening your bowels difficult, and worse the harder you strain.

Self-health

- The womb is held in position by pelvic muscles whose strength and flexibility can be improved by pelvic floor exercises (see separate entry). These exercises should be done by all women most days but especially after childbirth and as you grow older, when your muscles have a tendency to become lax.

- The more children you have the more likely you are to suffer from prolapse. But there are, of course, many women who have had large families and who never suffer from prolapse. Pelvic floor exercises after childbirth are an important way of helping to prevent prolapse.

- A difficult childbirth which tears muscles and ligaments makes you more likely to suffer a prolapse. The muscles should be carefully repaired surgically, after which you should start your pelvic floor exercises.

- Lose weight if you are overweight (see chapter on Understanding Weight Loss).

- Eat plenty of high-fibre foods to make sure your stools are soft and you do not need to strain.

- Stop doing work which involves a lot of heavy lifting.

- If you smoke, give up (see **Smoking**), because coughing makes prolapse worse.

- Lie down when you notice symptoms. This often helps temporarily but is not a permanent solution.

- If your symptoms continue or get worse despite your own efforts, consult your doctor. He or she may:
  1. Examine you to make sure the diagnosis is correct.
  2. Make sure your pelvic floor exercises technique is correct.
  3. Prescribe oestrogen cream for your vagina.
  4. Place a ring pessary into your upper vagina to keep the prolapse up (especially useful for elderly people).
  5. Refer you to a gynaecologist for advice on whether you need a surgical repair.

PROSTATE, BENIGN ENLARGEMENT

The prostate is a male gland lying below the bladder and surrounding the urethra (the tube that drains the bladder). Its function is unknown but it does add secretions to the semen, which may encourage the sperm to be active.

For reasons that are not yet understood it begins to enlarge after the age of forty-five and by sixty most men are affected, although only one in ten needs surgery. The troublesome symptoms are a desire to pass water more often than usual (interrupting sleep), difficulty starting to pass water and a weak stream once started, dribbling, and sometimes pain.

Self-health

- There is little you can do to stop the enlargement. Some doctors think continued active sex may help a little but this has not been proved.

- Eat a high-fibre diet to ensure constipation does not make your symptoms worse.

- To reduce dribbling when you have finished passing water, 'milk' the urethra from the base to the tip to remove all urine.

- Cutting down on the amount of fluid you drink will not help your symptoms. On the contrary, it is likely to encourage an urinary tract infection which will make them worse. So continue to drink about five or six cups of fluid a day.

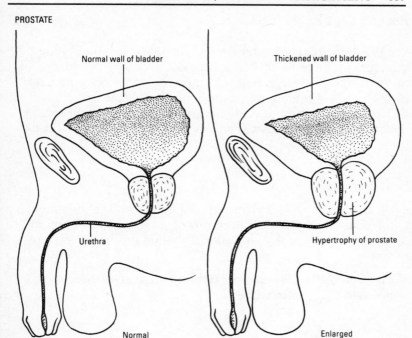

PROSTATE

Normal wall of bladder

Thickened wall of bladder

Urethra

Hypertrophy of prostate

Normal

Enlarged

- Avoid alcohol because it stimulates the kidneys and will make you want to pass water even more frequently.

- As soon as symptoms begin, see your family doctor, who will examine you and decide whether surgery should be considered. Results are usually excellent.

- If you suddenly find you cannot pass water despite your best efforts you should:

   1. Get into a hot bath. Relax and then gently attempt to pass water into the bath water. It often works.
   2. Take a tot of gin (or other spirit if gin is not available) which also helps.
   3. Do not strain as hard as you can; just start gently.
   4. See your doctor immediately if you have been successful because next time you may not be so lucky.
   5. Call your doctor or hospital immediately if you are not successful, because the pain of a full bladder is said to be among the worst known.

PROSTATE, CANCER

See **Prostate, Benign Englargement**, for an explanation of the structure of the prostate. The symptoms of cancer are similar to those of benign enlargement which is why your doctor may take blood tests and sometimes a biopsy of the prostate to differentiate between the two. Sometimes the cancer spreads to the backbone and the first symptom you notice is unusual back pain.

Self-health

- Clearly the earlier you can see your doctor and get treatment the better the outlook. The results of surgery and/or hormone treatment are usually very good provided the cancer has not spread.

- The self-health measures for benign enlargement of the prostate apply to cancer too.

PSORIASIS

Psoriasis is a skin condition in which the normal rate of skin cell production is speeded up. As a result a rash appears, consisting of pink, raised patches covered by white scales which flake off. The patches affect the knees, elbows and scalp mostly. They are rarely painful but sometimes itchy. About one in forty people is affected, usually between the ages of ten and forty.

Self-health

- Psoriasis cannot be prevented but it is possible to learn to live with it. There are numerous treatments and ointments, some of which can be very time-consuming to apply, so when deciding which one to use, you and your doctor should aim to strike a balance between the demands of living a full life and the demands of the illness.

- You may learn that certain stimuli (e.g. stress or a throat infection) trigger an attack and should therefore be avoided.

- Some people find careful sunbathing or ultra-violet rays from a sun lamp help.

- About seven per cent of sufferers develop arthritis, so do not ignore pain or stiffness in your joints, consult your doctor.

- Take good care of your hands and nails (see **Nails, Care of**) because psoriasis may affect them.

PULSE

The pulse measures the rate at which the heart beats. It is best measured by feeling the radial artery on the inner wrist near the base of the thumb. It can also be measured by feeling the carotid artery in the neck.

There are three important aspects to your pulse – its rate, its regularity and its strength.

RATE

The normal rate varies throughout your life. As an infant it may be 140 beats per minute, by ten years old it will have slowed to about ninety beats a minute and as an adult the average is seventy-two times a minute for men and eighty times a minute for women. The rate normally drops by about five to ten beats per minute when sleeping, or even lower if you are physically fit. Generally your pulse rate rises during any stress or illness, and particularly if your temperature is raised. It drops again when you are getting better. So the rate is often used as a guide to the progress you are making.

It is unusual for the pulse rate to drop dramatically and this usually only happens as a result of a heart attack, a stroke or thyroid disease.

REGULARITY

Your heart should beat regularly and any irregularity should be investigated. Irregularity may be perfectly harmless (e.g. certain inherited conditions) or it may suggest illness (e.g. heart attack, thyroid illness, or heart valve disease).

STRENGTH

Become familiar with the strength of your pulse – and that of members of your family – so you can tell when it becomes weak. The most common causes of weakness are blood loss, fever, fear, shock, and heart and blood vessel disease.

Self-health

- If you notice an unexplained change in your pulse (or palpitations) see your doctor immediately so that the cause can be found.

Screening

- Your resting pulse rate is a valuable guide to your health and is one of the measurements life insurance companies insist on.
- How quickly your heart responds to exercise and then returns to normal is also a valuable test of your health, and again is often used by life insurance companies. Sports coaches use this test to monitor athletes' progress.

R

RABIES

Rabies is mainly an animal disease caused by a virus, but it can be passed on to humans in whom it is often fatal if untreated. Symptoms start any time from two weeks to two years after a bite, scratch or lick from an infected animal, and include fever, headache, sore throat, muscle pains, and feeling unwell, followed by confusion, hallucinations, muscle spasms, stiffness of the neck or back, paralysis, or difficulty swallowing (especially fluids, which may cause intense terror). If it is untreated or treated too late, rabies is fatal.

Self-health

- Only those people at special risk of getting rabies (e.g. veterinary surgeons) should consider having routine vaccination, but everyone should be aware of whether they are in a rabid area and what to do in an emergency.

- You can catch rabies if you are bitten, scratched or even licked by an infected dog, cat, fox, monkey, bat or other animal. So be careful when touching animals.

- If you are bitten or scratched by an animal you think may be infected you should:

  1. Wash the wound immediately using soap as a detergent and flushing with clean water. Apply alcohol if available.
  2. Get medical attention fast from the nearest doctor or hospital. You may need vaccination which, if given soon enough after the injury, can prevent symptoms.
  3. If possible, arrange for the animal that bit or scratched you to be kept under observation for the next two or three

weeks. Exchange names and addresses with the person in charge of the animal so that you can be told if it dies or becomes sick. Find out if it has had the rabies vaccine or ask to see the certificate, although do not assume that its production means there is no risk.

4. Note the place, date and animal's description if it is wild or stray.
5. Inform the local police.
6. Tell your own doctor as soon as you get home.

• Help countries that are rabies free (including the UK) by never importing animals without a licence or consultation with the health authorities.

RAPE

A rape is a sexual assault, including intercourse, usually on a woman, against the persons' will. It is becoming more common in the Western world. Most are committed by a man known to the woman, often in circumstances which make it difficult for her to prove his guilt.

Self-health

• Many women are aware that a particular man poses a threat to them. If this is the case, try to make sure that he never has the opportunity to rape you, and avoid being alone with him. You can also contact your local rape crisis centre. They are very experienced and will give you sensible advice on what to do in your circumstances.

• Keep away from lonely places, especially at night. If this is not possible take someone with you or wait until someone else walks by and then follow closely behind.

• If possible, take taxis (from reputable companies) when going home late at night.

• Avoid going to areas where you know local gangs roam.

• Always lock your car doors. Park under a streetlight at night, and never get into your car without first checking the back seat.

- If you think you are being followed, have no hesitation in stopping someone else for protection.

- Check the security of your home. Make sure any windows left open at night cannot be reached by an intruder.

- Never open the front door to a stranger – always use the security chain, peephole or even letter box to check identities first.

- Be wary of false identities, especially among workers who come to the house. Be sure you know in advance the name of anyone who is due to spend time in your house.

- The question of whether to use force to counter sexual attack is a difficult one. Much depends on the circumstances of the attack and on your personality and physique. If you think you would want to resist an attack physically, go on an accredited self-defence course. Nothing is worse than being only half prepared and falsely believing you can take on any attacker.

- There are various items such as whistles, sprays and alarms which you can carry with you. But do not let them give you a false sense of security. Also remember that a good scream may scare away some rapists.

- If the rapist is determined and armed it may well be that you decide to take a passive role. Be particularly wary of an assailant who has been drinking, because he will be more dangerous and unpredictable.

  If you decide on a passive role try talking quietly to your attacker. Many a rape has been prevented by the man being made to realize you are an ordinary person. But it is difficult to stay calm enough.

  Whatever happens, try to remain as unemotional as you can. Unfortunately many rapists are so sick they will be encouraged if you let them know how much they are hurting you.

- If the man is unknown to you try to remember as many details about him as you can – height, weight, colour, hair, accent, clothes, unusual marks – which will help to identify him later. If he is caught you will feel safer, since many women are frightened that their rapist will return to terrorize them. It will also prevent him raping other women.

- After being raped, many women feel that they can tell no one, least of all the authorities, because they want no one to know about their humiliation and because they may not be believed anyway. Before taking this view consider these points:

  1. Attitudes to rape have changed greatly in recent years. In almost all cases nowadays you will be treated gently and sympathetically, your story will be believed, and every effort made to catch the rapist and get you back to normal life.
  2. You may have caught a sexually transmitted disease which will need treatment urgently, or be pregnant. Seek medical advice.
  3. You may need professional help to learn how to cope with the trauma you have been through. 'Going it alone' is not usually advisable.
  4. If you have been raped by someone you know and tell no one else, he will almost certainly think you are 'willing' and will try again.
  5. If you have been raped by a stranger he needs to be caught as soon as possible to protect other women.
  6. Police and their doctors are now specially trained to handle rape victims. But if you still cannot face going to them, contact your local rape crisis centre instead. You can be sure of experienced and sympathetic care.

REFLEXOLOGY

Reflexology is a system of healing derived from the ancient Eastern technique of massaging special points on the feet to treat other, apparently unconnected, parts of the body. An American, Dr William Fitzgerald, probably did most to outline the principles of the system.

Reflexologists believe that stress and illnesses are reflected in the zones of the feet. They believe that deep massage of the zones using the thumb will stimulate the body to heal itself.

Self-health

- Like many 'complementary' therapies reflexology does not harm you, although some people may find the treatment unpleasant; most, though, find it a pleasant experience.

- There is so little research into reflexology that it is impossible to say how successful it is. It should certainly never be the main form of treatment for serious illnesses.

RESTLESS LEGS

Restless legs is the name given to an unpleasant creeping sensation which some people feel deep in their calves (and occasionally feet and thighs). Sufferers find it difficult to describe the feeling. 'Ants running up and down my legs' or 'my whole leg felt as if it was full of small worms' are two descriptions. The feeling usually starts in the evening, often after sitting for a while. Men and women are equally affected. There is no known cause for restless legs, which of course makes preventing and treating them difficult.

Self-health

- Most people find getting up and walking about will prevent symptoms coming on or will help them go away. Massaging the calves and thighs also helps.

- Some people find going to bed and sleeping is the only way to help themselves. Others, though, find the feeling so unpleasant it stops them sleeping.

- Others find restless legs start when they are tired or have been standing a long time. If you are prone to restless legs try avoiding both.

- If the symptoms persist see your family doctor. There are one or two conditions (such as iron-deficiency anaemia) which are linked with restless legs and which can be treated, and there are medicines that will help some people.

S

SALMONELLA FOOD POISONING

Salmonella are bacteria often present in the bodies of farm animals and birds. They can infect food if precautions have not been taken and cause gastroenteritis, which may be dangerous to young children, elderly or sick people.

There has been a recent rise (some would say an epidemic) in the number of people suffering from salmonella food poisoning in all Western countries. Poor hygiene and food handling, a rise in sales of ready-prepared and frozen food, and the increasing use of low-dosage antibiotics for farm animals and poultry which encourage salmonella to become resistant are some of the reasons.

The main symptoms are diarrhoea and vomiting starting about twelve to thirty-six hours after the infected food has been eaten. Fever and stomach pain are often present as well. In young babies, elderly or already sick people the fluid losses can be so dramatic that they become dehydrated and die. Sometimes the

---

Rules for refrigeration

1. Hot food must cool to room temperature before you put it into the refrigerator.
2. Do not cram every available space in the refrigerator with food because this will make it less likely that all the food will be kept adequately cold.
3. Make sure the refrigerator is cooling to 3–5°C. A common fault is to open and close the refrigerator too often, or to have inadequate seals on the door so it does not shut efficiently. Defrost it regularly.
4. Keep uncooked food away from cooked food so that they cannot contaminate each other.
5. Do not keep cooked food for more than three days in the refrigerator.
6. Keep the refrigerator scrupulously clean, both inside and out.

bacteria may spread from the gut into other organs such as the gall bladder or kidneys, causing serious infections there too.

In most people the illness lasts twenty-four to forty-eight hours before the symptoms disappear. Occasionally it can last longer, in which case you should see your doctor.

Self-health

- Salmonella are not killed by deep freezing but they are killed by being thoroughly cooked. So meat must be thoroughly defrosted before cooking and cooking must be long enough to ensure all parts of the meat are cooked. Two of the most common mistakes are not defrosting chicken (many of which are infected with salmonella because of overcrowded battery conditions) adequately, and failing to cook it for long enough (see below).

- See **Food Poisoning** for advice about handling and preparing food. Salmonella is easily passed on by hands so food handlers and cooks should take special precautions if there is any possibility they have the illness.

- Eggs are a common source of salmonella infection. This can be partly avoided by choosing free-range eggs which are less likely to have salmonella. Infection can be entirely avoided by making sure all eggs are cooked hard before eating. So, raw eggs or soft-boiled eggs (in sauces for example) must be avoided.

- Never merely warm leftover meat, because warming encourages the bacteria to multiply and makes you more likely to get the infection. Always eat meat directly from the fridge or thoroughly heated.

- If the symptoms last longer than forty-eight hours, or if you become weak, confused or dehydrated contact your doctor immediately.

SALT

Salt contains the minerals sodium and chloride, both of which are found in all cells of the body and are essential for life. In ancient times it was a very precious commodity over which countries fought. It still is in such countries as India and Ethiopia where it is in short supply.

Changes in taste, and in preserving and manufacturing techniques have resulted in much more salt being added to modern Western foods. This has caused some health problems, particularly for those with a tendency to high blood pressure (see separate entry).

Self-health

- Because of the dangers of high blood pressure (e.g. stroke) it is generally agreed that the current average daily consumption of salt in Britain and America of 12–24 g is too high. The National Institute of Health in America has recommended that Americans should reduce their salt intake to 5–6 g daily. In Britain the NACNE report recommends a daily maximum of 9 g.

  Cutting down on how much salt you eat will not necessarily lower your blood pressure. In fact studies show that only ten to fifteen per cent of people are affected. The problem is that it is impossible to predict whether you are one of those people. So just in case you are, and as a sensible precaution, it is worth keeping within the recommended guidelines, particularly as it need not affect your enjoyment of food.

- Do not encourage your children to develop a taste for salt. When cooking do not add salt to foods (especially vegetables). Banish the salt cellar from the dinner table. Avoid foods with a lot of salt such as bacon, salted fish, crisps and peanuts. Beware of 'hidden' salt in processed foods – it is now possible to buy low-salt varieties of most popular foods, e.g. baked beans, sauces, butter and margarine. Cereals can be a source of 'hidden' salt; for example, weight for weight cornflakes have twice as much salt as salted peanuts. However, a large takeaway hamburger has up to five times as much sodium as 25 g of cornflakes, so should be eaten as an occasional treat only.

- Use herbs and spices as alternatives to salt to make your food tasty, and avoid overcooking food. For example, add a bay leaf, garlic and onion powder to roast meat, use ginger, cloves and peppercorns for chicken; mint or rosemary go well with veal and lamb. Add flavour to mashed potatoes with parsley, garlic, a little cayenne and paprika, and try adding vinegar, wine or lemon juice to vegetable and meat soups.

- In your efforts to reduce your salt intake do not forget that salt is essential for life. If you already have low blood pressure a low-sodium diet may be dangerous. In hot countries where you sweat a lot (and therefore lose a lot of sodium) you may need extra supplements to prevent cramp, low blood pressure, dizziness and fatigue.

SCABIES

Scabies (also known as 'the itch') is a highly contagious skin disease caused by a mite, *sarcoptes scabei*, which burrows into the skin. It usually affects the insides of the wrists, the palms, fingers, soles of the feet, and occasionally the penis. The symptoms include a rash of itchy pimples which itch more at night.

Self-health

- The mite lives only on human skin so avoid close contact with an infected person. Clothing and bedding may also harbour the mite for a short time (about twenty-four hours).

- If you suspect you may be infected see your family doctor as soon as possible so that you can start treatment and do not infect other people. All members of your household will need treatment regardless of whether they have the symptoms. A course of benzyl benzoate emulsion or gamma benzene hexachloride ointment is usually used.

- Launder all clothes and bedding to kill mites and larvae which might start a fresh infection.

SCOLIOSIS (CURVATURE OF THE SPINE)

Abnormal sideways curvature of the spine is known as scoliosis.

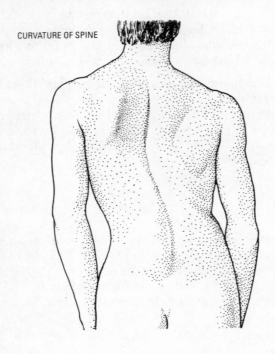

CURVATURE OF SPINE

It may be present at birth or start in childhood – or more commonly adolescence – and gradually get worse till growth stops.

Self-health

- Even slight curvature should be seen by a doctor because it may be possible to prevent it getting worse. Physiotherapy may help to strengthen muscles or the child may need to wear a brace for a year or so. Occasionally an operation may be necessary.

SCURVY

Scurvy is a disease caused by not eating enough vitamin C. It used to be common in overcrowded, poor inner cities and in armies and navies but is now rare except in a few Third World countries. The symptoms include poor healing, easy bleeding and bruising, poor resistance to infections, tiredness and tooth loosening. In very bad cases death may result from uncontrollable bleeding.

Self-health

- 10 mg of vitamin C daily is all that is needed to prevent scurvy.

- Sources of vitamin C include fruit and vegetables. Most people's diet contains more than enough vitamin C to prevent scurvy so no special dietary measures are usually necessary.

- There may be special circumstances (e.g. after a gastro-intestinal operation or being on a special diet) when you need vitamin C supplements to be sure of absorbing enough. Consult your doctor or nutritionist.

SEX, AFTER A HEART ATTACK

Most people are worried about sex after a heart attack so there is no need for you to feel shy about asking your doctor.

Self-health

- Researchers have found that the average amount of energy used up during sexual intercourse is similar to climbing one or two flights of stairs. So it is significant exercise but within six months almost everyone gets back to enjoying as much sex as they did before the heart attack.

- Depending on how bad your heart attack was most doctors recommend starting to have sex again four to six weeks after going home from hospital. The advantage of knowing that intercourse is not recommended to start with is that it takes the pressure off both partners to perform. But caressing and kissing each other is excellent therapy and masturbation may be a gentle way back to intercourse.

- In the past doctors used to recommend lying on your side for sex or suggest that the heart attack sufferer should be below his or her partner. Nowadays, though, it is generally thought the position does not affect the stress placed on the heart so use the positions you enjoy most.

- Don't eat a heavy meal just before sex because a great deal of blood will be directed towards your stomach and away from your heart, which needs it during the exercise.

- Avoid alcohol for about three hours before sex because it quickens the heart and makes it work harder.

- Try to have sex when you're rested and happy – avoid it when you're worried or angry, because stress puts your heart under an extra load.

- Perhaps the most stressful experience is having extramarital sex with a much younger partner. One study of partners of thirty-four people who died during sex showed that on average the partners were eighteen years younger, and thirty were not marriage partners.

- If you notice chest pain (angina) during sex you should tell your doctor so you can decide together what needs to be done.

SEX, AFTER CHILDBIRTH

Self-health

- If you have had an uncomplicated delivery there is no reason why you shouldn't start having sex as soon as you feel like it (perhaps using a lubricant like KY jelly to start with). But be warned; you may not feel like it for a few weeks. Some couples wait until after the postnatal check at six weeks.

- If you have had a difficult birth or your vagina has had to be cut to let the baby out (episiotomy) your vagina may be sore for a few weeks, making intercourse uncomfortable. So avoid it until you heal, usually after a few weeks. If sex is still painful when you go for your postnatal check at six weeks tell your doctor so he or she can examine you and discover the cause.

- A painful episiotomy is a common problem after childbirth, although the number of episiotomies performed is slowly decreasing. There are creams which can soften the scar when rubbed into it and your doctor can advise on whether surgery will help.

- Some couples worry that sex will not be so enjoyable after childbirth because the woman's vagina will have been stretched too much by the baby (or occasionally that the woman will have been stitched up too tightly after an episiotomy). Don't worry, because very few couples notice any difference after childbirth. Feeling and muscle tone, though, can be improved by doing pelvic floor exercises (see separate entry) and many midwives recommend these routinely.

- Looking after a new baby is very tiring, physically and emotionally and may leave a mother little energy for sex. One solution is to involve the father in the care of the baby as much as possible. Not only will this stop him feeling left out but it may save the mother a little energy which she can use for sex!

- The fact that you are breast-feeding does not stop you becoming pregnant, nor does not having periods mean you cannot become pregnant. So you will need to use a contraceptive method to suit you (see **Contraception**). Most doctors don't fit an intra-uterine device (IUD) until some months after birth and don't recommend vaginal methods of contraception until all the tissues are healed. The sheath is a good choice at this time.

SEX, ARTHRITIS

For some people with arthritis even the gentlest hug may bring on pain. However, most can enjoy sex, making allowances for their disabilities.

Self-health

- Plan to have sex at the time of day when you generally feel best.

- Time your painkilling and anti-inflammatory drugs so that

they are working best while you are having sex.

- A warm bath or shower may relax and soothe you before sex.

- Experiment with different positions to find the ones that suit you best.

- Save your energy for sex so you can enjoy it to the full.

SEX, BOREDOM

After five or ten years together many couples experience sexual boredom some, if not all, of the time. This boredom, however, is not inevitable and can be prevented.

Self-health

- If your sex life gets off to a good start you are more likely to enjoy sex throughout your life. See **Sex, Good** for some tips.

- Boredom with your sex life often reflects boredom with yourself, your work or life in general. So take a fresh look at yourself and your partner and think of new ways to inject excitement or interest into your life. Take up a new hobby (not necessarily with your partner), visit friends more, go to evening classes, try a holiday with a difference.

- Boredom often happens because you do not have the courage to let go of your inhibitions and tell your partner what you really want out of sex. So communicate with your partner and, if necessary, get professional help to unlock those problems that are holding you back. You may be pleasantly surprised by how exciting your partner finds your revelations after all those years of keeping silent.

- Have another look at your partner and discover again what it was that first attracted you. Take the time and trouble to share your dreams and hopes (not necessarily sexual) so that you start building a relationship again. Remember that the mind is the most exciting sexual organ of all.

- Think about the place where you make love. Does it need a spring clean, perhaps a coat of paint, some new curtains and cushions, a firmer, better bed, a new TV or video on which you can play erotic films? Perhaps some erotic literature or sex aids might help.

- Make love in different places – at home and away from home. Some couples enjoy places where there is a tiny chance they might get caught, such as the open air, a boat or the sea.

- Make love in different ways. Get advice and help from sex manuals, magazines or books. Try reversing your customary roles so each partner has to make different moves. You may find that your partner reveals inner longings and needs by doing to you what he or she has always hoped you would do to him or her.

   Get away from stereotypes so that your lovemaking is special to you as a couple. Something good between you, something unique, can be thought about and enjoyed even when you're doing the most ordinary things like washing up or getting on a bus and will fill you with enthusiasm for the next encounter.

- You don't have to be feeling romantic or happy to enjoy sex. This will limit the times and places. Try it when you're in different moods – feeling angry, tense, miserable – you may surprise yourself how much you enjoy it and it will break the mood you're in.

- Try stopping having sex if you both agree it is boring. Go back to the days when you were courting, when you kissed, touched and petted each other but didn't necessarily have intercourse. Rediscover the joys of other forms of sexual stimulation and it won't be long before you start wanting intercourse again.

- Finding something new and exciting, and rediscovering old pleasures are ways of getting your sex life going again but don't 'throw the baby out with the bath water'. In other words, there may be much about your old sex life that is good, secure and enjoyed by both of you which should not be lost in your search for adventure. Too much sudden change can be a sexual turn-off.

- There may occasionally be a physical cause for your loss of interest in sex. It may be the first sign of illnesses such as diabetes or thyroid disease. Depression (see separate entry) is a very common cause, as are fatigue, stress, pain and sexual problems such as premature ejaculation, impotence and vaginal infections (see separate entries).

- Certain medicines may cause loss of interest in sex. The contraceptive pill is the best-known cause but others include steroids, and medicines for reducing blood pressure. If you lose interest in sex and have recently started some new medicines consult your doctor about whether this may be the cause.

- If your own efforts to improve your interest in sex do not seem to be working, get professional help before it causes serious damage to your life. Your family doctor may be able to solve the problem or it may be more deep-rooted and need specialist help.

  Marriage counsellors are often able to give excellent advice about sexual problems. They are very experienced, completely unshockable and able to give unbiased opinions.

  Sex therapists (often psychologists) are another source of help. They will not expect you to perform in front of (or with) them so do not be alarmed if you are referred to one. They will discover whether you have any deep-rooted problems, arising perhaps from your childhood, which can be unearthed and solved. They often also use the technique of asking you to stop having intercourse for a few weeks and going back to caressing and petting only, at an increasing level of intimacy, until you are allowed to have intercourse again.

SEX, GOOD

Until the Kinsey reports on sexual behaviour in men (1948) and women (1953), sex was hardly ever discussed openly. These reports showed the enormous differences between people's sex lives and provided reassurance for the first time for many people that their own sex lives were 'normal'.

In 1965 Masters and Johnson published their research into sexual responses and biology. For the first time people began to understand how their bodies worked and how their pleasure in sex could be improved. For example Masters and Johnson dismissed earlier, vague theories about two types of female orgasm and showed that there was probably only one, arising from the clitoris, and that stimulation of the clitoris by their lover is what most women find makes them have an orgasm.

At the same time there had been important medical advances. The discovery of antibiotics meant that for the first time the feared sexual infections (e.g. syphilis, see separate entry) could be reliably treated. And the invention of the Pill and the intra-uterine device (IUD) allowed women, for the first time, to control their own contraception reliably. A new sexual freedom and liberation seemed possible.

Nowadays we are more cautious. The emergence of AIDS and the antibiotic-resistant sexually transmitted diseases has warned us that not all diseases can be automatically cured. Long-term use of some contraceptives has shown that some of them have their own dangers (see **Contraception**). And attitudes to sex and promiscuity have changed so that many people now believe their chances of a good sex life are best if they concentrate on good sexual technique within just one or two warm, loving, emotionally satisfying relationships.

Others have also pointed out that sex is not essential for everyone and that it is perfectly possible to live a full and satisfying life while remaining celibate.

Self-health

- Before you can learn to make love skilfully to someone else's body you need to learn about your own. It is easier for boys because their sex organs are more prominent but it is just as important for girls to explore themselves and their responses.

  Masturbation is one effective and safe way and many people find they continue to enjoy masturbation throughout their lives, either alone or by or with their partner. It is a normal part of sexuality.

- For most people the next stage is learning to kiss, caress and 'pet'. This is an important stage which parents in particular should not discourage because it teaches children about sexual arousal and responses. It also shows that it is perfectly possible to have very pleasurable sexual experiences without proceeding to full sexual intercourse.

- Finally most people learn to have intercourse. Do not imagine that this will necessarily be an instinctive and natural act which will give you great pleasure immediately. Many people make a slow, even painful, start which is only made bearable because they are sharing it with someone they care for.

  Eventually, though, most people find intercourse a satisfying experience which they can enjoy into their seventies and eighties. Do not be shy about using a sex manual to speed your learning, to help you with difficulties or to suggest new techniques and positions to keep your lovemaking fresh and fun.

  Some people, however, never find intercourse particularly enjoyable however experienced or skilful they may become. If you are such a person do not worry – you are not abnormal. You will need, though, to find alternative ways of making love and then work out a compromise with your partner which makes both of you happy.

- It is not the place of a book such as this to go into detail about how to become a skiful lover but here are some tips to get you started:

  1. Ignore most of the so-called facts and statistics about sex which you may read in some books and specialist magazines. They are often so fantastic and far from reality that, if you were to take them seriously, you would immediately fall into such a depression you would never recover. Your purpose is not to match these heroics but to find the sexual level that suits you and your partner. For example there are some couples who have sex every day (sometimes twice), most have it twice a week and some once a month. All are perfectly normal provided they are sexually satisfied.
  2. Keep a sense of humour whatever happens. There will be times when everything goes horribly wrong but seeing the funny side will help, even turning a disaster into a triumph. A sense of humour will also make you a better lover, more spontaneous, imaginative and fun.
  3. Keep communicating with and thinking about your partner – a selfish lover can never be a skilful lover. Your communication can be verbal – explaining to your lover what you enjoy and finding out what he or she enjoys – or

it can be by example – most people do to other people what they want done to themselves, so if your partner does something special to you you can be almost certain he or she wants you to respond similarly.

4. Don't imagine that sex should always be the same. It is a delicate balance between keeping your partner's confidence that you are not suddenly going to do something unexpected which he or she may not like and introducing an element of the uncertain or unexpected which makes sex more exciting. Reverse the normal routine of your lovemaking, for example, or try oral sex, or find out whether your partner likes multiple orgasms.

5. See **Orgasm, Lack of** for common myths about the need for orgasm, frequency of orgasm, simultaneous orgasm and methods of achieving it. One common myth is that the 'right way' for a woman to have an orgasm is by the thrusts of her partner's penis alone. Many women will never have an orgasm this way and need stimulation by hand by their partner or themselves before, during or after intercourse, or oral stimulation.

6. Another myth, which many doctors, counsellors, books and magazines, try to perpetuate is that the size of a man's penis makes no difference to his capacity to give his lover

---

Are you in tune with your partner's sexuality?

1. Are you satisfied with your sex life with your partner?
2. Is your partner satisfied with your sex life?
3. Do you know what turns your partner on?
4. Do you respect your partner's right not to do things she or he dislikes in bed?
5. Are you able to tell your partner what you like?
6. If your partner objects to some aspects of your lovemaking, do you take this seriously?
7. Do you take time to show affection to your partner both in and out of bed?
8. Do you still fancy your partner more than anyone else?
9. Do you take time to have candle-lit dinners or have a romantic evening together?
10. Is your sex life fun?

If you answer 'no' to more than one or two of these questions, beware – you could be headed for trouble.

pleasure. In fact, if his penis is small it may be more
difficult for him to give pleasure. But there will be few
women who will not agree that size is no substitute for
skill, consideration and care and it is these qualities which
they value most in their lovers.

7. Enjoy your fantasies, never be ashamed of them, they will
make you a better and more imaginative lover – and share
them with your partner if he or she likes this sort of thing.

8. Above all else, remember that everyone is different and
what may turn one person on, may do the opposite for
someone else. And remember, too, that everyone changes
from day to day and that the skilful lover adapts to new
moods, needs and situations as they arise.

SEX, MENOPAUSE

Many women imagine that the menopause (see separate entry)
marks the end of their sex lives. This is far from the truth, and in
fact some women find that the release from worries about
childbearing and rearing brings them a new sexual energy.

Self-health

- There are no norms about the frequency of intercourse so feel
comfortable with whatever best suits you as a couple. Once a
day is fine, a slow decline in interest is fine, complete
abstinence is fine, provided both partners agree. If not you will
need to find a happy compromise.

- Some women experience vaginal dryness which makes
intercourse painful. Plenty of skilful foreplay helps, as does a
lubricant like KY jelly. You can also discuss with your doctor
whether you need an oestrogen cream for the vagina to replace
the lost hormones.

- Some women find hormone replacement therapy (see separate
entry) helps their symptoms and restores their interest in sex.
Some doctors also believe a small amount of the male
hormone, testosterone, stimulates your interest while not
affecting your femininity.

- Medicines and sex aids have their place but ultimately you will enjoy sex only if you continue to believe in yourself as an attractive person who your partner desires sexually.

SEX, PAINFUL, FEMALE

Many women suffer from painful sex (dyspareunia) at some time in their lives. There are two types, superficial and deep.

Superficial pain is usually described as a burning or itching of the vulva or vagina.

Deep pain is less common and is felt as pain in the back or pelvis during or after sex. Women often say it feels as if the penis is hitting a tender spot deep inside themselves.

Self-health

SUPERFICIAL PAIN

- The most common cause is lack of sexual arousal. As a result the tiny glands that lubricate a woman's vagina are not stimulated and it remains dry. So men need to learn that women take longer to become aroused than they do and that it takes care and skill (see **Sex, Good**). A woman should also be ready to show she is not yet aroused, to slow her partner down and help him understand the things that arouse her.

- It would be impractical to expect a woman to be fully aroused and lubricated every time she has sex. Indeed that expectation might be enough to put her (and her partner) off. There will be times when a lubricant like KY jelly is needed and its use should not be regarded as a 'failure' either of the woman or her partner. There is no reason, too, why sex using a lubricant should not be as enjoyable for the woman as if she had lubricated herself naturally.

- Occasionally a long-standing inability to become aroused, or difficulty with intercourse (vaginismus), has such a deep-seated cause that your family doctor may think sex therapy is needed. Do not be alarmed (see **Sex, Boredom**).

- Other conditions that can cause pain include sexually transmitted diseases (e.g. herpes, syphilis, or gonorrhoea – see separate entries), cystitis (see separate entry) and surgical scars (see **Episiotomy**). Treatment of each will stop the pain.

- Try stopping or changing any douches, deodorants or spermicides you use because they are a common cause of allergy which results in pain.

DEEP PAIN

- Deep pain is difficult to identify, prevent or treat yourself so you will almost certainly need a doctor's help.

- The most common cause is pelvic infection caused by sexually transmitted diseases such as gonorrhoea (see separate entry). Treatment with antibiotics may help but some pain often remains.

- Other causes include fibroids of your womb or your womb being in an unusual position. Sometimes changing the position of your lovemaking helps but surgery is usually needed.

- Occasionally abnormalities of your ovaries or endometriosis will cause pain. Both conditions need your doctor's advice and help.

SEX, PAINFUL, MALE

Sex is rarely painful for men and when it is, the cause is usually more obvious than for women.

Self-health

- Avoid sexually transmitted diseases because they can cause painful ulcers or raw skin.

- Spermicides and douches used by your partner can irritate the skin of your penis. A change of contraceptive method may solve this problem.

- Some men are allergic to the rubber in condoms so avoid them if your penis develops a painful rash after use.

- The threads of your partner's intra-uterine device (IUD) may cause pain, in which case it will need trimming by a doctor.

- Avoid lovemaking when your partner's vagina is not well lubricated, either naturally by her own secretions or by a lubricant like KY jelly.

- Some men's foreskins become very tight when they have an erection and may need surgical removal (circumcision).

- Occasionally men notice pain while they are ejaculating. There is nothing you can do yourself to solve this problem so see your family doctor who may diagnose inflammation or narrowing of your urethra (the tube which runs from the bladder to the outside) or problems with your prostate gland.

- Occasionally the cause of the pain is difficult to pinpoint and your family doctor may refer you for a specialist opinion to a urologist, or for sex therapy.

SEX, PREGNANCY

Self-health

- If your pregnancy is normal there is no reason why you cannot have sex throughout. Some couples find their interest in sex increased, others find they lose the desire altogether. Both reactions are quite normal and will not affect your feelings about sex after childbirth when almost all couples return to the same level of activity as before the pregnancy.

- If you have had miscarriages in the past it is probably wise not to have sex until about the fourteenth or sixteenth week. Consult your doctor about when you can start again. If you have had any bleeding from the vagina (threatened miscarriage) you should avoid sex until your doctor advises you it is safe to resume.

- Towards the end of your pregnancy you may find it more comfortable to have sex lying on your side. The other advantage of this position is that the penis cannot penetrate quite so deeply into the vagina and is therefore less likely to start premature labour.

- Pregnancy is a surprisingly common time for male partners to be unfaithful, perhaps partly because they are enjoying less sex. Both partners should be aware of the dangers and take steps to avoid the pitfalls. Alternatives to vaginal sex, such as oral sex or masturbation, may help relieve tensions until after childbirth.

SEX, SAFE

All sexually active people should know about safe sex so that they know what to do if their sexual partner(s) falls into one of the AIDS high-risk groups (see **AIDS**). These groups include homosexuals, bisexuals and drug addicts. Never forget when you are making love to someone that you are making love to their past too.

The purpose of safe sex is to prevent body fluids (especially blood and semen) containing the AIDS (HIV) virus from an infected person getting into an uninfected person's body through the vagina, rectum, mouth or breaks in the skin such as grazes, cuts or ulcers.

Self-health

- If in doubt about whether you are at risk, always use a condom as a barrier:

    1. For heterosexual sex, both vaginal and anal.
    2. For homosexual anal sex (when a strong condom is necessary).

- Spermicides such as Duragel or Delfen may partially protect provided they are used with a condom. But they should not be used for anal sex because they may irritate the lining of the rectum.

- Grease-based lubricants such as Vaseline, cooking oils or butter should be avoided because they quickly damage the rubber of the condom. Instead use water-based ones such as KY jelly.

- No-risk sexual practices include:

    1. Solo masturbation.

2. Stroking or caressing away from the genital area (e.g. away from the penis, anus or vagina).
3. Ejaculation of semen on to the body away from the genital area.
4. Using your own sex toys.
5. Kissing is safe because saliva is thought not to contain the HIV virus, but beware of blood in the saliva from enthusiastic lovemaking, bleeding gums or mouth ulcers.

- Very low-risk sexual practices include:

1. Mutual masturbation.
2. Bondage, provided the skin is not broken.
3. Urination (often called 'water sports').

- Low-risk sexual practices include:

1. Oral sex, be it woman to man, man to woman (more risky during her period), man to man, or woman to woman.
2. Direct contact with the genital area.
3. Contact with an infected person's urine or faeces if the uninfected partner has open cuts, sores or grazes of the skin.

- High-risk sexual practices include:

1. Vaginal intercourse without using a condom. Withdrawal before orgasm may help a little, but not enough to make it safe.
2. Anal intercourse without using a strong condom and plenty of water-based lubricant. The rectum is easily damaged.
3. Any act which draws blood (especially from the genital area).
4. Enemas or douches used before or after anal or vaginal sex because they may damage the skin and cause bleeding.
5. Vaginal sex during menstrual periods because the blood may contain the HIV virus.

SHINGLES

Shingles is a very painful condition in which a crop of blisters appears over an area of skin supplied by a single nerve.
It affects only people who have had chickenpox. In the course

of the chickenpox the herpes virus gets into the root of a nerve where it usually lies quietly for years. But eventually it may become active again and cause symptoms.

Symptoms include pain, usually on one side of the body only and affecting the chest, face and eye especially. The rash appears a few days after the pain and may last about seven to ten days before disappearing, sometimes leaving a scar. The pain may last long after the rash has faded.

Self-health

- Take measures to make sure chickenpox (see separate entry) is not spread about, especially by children.

- No one knows why the virus becomes reactivated to cause shingles but emotional or physical stress, any illness (e.g. flu) and radiotherapy may trigger it off.

- Take painkillers in frequent small doses to ease the pain.

- Wear loose-fitting clothes to ease the pressure or rubbing on the affected skin. Cool bathing may also help.

- Avoid applying powdery lotions to the skin because they may irritate the blisters.

- See your doctor as soon as you suspect the diagnosis, because there is an anti-viral medicine which is most effective if used as soon as possible. Your doctor will also show you how to look after your eye if it is affected because shingles may permanently damage your cornea if care is not taken.

- Sometimes the pain lasts for many months (even years) after the rash has disappeared. All sorts of painkillers have been tried and there is no doubt acupuncture can be very effective.

SHOULDER, FROZEN

A frozen shoulder is caused by inflammation of the lining of the shoulder joint. The shoulder feels stiff and painful to move, particularly away from the body. It tends to affect people aged between forty and sixty.

Self-health

- Very often the symptoms come on gradually and cannot be linked to a particular injury. Prevention is therefore impossible but your symptoms can be helped if you see your family doctor soon and take advice on reaching a compromise between resting and moving the shoulder and taking painkillers and anti-inflammatory medicines.

- This condition can follow a stroke (see separate entry), a fracture or any kind of injury to the shoulder. Prevention may be possible if you exercise your shoulder by moving it gently in all directions regularly (e.g. three times a day) under the direction of your doctor.

- Once treatment has begun, be patient. This condition may take up to one year to heal but almost all sufferers are completely cured eventually.

SICKLE CELL ANAEMIA

Sickle cell anaemia is an inherited condition which almost always affects people of African origin. About one in 1,000 black Americans has the disease in a severe form. The symptoms are similar to other types of anaemia (see separate entry) and include tiredness, paleness, shortness of breath, dizziness, headaches, difficulty sleeping, palpitations, and chest pain in older people. It is caused by abnormal haemoglobin, the oxygen-carrying part of the red blood cells. As a result the cells do not flow well and become stuck or destroyed in tiny blood vessels. This may cause anaemia, or even long-term damage to vital organs like the kidneys, heart or brain. If many cells become stuck or destroyed, what is known as a 'crisis' may occur, resulting in severe joint, abdominal or head pains, and even death.

Self-health

- If you have a close relative with sickle cell anaemia you should consult your doctor so blood tests can be carried out to discover whether you also suffer from it. This information will enable you to avoid making the condition worse.

- If you have sickle cell anaemia you should ask your doctor for genetic counselling before planning to have children. The counsellor will discuss with you your chances of having a normal baby so you can decide whether to go ahead.

- Be wary of any infection because you are more prone to them than other people and they may bring on a 'crisis'. Take avoiding action whenever possible.

- As soon as you get an infection have it treated with an antibiotic to minimize any damage it may do. Some doctors believe low-dose antibiotics should be taken regularly throughout childhood to prevent infection.

- Avoid becoming dehydrated because this may bring on a 'crisis'. Do not forget that exercise is a common cause of unrecognized dehydration, and remember also to drink plenty in hot weather.

- Travelling by plane makes you more prone to a 'crisis' because it is thought to drop the oxygen saturation of the cells, so consult your doctor before flying.

- During 'crises' take painkillers freely to prevent pain, but follow the principles of 'few often' rather than 'many occasionally'. You will need the constant supervision of a doctor.

SINUSITIS

Sinusitis is inflammation of the lining of the sinuses (bony cavities connected to the nose), and is usually caused by bacteria or viruses.

Acute sinusitis happens suddenly two or three days after a cold or flu, just as you are expecting to get better. It may cause a greenish discharge from the nose, a stuffy nose, forcing you to breathe through your mouth, pain above the eyes (frontal sinuses) or below the eyes (maxillary sinuses), headache and a general feeling of being unwell.

Chronic sinusitis is a persistent inflammation of the sinuses without necessarily a viral or bacterial cause. Allergic rhinitis (see separate entry) may be one cause. The symptoms are usually less severe than acute sinusitis and include persistent blockage of the nose, a discharge from one or both nostrils, facial pain made worse by lying or stooping, and a poor sense of smell or taste.

Self-health

ACUTE SINUSITIS

- Blow your nose correctly while you have a cold or flu (see **Nose, Stuffy**).

- Avoid dust and smoke, which irritate the lining of the sinuses.

- Rest and painkillers will help control your symptoms.

- Inhale steam from a basin of boiling water (be careful not to scald children). Sometimes adding crystals of menthol or eucalyptus, available from the chemist, makes the steam more effective in loosening the mucus so it drains better.

- See your doctor if pain and high temperature last longer than twenty-four hours after you have started your own treatment.

CHRONIC SINUSITIS

- Avoid irritants like dust or tobacco smoke.

- See **Allergic Rhinitis**.

- Avoid the temptation to use sprays or drops (unless prescribed by your doctor) because some may make the condition worse.

- See your doctor as soon as you suspect the diagnosis, because antibiotics or surgery may be needed. Do not delay with children because the constant discharge down the back of their nose may cause lung damage.

SKIN, AGEING

Skin ages for many different reasons. One may be that as you grow older your skin cells lose the ability to reproduce themselves perfectly and thus cannot maintain the beautiful, healthy skin of youth. This ability to reproduce perfectly is partly controlled by your family genes and partly by environmental influences such as wind, sun, pollution and dryness.

Ageing mostly affects the inner layer of the skin rather than the outer layer (epidermis). In youth the network of collagen fibres in the dermis stretches in perfect harmony with underlying muscles, especially the facial muscles. But with age these fibres lose their elasticity and so wrinkles appear.

Older skin also loses the ability to sweat, so the surface becomes dry and itchy and less attractive.

Self-health

• Avoid the damage caused by sunburn (see separate entry) and windburn because this is one of the quickest ways to age your skin.

• Avoid exposing your skin to extremes of hot and cold. A fresh, cool environment is ideal for the skin. For the same reason do not have long baths using highly perfumed bath salts.

• It is tempting to hope that creams applied to the surface of the skin might prevent ageing. Unfortunately the important ageing changes are taking place deeper in the dermis which is not reached by these substances. So most of the substances which claim to prevent ageing cannot do so.

Some recent research, however, has suggested that hormone preparations may have a beneficial effect on skin. Ask your doctor for advice.

• Experiment with moisturizers and conditioners to find one that suits your particular skin. It should be emphasized that these do not prevent ageing but they can make the skin look younger and better. They prevent water escaping from the horny layers of the skin, which makes it feel softer and smoother and look more shiny. They will also prevent fine lines developing caused by excessive dryness and flakiness.

• Cosmetic surgery can also make the skin look younger by removing unwanted folds and stretching it tighter. It is particularly effective round the jaw and eyes. Consult your doctor if you would like more advice.

SKIN CANCER

Skin cancer is the most common type of cancer, but it is generally less dangerous than other types (e.g. lung and breast cancer).

There are three main types of skin cancer:

BASAL CELL (RODENT ULCER)

Basal cell cancer is the most common and least dangerous type. It appears as a small, flesh-coloured, pearly-looking lump, usually on the face near the nose. It grows slowly and does not usually spread to other organs. Death from it is extremely rare. Older people with light-coloured skin are most affected.

SQUAMOUS CELL

Squamous cell cancer is more serious than basal cell cancer because in about fifteen per cent of cases it spreads to local lymph glands or other organs (less likely). It can be either a firm, fleshy skin lump or a skin ulcer which doesn't heal, despite your efforts, usually on sun-exposed parts like the face, tips of ears, and hands. Older people with fair skin are most affected.

MALIGNANT MELANOMA

Malignant melanoma is the most dangerous form of skin cancer because it spreads quickly and easily to local lymph glands and other organs (e.g. liver and lungs) even though the original tumour may still be small. Usually a mole (or freckle) you have had for a long time starts to change its colour or shape (see below). Sometimes an entirely new brown or flesh-coloured tumour may appear on the skin. Generally tumours that appear on the arms and legs are less dangerous than those on the head and neck. Melanomas on the body, soles of feet, scalp and vulva are the most dangerous. Women have a better chance of survival than men and young people fare better than old.

Self-health

- People with fair or red hair and fair colouring are most likely

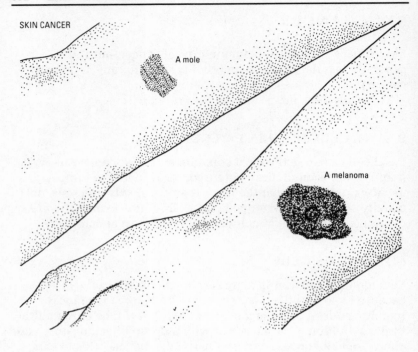

SKIN CANCER

A mole

A melanoma

to be affected by skin cancer if they overexpose themselves to strong sun. They should take special precautions.

- See **Sunburn** for ways to reduce your exposure to sun. In the past it has always been known that long-term exposure is dangerous (e.g. Australian or Texan farmers, sunbathers from California to Bondi Beach) but recent research has shown that two or three severe episodes of sunburn on an unprepared skin can also be dangerous so be careful on your annual holiday to sunny beaches.

- The more moles and freckles you have the greater your chance of skin cancer. It is important, therefore, that you watch carefully and tell your doctor if you notice any of the following changes to a mole or freckle:

  1. It has become larger or changed from being flat to raised.
  2. Its colour has changed, especially if it has become darker or developed little moles round it.

3. It has started to bleed.
4. It has become ulcerated.

- You should also show your family doctor any new moles.

- There are many different treatments for skin cancer,
  depending on its site and type. These include surgery,
  radiotherapy, cryotherapy, and occasionally drug treatment. It
  is a good rule that the earlier treatment is started, the better
  your chances of recovery.

SKIN, CARE OF

Skin is the biggest of the human organs. Its surface area can
measure up to two square metres and it weighs between seven
and twenty per cent of your total body weight.

Skin has several layers. The outer layer – the epidermis – is
thin and constantly being renewed. Below, the dermis has
connective and elastic fibres, hair roots, blood vessels, sebaceous
and sweat glands, nerves and sensory organs for temperature,
touch and pain. The lowest layer of the dermis merges into the
subcutaneous tissues which act mainly as a fatty pad, storing
about two-thirds of the total body fat.

Skin is a complicated structure. If you look under a
microscope, for example, you will find that within one square
centimetre there are about six million cells, 5,000 sensory
organs, four metres of nerve fibres, one metre of blood vessels
and 100 sweat glands.

Self-health

- There are two secrets of successful skin care. One is to avoid
  excesses such as too much sun, wind, cold, make-up and
  cleansing. The second is to live a healthy lifestyle: plenty of
  fresh air and exercise, a balanced diet, avoiding smoking and
  sufficient sleep will keep your skin looking good.

WASHING

- The purpose of washing is to get rid of grease, dead skin cells,
  dirt and germs.

- Most people can use the soaps of their choice. There is normally no need for special 'neutral' or 'medicated' soaps. Perfumed or 'superfatted' soap is acceptable for normal skin.

- People with sensitive skins should avoid washing their hands often and should select a soap with minimum capacity for irritation (e.g. Neutragena, Pure Soap or Simple Soap).

- People with oily skins can use more soap and water, especially in areas where the skin is particularly greasy. Spirit solvent (found in toners and fresheners) is helpful for clearing grease.

- Use soap sparingly or not at all if you have dry skin. A cream cleanser or baby soap will clean the skin. Particularly avoid bubble baths which have an additional detergent drying effect.

- After washing make sure you rinse the skin thoroughly using warm water.

MOISTURIZERS AND CONDITIONERS

- These products do not penetrate the skin so they cannot have any long-term effect upon its quality. What they do is slow the evaporation of water from the skin. So the skin retains water and feels more supple and soft. In addition the film of grease removes any feeling of dryness or superficial flakiness, and makes the skin feel smoother (like oil on any object does). Experiments using panels of observers to decide whether these products make the skin look more attractive confirm that they do, but sadly they cannot slow ageing.

SLIPPED DISC

Discs are the 'shock absorbers' that lie between each of the vertebral bones in the spine. They are made of jelly-like material which provides some 'give' during normal jarring of the body when moving, walking and running.

It is very common, especially in young people, for a disc to 'slip' out of place. What happens is that a previously damaged or worn disc bulges out of place, often for no obvious reason, irritating one or more nerves that run close by from the spinal

cord. This causes pain and sometimes numbness in the skin area
from which the nerve runs. In the leg this is called sciatica, but
similar symptoms can occur in the neck and arms.

The lower part of the back is the commonest place to develop a
slipped disc and the pain often runs down the leg as far as the
knee, ankle or toes. It is made worse by bending, sitting, lifting,
laughing or sneezing and is usually relieved by lying down.

Self-health

- The good news is that most episodes of back pain and sciatica
  will get better on their own, though occasionally it takes
  weeks or months. Lying down, not necessarily on your back
  but whichever way is most comfortable, preferably in bed and
  not on the floor, will help.

- Take painkillers such as aspirin or paracetamol and apply
  local warmth such as a hot-water bottle.

- You need to see the doctor urgently only if one of your legs
  starts to get weak, or if you notice any numbness around your
  bottom, or difficulty passing water or opening your bowels.

- To help look after your spine it is worth avoiding becoming
  overweight, avoiding heavy lifting, and making sure you take
  plenty of regular exercise such as swimming or walking.

- If you must lift something heavy, bend your knees rather than
  your back to reach the object if it is low down, and hold it
  close to you.

- A firm mattress on your bed and sitting in firm upright chairs
  will help.

- Avoid long hours driving. Stop the car every hour or so and
  take a walk for five or ten minutes.

- If symptoms do not settle despite your own efforts, see your
  doctor. He or she may suggest a surgical corset to support the
  joints in the back when they are sore and inflamed, and if the
  symptoms are slow to settle may recommend manipulation,
  traction, or occasionally surgery.

- Fortunately most problems from slipped discs settle on their
  own although a proportion recur, often for no obvious reason.

SMELLY FEET

Everyone will have smelly feet if they do not wash them
regularly. However some people seem to have smelly feet despite
regular foot care. No one is certain about the cause of this
condition, but it may be due to the action of certain bacteria in
sweat. If you are one of these people take the following advice.

Self-health

- Check the soles of your feet and between the toes to make sure
  you do not have a fungal infection, as this will cause smelly
  feet. If you have a tendency to infections, use an anti-fungal
  powder or ointment to prevent them.

- Wash and dry your feet carefully each day. Use cottonwool to
  spread surgical spirit all over the feet – this tones up the skin
  and makes it less soggy.

SMOKING

About 100,000 people in Britain and 300,000 people in the USA
die from smoking-related diseases each year. They die because
they inhale three dangerous substances contained in cigarettes –
nicotine, tar and carbon monoxide.

Since 1978 the number of smokers in the UK has gradually
declined (especially men) from over forty per cent to thirty-five
per cent of men and thirty-one per cent of women (1986). But in
1988 there was a rise which was particularly worrying, because
it is young people who are increasingly smoking and there is a
direct link between the length of time you have smoked and the
increased risk of death. In 1986 ten per cent of children aged
eleven to fifteen in England and Wales were regular smokers (i.e.
one or more cigarettes a week) and among fifth-form pupils thirty
per cent of girls and nineteen per cent of boys smoked regularly.

One argument used by smokers to justify their habit is to point
out that no research has shown that smoking directly causes
such diseases as lung cancer, heart disease and bronchitis. This
is true but the evidence against smoking is overwhelming:

- About 30,000 people die from lung cancer in the UK each

year, of whom ninety-five per cent are smokers.

- A smoker is roughly twice as likely to die of a heart attack (about 40,000 British deaths each year) than a non-smoker.

- Smokers are about seventeen times more likely to die of bronchitis than non-smokers.

- Smokers are four times more likely to die of cancer of the gullet than non-smokers, and twice as likely to die from bladder cancer.

- A pregnant woman smoking fifteen to twenty cigarettes a day is twice as likely to have a miscarriage than a non-smoker, and after birth her baby may have up to thirty times greater risk of dying.

Self-health

- The best way to avoid all the problems of smoking is never to start in the first place:

  1. As parents, try not to smoke. Research has shown that children with smoking parents are more likely to smoke than those with non-smoking parents.
  2. Some parents have tried banning cigarettes from the home but the problem is that this may make smoking seem exciting and rebellious instead of a nasty, dangerous, smelly habit.
  3. Other parents have tried bribing their children with promises of a large present if they reach, say, the age of eighteen without smoking. The advantage is that it persuades your child not to smoke until at least a reasonable age and research has shown that the younger you are when you start smoking the more likely you are to become a heavy smoker. The disadvantage is that it may encourage your children to lie to you, or they may find the temptation to try smoking once they have reached the necessary age overwhelming.
  4. The best approach is to discuss the dangers (and pleasures) of smoking calmly and rationally without making it a confrontation between you and your children. In many cases your children will accept your (and hopefully your

friends') arguments to refrain. If not, make one room available for smoking, where at least you can keep an eye on how much smoking is taking place and insist all the mess and unpleasant smell is cleared up by them. Hopefully your children will soon learn it is not a glamorous addiction.

5. For yourself, try to avoid social pressures to smoke. One way is to take up hobbies or go to places where smoking is unpopular.

6. If you are a smoker do not put pressure on young non-smokers to smoke by repeatedly asking them to join you or by constantly smoking in their presence.

- A thousand and one different ways of stopping smoking have been tried but ultimately they all depend on whether, deep down, you want to stop. If you are truly committed almost any method will work. If not, no method will work. Here is one well-tested and successful method:

  1. First, think about all the advantages of not smoking:
     a. You'll be free of the worry you may be killing yourself.
     b. You'll have more money to spend on yourself, your family and friends.
     c. You'll smell fresh. Remember the slogan 'kiss a non-smoker and taste the difference' or the comparison between kissing a smoker and kissing an ashtray.
     d. You'll feel healthier and more energetic.
     e. You'll lose your smoker's cough (although it may get worse for the first two or three months).
     f. You'll suffer fewer coughs, colds and flu.
  2. Next pick a day in the future when you will finally stop smoking. Make sure it is a time when you will be under as little pressure as possible. Stress will drive you straight back into the habit.
     You can start cutting down on the number of cigarettes you smoke before 'the big day' but never let this be a substitute for stopping altogether.
  3. After your last cigarette the day before you give up, get rid of all remaining cigarettes, ashtrays and lighters.
  4. Make 'the big day' rather special by, for instance, getting up late, going for a run or cycle, having a hot bath, having grapefruit for breakfast. Later reward yourself with a

present if you manage to get through the day without
smoking.

5. Work out a routine for your day which avoids, so far as it
   is possible, those situations (e.g. after a meal, while
   drinking, after sex) when you know you will want a
   cigarette. Instead do something else quite different, e.g. do
   all the washing-up immediately after a meal if that is
   going to be a difficult time for you.

6. Distract yourself from the desire to smoke and it will go
   away. Some people find it helps to do something with
   their hands, such as knitting or playing with keys, others
   find they have to chew or suck something, or drink a glass
   of water every time they want a cigarette.

7. Get help from your family and friends:
   a. Tell them why and when you are going to stop
      smoking.
   b. Make a bet with someone that you will succeed,
      preferably someone else also trying to stop with whom
      you can share your experiences.
   c. Get sponsorship for your attempt.
   d. Use the expertise of a local self-help or non-smoking
      group.

8. The first six to eight weeks after stopping smoking will be
   difficult. You may be tense, irritable, shaky, have
   headaches, feel sick and have an intolerable urge to
   smoke. The pressure to start again will be great but
   remember that each day will be a bit better than the last
   and that in time you will get over the craving (although
   some hardened smokers admit they never get over it
   completely).
      If nicotine-flavoured chewing gum (or nasal spray),
   hypnosis, acupuncture, group therapy or even aversion
   therapy seem a good idea to you try it during this difficult
   time – you will need all the help you can get.

9. Give yourself a treat for every day you manage not to
   smoke. Because many people's appetite is stimulated by
   not smoking they tend to give themselves food treats. This
   is not a bad thing during the first few days but it may
   make you overweight so when you lose the intense
   craving for cigarettes (after about eight weeks) you will
   have to start cutting back on the food.

10. Don't be tempted to try a cigarette after several months to prove to yourself you've beaten the habit or to see what it's like. Many people start again like this so it is an unnecessary risk.

• Some people find that for one reason or another they can never give up smoking. For such people it is sensible to smoke as few cigarettes as possible and select a low-tar brand. However, research has shown that many people compensate for low-tar cigarettes by inhaling more deeply and smoking the cigarettes right down to the butt. So beware of deluding yourself about how much damage you are doing to your health.

• Substituting cigar or pipe smoking for cigarette smoking is something many people try. It is worthwhile for some people because cigar and pipe smokers get fewer cancers and heart disease than cigarette smokers, mainly because they inhale less. But for others it is the start of a slippery slope down to or back to cigarettes.

• Smoking is often a response to stress or tension. Learn to cope with (even enjoy) stress and use relaxation techniques (see chapter on Stress and Mental Health) to avoid smoking.

SNORING

Snoring is due to vibration of the uvula or soft palate. This lies at the back of the throat and acts as a valve, shutting off the throat from the nose when needed, for example when eating. If you sleep with your mouth open, the muscles of the throat relax and allow the soft palate to fall back, partly blocking the free flow of air up and down your throat and thus causing the vibration. Snoring is more common in men than women and usually gets worse as you grow older. Recent research has suggested that people who snore may suffer from a sleep disorder known as sleep apnoea, during which the sleeper stops breathing for up to a minute. The resulting fall in the level of oxygen in the blood may be linked to heart disease and poor concentration during the day.

Self-health

- Lose weight if you are overweight because this is associated with snoring.

- Smoking and excessive drinking of alcohol also make snoring worse.

- Sleep on a firm bed that supports you well.

- Get your partner to turn you on your side (or wake you up!) if your snoring troubles him or her. Another way to prevent you lying on your back is to sew a hard object such as a cotton reel into the back of your pyjama jacket.

- It is possible to buy electric alarms that detect the sound of your snoring and wake you.

- If your marriage is threatened or your sleep very disturbed by your snoring, consult your family doctor. Occasionally surgery can be helpful.

SPEECH DIFFICULTIES

A child starts to learn to speak long before actually uttering a word. Your child listens to you, babbles, and learns primitive forms of communication such as shouting or crying to attract your attention.

Children vary greatly in how quickly they learn to talk. Some are talking fluently by eighteen months, others (especially boys) manage only a few words by two years. Progress is often in spurts, with weeks in between when nothing much seems to be happening. Don't worry if your child keeps repeating one word – it is a normal stage of speech development while he or she searches for the right word.

Self-health

- You should consult your family doctor or ask for advice on contacting a speech therapist if:

  1. At eighteen months your child is making no attempt to learn or use words.

2. At two and a half years your child has not put two words together.
3. At three years your child cannot make him or herself understood.

- If your child has constant colds and coughs it is quite possible that their ears may be infected (often without obvious symptoms such as pain). So ask your GP to examine your child's ears, especially if speech is slow to develop.

- You can help your baby learn to speak by:

  1. Talking naturally about everyday things, without oversimplifying or using a special voice. Your baby won't understand but he or she needs to hear you talk.
  2. Naming objects in your house, garden and in picture books.
  3. Explaining to your baby what you are doing to him or her, e.g. dressing, feeding, bathing.
  4. Listening to your baby and trying to answer so that he or she learns that speech is all about communication.

- You can help your toddler's speech by:

  1. Trying to spend some time every day helping with speech.
  2. Talking directly with your child. Avoid having the TV or radio on all the time; try to answer questions and to ask them yourself. Teach your toddler good speaking habits by persuading all members of the family to set a good example.
  3. Letting your toddler see what you mean by matching words to actions (e.g. 'Let's have a hug'), and matching facial expressions to feelings (e.g. smiling when hugging him or her).
  4. Encouraging your toddler by acting as his or her interpreter, especially when talking with other people.
  5. Quietly correcting your toddler if he or she constantly makes a mistake, but not getting angry or discouraged if the mistake continues to be repeated. It will come right soon.
  6. Providing lots of interesting things to talk about at home and on trips to the park, supermarket, zoo, friends' houses.
  7. Teaching your toddler that a lot of communication is non-verbal, e.g. putting on your child's outdoor jacket is a sign that you are going out and he or she can run to the front door without wasted effort.

- Speech is a vital part of a child's development. As a parent you can play your part by providing the right environment and making sure your baby/toddler/child does not fall behind seriously both in the way words are used and how they are pronounced. For special problems see **Stammer** and **Dyslexia**.

- Loss of speech is a common and devastating result of a stroke (see separate entry) damaging the part of the brain that controls language. Sometimes people's ability to speak words is affected but their understanding is normal (dysarthria); others have no difficulty saying words but forget them or use them inappropriately (dysphasia).

  Many people recover speech within twenty-four to forty-eight hours of a stroke. Thereafter recovery will be slower and for some it is an exhausting and frustrating process. The key in all cases is expert tuition, preferably from a speech therapist, and patient, calm encouragement from friends and relatives on the basis of 'a little and often'.

- Difficulties with speech are part of a number of other conditions, especially Parkinson's disease (see separate entry). In many cases you will not be able to cope alone and will need professional help.

SPINA BIFIDA

A child born with spina bifida has vertebrae (bones of the spine) that have not joined up properly. This leaves a gap (large or small depending on how bad the condition is) through which the vital nerves of the spinal cord may be exposed. The causes are unknown but are probably partly environmental, partly genetic.

The condition should be noticed at birth. In the mild form there may be an unusual tuft of dark hair at the base of the spine or a dark mole or fatty lump. In more severe forms there may be a large swelling covered either by skin or a red membrane (the worst kind). In the severe form the child will be paralysed from the waist down, suffer from incontinence, have a swollen head (hydrocephalus), and limited intelligence.

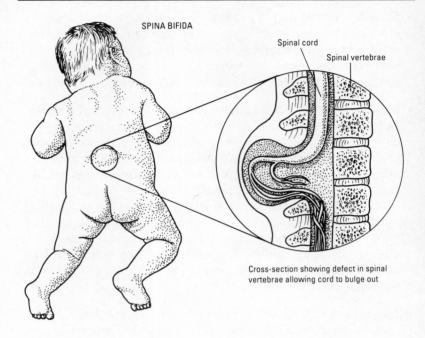

SPINA BIFIDA

Spinal cord

Spinal vertebrae

Cross-section showing defect in spinal
vertebrae allowing cord to bulge out

Self-health

- Parents who have already had a baby with spina bifida should
  realize they have a one in twenty chance of another affected
  baby. Unfortunately nothing can be done to lessen this risk.

- Decisions about how to look after a child with spina bifida
  must be made by the parents guided by expert medical advice.

- In the mild form a small cosmetic operation will be all that is
  needed, the child will have normal intelligence and develop
  normally at an ordinary school.

- In more serious forms operations and medicines (e.g.
  antibiotics) will prevent the child dying although he or she
  will always have difficulties (e.g. walking), may have below-
  average intelligence and need to go to a special school.

- In the most serious forms it may be kindest to allow the child
  to die peacefully, as he or she will do within a few weeks.

Screening

- About one in 700 babies in the UK has spina bifida in one form or another, so it is a condition that is worth searching for before birth so that parents have the choice of whether to terminate the pregnancy.

   A mother who has already had a baby with spina bifida will need specially careful screening because of the increased risk of her having an affected baby.

- Most mothers in the Western world now have an ultrasound examination (from the twelfth to eighteenth week of pregnancy usually) which will show the serious spina bifida changes that might make a termination worth considering. The diagnosis can be confirmed by finding high levels of a substance called alphafetoprotein in the mother's blood and amniotic fluid round the baby. This fluid is taken during a procedure called amniocentesis, which itself has a two or three per cent chance of causing a miscarriage.

SPORTS INJURIES

Since most people take up sport for pleasure the last thing they want is an injury that causes them pain, inconvenience or long-term problems like osteoarthritis (see separate entry). The risk of a serious injury depends on the sport, with horse riding and motor cycle racing carrying the highest risks of fatal accidents.

Many sportspeople would agree that the element of risk is an important part of their enjoyment. But they would also agree that it is sensible to minimize the risks by preparing themselves correctly and, should an injury occur, limiting the damage as much as possible.

Self-health

- **Correct equipment**. It is easy to be deceived by bogus and unscientific claims made by sports equipment companies on behalf of their particular models. Nevertheless it is important you make sure your equipment gives you the best chance of enjoying your sport.

- **Correct training:**
  1. Anyone taking up a sport should be taught the correct techniques from the start. Thereafter these techniques should be constantly practised and checked so that you do not put unnecessary strains on muscles and joints.
  2. The fitter you are the less likely you are to injure yourself. Fitness involves strength, stamina, and suppleness.

     Training strengthens muscles and probably tendons too, so they are less likely to tear under stress. Strong muscles will also protect vulnerable parts of the body like the back or knees. Overall strength is important but generally the muscles that are used in the sport are the ones that should be trained, e.g. swimmers should swim and runners run. Weight-training is useful but never start without proper coaching.

     Stamina (the ability to maintain your level of performance for a long time) is important because it reduces the time when injuries are most common (i.e. when you are exhausted). It may also reduce your chances of a serious illness like a heart attack.

     Suppleness helps prevent injuries in all sports but is often neglected. If nothing else, learn and practise a few basic routines at least three times a week. A little often is better than a lot once a week. Yoga is an enjoyable way of keeping supple.

- **Correct preparation before the sport**. A 'warm-up' period before starting your sport is important. Stretching muscles will make them less likely to tear under strain later on. Concentrate on the muscles you will use most in your sport, but a general 'limbering-up' is useful.

- **'Warming down' after the sport**. Do not stop hard exercise suddenly – wind down gradually with gentle exercises, including stretching. This will help reduce pain and stiffness afterwards.

- **Coping with an injury**. There are three main types of sports injury: breaks, pulled muscles, and sprains. In each case stop playing the sport immediately. Adrenaline may encourage you to 'play through' an injury but you will suffer afterwards and you will always make the injury worse.

1. A break should be moved as little as possible and medical treatment sought immediately. Be very wary of possible fractures of the spine because even the slightest movement can cause permanent paralysis.
2. Early treatment of pulled muscles will speed recovery:
   a. Apply ice-packs (e.g. a frozen pack of peas, ice-cubes wrapped in a tea-towel) over the injury for about twenty minutes two or three times a day.
   b. Gently bind the injured part. The bandage must be elastic so it can stretch to accommodate more swelling.
   c. Keep the injured part raised so fluid flows away from it.
   d. Rest the injured part, preferably until the pain has stopped.
3. For sprain, see separate entry.

SPRAIN

A sprain occurs when the ligaments supporting a joint tear because of excess strain upon them. The injury may be mild with some local pain and swelling or it may cause so much pain, swelling and deformity that it is difficult to distinguish from a break. Ankles, wrists, thumbs and backs are most commonly affected.

Self-health

- See **Sports Injuries** for ways to prevent a sprain.

- Active, early movement is now recommended to get the ligaments and joint back to normal as quickly as possible and prevent long-term weakness. Keeping off the joint, repeated non-weight-bearing exercises, ice and elevation are the secrets of success.

- Do not ignore pain and a feeling of weakness when returning to a sport or you may find your joint never gets back to normal. Far better to get it strong first and then return confidently to the stresses of the sport.

STAMMER

All children between the ages of two and four go through a stage of stuttering or stammering, when their ideas run ahead of their ability to put them into words. This is normal but difficulties arise when the stuttering continues into school age, adolescence and beyond. About four per cent of the population stammer, men four times more commonly than women.

Self-health

- Stammering is not genetic. It runs in families but this is 'learned' from other family members rather than inherited. Relatives may have (or have had) a speech problem themselves and so are over-anxious about a child showing any speech difficulties. This creates tension and insecurities within the child, who responds by continuing to stammer. This sequence of events must be recognized and avoided at all costs.

- Parents should also be aware of other insecurities that can trigger stammering, such as a major illness, the birth of a younger brother or sister, or self-doubts about the ability to live up to their parents' ambitions and hopes.

- Try to listen to what your child is saying, not how he or she is saying it. Particularly don't rush your child, don't finish off your child's sentences, or scold him or her for not speaking more clearly or slowly.

- To make your child feel secure, say how much you enjoy his or her company and speech. Give your child a chance to say things, even if it means clearing other noisy children out of the room.

- Consider whether you can reduce other areas of stress, e.g. at school.

- If you continue to be worried about your child's speech despite your own efforts you should see your family doctor or arrange to see a speech therapist. It is rare for there to be a physical cause for stammering but this will be excluded before treatment begins, and then a personal programme planned. This may include relaxation techniques, speech exercises, headphones to cut out the sound of the child's own voice, and systems of reward and punishment. Residential courses in speech-therapy units are also effective.

STERILIZATION, FEMALE

Sterilization is the most popular, safe and permanent method of birth control for women who have had all the children they want or who don't want to have children at all. It was first described by doctors in 1834 and since then millions of women have benefited.

The purpose of the operation is to close the Fallopian tubes so that the ovum (egg) and sperm cannot meet and start a pregnancy. It can be done under general anaesthetic, which means you are unconscious throughout the operation, or it can be done under local anaesthetic when you are drowsy but awake at all times.

Self-health

- You must accept that sterilization is permanent, so if there is any chance you may change your mind and want children you must not choose this method of birth control. Remember that your family circumstances may change.

- It is wise to discuss sterilization with your partner and your family doctor. Many clinics have special counsellors who are trained to help you. In the end, though, it is you who must decide because it is you who will have to live with the consequences for the rest of your life.

- You should tell the doctor or clinic if you have had any pelvic infections, a ruptured appendix or an ectopic pregnancy. Diabetes, heart disease, epilepsy, ovarian cysts, and raised blood pressure are also conditions your doctor will want to know about. They are important because they may affect whether or how the sterilization is performed.

- Five or six days after the operation you will be able to resume sex as before. You will notice no physical or emotional change except that many women find they can enjoy sex more because the problems of other methods of birth control or the possibility of an unwanted pregnancy have been banished for ever.

STERILIZATION, MALE (VASECTOMY)

Vasectomy is an increasingly popular method of contraception for men and couples who do not want to have children or who feel they have enough children.

The purpose of the operation is to tie the two tubes (vas deferens) that carry the sperm from the testes to the penis. It is usually done under local anaesthetic and takes about fifteen to twenty minutes.

Self-health

- You must accept that a vasectomy is permanent so do not consider this method of contraception if you think there is a chance, however remote, you may want more children. Remember your family circumstances may change.

- It is sensible to discuss vasectomy with your partner and your family doctor. Many clinics have special counsellors who are trained to help you. In the end, though, it is you who must decide because it is you who will live with the consequences for the rest of your life.

- After the pain and swelling caused by the operation have disappeared (usually seven to ten days and helped by a scrotal support) you can resume sex as before. But you must continue to use contraception until at least two specimens of semen obtained by masturbation have been proved to contain no sperm. This usually takes three or four months. You will notice no physical or emotional change in your sex life after the operation except that many couples find sex more enjoyable once the fears and worries of other methods of contraception have disappeared.

- It is important that you realize you are no less male, virile or attractive for having had a vasectomy. It does not affect your erection or how long or how often you have sex. Nor does it change any of the other characteristics that make you male.

- A few men may find problems with their sex lives after a vasectomy. This is always due to psychological reasons. For example, the operation may uncover deep-rooted fears or anxieties which the person never consciously knew existed before. If you are one of these few men, get professional treatment soon because you can be helped – the sooner the better.

STROKE

If something goes wrong with the circulation of blood to a part of the brain it may become damaged and stroke (cerebrovascular accident) may result. One common cause, occurring in seventy per cent of cases, is a blockage in an artery caused by a blood clot. This often happens within an artery that has been narrowed and hardened by a build-up of fatty deposits known as atheroma. The other common cause is a bleed (haemorrhage) from an artery, forming a blood clot which itself presses on the brain, damaging it and perhaps further cutting off its blood supply.

The symptoms include drowsiness or loss of consciousness, and partial or complete loss of movement in the limbs of one side, the arm being more commonly affected than the leg. The person's face may also be paralysed on one side, giving it an awkward twist.

Sometimes the patient has difficulty understanding what is being said and difficulty talking, reading or writing. Some people find they have difficulty seeing or are blind when looking in one direction. Often there are emotional changes so that the person may become unusually depressed, aggressive or easily offended.

The effects of a stroke vary greatly. One-third of sufferers die. In England and Wales this amounts to about 70,000 people a year or twelve per cent of all deaths, which makes stroke one of the three main causes of death (the others are heart disease and cancer).

One-third of affected people make a full recovery. These are usually people who notice an improvement shortly after the stroke. The earlier and quicker the recovery the better the final outlook. Certainly recovery is slow after six months have passed.

One-third of people make some recovery but are left with disabilities which they and their carers have to cope with.

Self-health

* **Prevention**
  1. Making sure your blood pressure is within the normal range for your age is the most important thing you can do to prevent yourself having a stroke (see **Blood Pressure**). The higher your blood pressure, the greater the risk: high blood pressure will treble your chances of dying from a stroke. In fact forty-five per cent of people with high blood pressure die from a stroke, compared to thirty-five per cent from heart disease.
  2. If you smoke, try to stop. Studies from New Zealand, Honolulu and Framingham, USA show that smokers are at two or three times the risk of stroke compared with non-smokers. And the more you smoke, the greater the risk.

     If you do stop smoking your chances of having a stroke will fall within five years to those of a non-smoker.
  3. Diabetics are at risk of stroke, especially women. Although doctors have not yet proved that good control of the diabetes (see **Diabetes Mellitus**) reduces the risk, it seems good sense.
  4. Doctors have been uncertain for over twenty years about whether women taking the contraceptive pill are at greater risk of stroke. Overall it seems they are, particularly if they smoke, are diabetic or overweight, or have high blood pressure. Low-oestrogen pills may carry less risk.
  5. Studies have shown that heavy drinkers (see **Alcoholism**) have up to four times the risk of a stroke compared with non-drinkers.
  6. Many doctors feel that being overweight carries an increased risk of stroke, although again this has not been proven beyond doubt.
  7. A diet which is high in fat (see **Cholesterol**) may carry an increased risk of stroke.
  8. Regular exercise may help reduce the risk of stroke. It certainly helps keep your weight down and stimulates interest in other activities.

* If you have made a full recovery from a stroke you will need to consider whether there is anything in your lifestyle that needs changing. Your doctor may be able to advise you. Many people imagine that stress is an important cause of stroke. There is no

proof this is so, in fact many people thrive on 'stress' (see chapter on Stress and Mental Health). So do not feel you have to change your job, or home, or exciting hobbies automatically just because you have had a stroke.

- If you have made only a partial recovery from a stroke it is vital that you learn to accept that your lifestyle may have to change but that it is still possible to live a full life within the limits of your disabilities. Nowadays there are many services and aids which will help the quality of your life:

  1. In the early days physiotherapy will help to keep paralysed limbs flexible. After you come home make sure your carers help you do the exercises you have been shown.
  2. Early speech therapy will help you develop new communication skills. Recovery may be painstakingly slow but you will be surprised at how much you can improve if you persist.
  3. There are all sorts of aids to help you in your home (see **Gadgets for Disabled and Elderly People**). Make full use of them.
  4. Incontinence is a problem for some. In most cases you will recover completely. If not, there are all sorts of aids (see **Incontinence**).
  5. Try to make a plan for each day. Unless you are very disabled you should try to dress every day. Plan short periods of activities such as walking, practising speech, buttering bread, tying shoelaces. Try to include a hobby every day. Swimming is excellent for many people and there may be a disabled club at your local pool.
  6. If you enjoyed sex before your stroke, there is no reason why you should not resume afterwards. There may be some initial difficulties and you will need an understanding partner, but for most people there is no risk. Discuss any problems or fears you may have with your doctor.

- If you are the carer of someone who has been severely disabled by a stroke it is easy to get bogged down in the extra work and responsibilities. Here are some tips:

  1. Make use of all the services (e.g. doctor, physiotherapist, occupational therapist, speech therapist, social worker, self-help groups) that you can.

2. Involve friends and other family members. You may wish to set up a rota. You will be surprised how often sufferers respond to positive suggestions from friends which they would not have accepted from you!

3. Do not be surprised if your friend or relative becomes depressed – it might be surprising if they didn't sometimes. Be encouraging without being unrealistic and try to shift the mood by focusing on interesting activities and friends' visits, and showing you care. If the mood persists, consult your doctor who may suggest a short course of anti-depressive medicine.

4. Finally, never neglect your own life completely in your efforts to care for your loved one. If you do it could destroy you and be the worst possible thing for both of you. Always keep some time and activities for yourself. And do not feel guilty if you sometimes feel resentful; it happens to most carers, is quite natural and usually passes. But if you do get to the point where you think you might neglect or damage your charge, do not be ashamed to tell someone responsible so the pressure can be taken off you for a while.

- Some victims of a stroke start to rethink their ideas about life, morals and religion. These thoughts can have as important an effect upon the person as the physical problems, and may need expert guidance from a minister of religion or a counsellor.

- Never underestimate how important a pet can be (see **Pets**) to help alleviate the feelings of frustration so many victims experience.

SUGAR

Table sugar is sucrose, a refined carbohydrate (see chapter on Healthy Eating). It consists of two simple sugars (glucose and fructose) joined together. It is found naturally in cane sugar (particularly used in the Western world), beetroot, dates and figs. After being eaten the sugar is broken down in the gut into glucose and fructose which are then absorbed into the bloodstream and carried to the body's cells to provide energy.

UK consumption has risen fast since the sugar tax was

removed in the mid-nineteenth century and is now about 36 kg
per head a year. In America it is about 54 kg per head a year.

Many nutritionists have now identified sugar consumption as
excessive. For example the influential 1983 NACNE Report
recommended that all Britons should cut their sugar
consumption by half. At the same time, though, there are plenty
of myths about the dangers of sugar consumption.

Self-health

- Since one teaspoon of sugar contains 30−40 calories and no
  other nutritional value such as vitamins, fibre or minerals, it is
  an 'empty' source of calories which should be avoided,
  particularly by people with a tendency to become overweight.
  Obesity and all the harm it causes is probably the most
  dangerous result of eating sugar.

  So, instead of eating empty calories in the form of sugar,
  choose foods that contain plenty of vitamins, minerals and
  fibre, such as fruit and vegetables. If you have a 'sweet tooth'
  you will be surprised by how sweet such foods can taste.

- The other main problem caused by eating sugar is tooth decay.
  Sugar does not directly damage teeth but bacteria living in
  plaque on teeth are able to convert it into acids which attack
  the enamel, causing decay. To minimize this decay it is worth:

  1. Trying not to eat sweet foods between meals so there is less
     opportunity for bacteria to get to work.
  2. Being careful about the source of the sugar. For example
     raisins or dried fruits (which might seem 'natural') are more
     harmful to teeth than chocolate, probably because they
     cling to teeth providing a growing surface for bacteria while
     fat in a chocolate bar coats the enamel making it difficult
     for the bacteria to get close.

- There are some useful tips for cutting down on sugar:

  1. Try not to let your children develop a sweet tooth. Some
     children are naturally more inclined to this than others, but
     try to satisfy them with sweetness from other sources, such
     as fresh fruit and vegetables.
  2. Don't have sugar routinely on the table as your children
     grow up. It will encourage a sweet tooth.

3. Remember invisible sugars in food. They are found in processed foods (e.g. soups, ice-cream, fizzy drinks), sauces, cakes, biscuits and cereals.
4. Check food labels for sugars – remember fructose, maltose, glucose and dextrose are all sugars. If any appear within the first three or four ingredients on the label it is worth considering buying an alternative.
5. If you have a craving for something sweet immediately fill yourself up with fresh fruit and vegetables, or do something active or useful as a distraction.
6. Consider artificial sweeteners, e.g. saccharin or aspartame. These are often as much as 600 times sweeter than sugar but the problem is no research has been done on the long-term effects of these substances on the body (e.g. saccharin has been linked with bladder cancer but no proof has been found). Certainly pregnant women should, as a matter of principle, avoid artificial sweeteners.

   Research has also shown that taking artificial sweeteners makes no difference to many people's total calorie intake – they simply consume the calories in another form. Other people also find that sweeteners stimulate their appetite for sweet things without satisfying it.

- Don't let your love for sugary foods trap you into avoiding sugar but eating other high-calorie products (e.g. fatty food) which may be bad for you for other reasons.

- Brown sugar is no more healthy than white sugar – it is simply white sugar with a coating of molasses.

- Honey is only slightly more useful as a food than sugar. It is made of sugar and water with traces of a few vitamins.

- Sugar does not cause heart disease. Its only connection is that it may make you overweight which itself is linked with heart disease.

SUICIDE

In the UK 4,000 people kill themselves (suicide) each year, and 200,000 try to kill themselves (para-suicide).

Self-health

YOURSELF

- If you feel desperate, talk to someone. Often a good talk and a cry is all you need. Sometimes, though, you may feel so bad that you need professional help from a psychiatrist, psychologist or trained nurse.

- Recognize the warning signs of depression (see separate entry) and get help before your symptoms start clouding your judgement. Sadly many people have had unrecognized, untreated depression for some time before committing suicide.

- Avoid loneliness, especially after the death of a loved one, because it provides the opportunity to brood – and to plan suicide.

- Be practical – don't have the means to kill yourself easily to hand, e.g. have as few pills in your house as you can.

- Make sure any physical problem or stress is treated. Being in constant pain can make you consider suicide seriously but modern treatment is so good you don't have to be in pain.

- Seek help from the Samaritans (twenty-four hours a day, telephone number in your local directory), your priest or religious adviser, your analyst or family doctor. Many people find the Samaritans particularly valuable because they provide compassionate yet disinterested advice.

SOMEONE CLOSE

- Severe depression (see separate entry) is the most common cause of suicide. These are some suicidal signs that you should watch out for (and get help for) in anyone who is depressed:
  1. Making a will, giving away loved objects, setting affairs in order.
  2. Discussing suicide. There is no truth in the old wives' tale that if someone talks about suicide he or she need not be taken seriously. Eighty per cent of successful suicides have discussed it earlier. And never joke, bluff, threaten, or argue – just listen to start with.

- Someone who has already tried to commit suicide, is at greater risk than someone who has not, even if it appeared to be a half-hearted attempt.

- Make use of the Samaritans. They have great experience, and are available twenty-four hours a day. Their telephone number can be found in your local directory.

- Feel free to contact the person's GP and explain your worries. You will be listened to sympathetically.

- Self-help groups can be a useful source of support.

SUNBURN

There is no doubt too much sun is a danger to your skin. Small amounts are needed by the body to make vitamin D but more irritates your skin, making it hot and red. Longer exposure to the sun causes it to become inflamed and swollen, and longer still causes it to blister and peel.

The damage is caused by shortwave ultra-violet rays. We are partially protected from these rays by the ozone layer which surrounds the earth at a high altitude. But clouds offer little protection, allowing as much as eighty per cent of the ultra-violet rays that have got this far to pass through.

The ultra-violet rays particularly attack the collagen in skin, which is responsible for making it soft and supple. This causes the premature ageing of skin seen in people who have sunbathed too much. It also affects the skin cells themselves, making them more likely to become cancerous (see **Skin Cancer**).

Tanning is the body's reaction to sunlight. The tan absorbs the ultra-violet light and so prevents it damaging the delicate skin cells. The skin also protects itself by increasing the thickness of the outer layer of skin so that there are more dead cells for the rays to pass through before they reach the living cells beneath (which is why our thick-skinned palms rarely get burned). Tanning needs time to establish itself, especially in fair skins.

Self-health

- If you live in a hot country be sure to protect yourself from the sun with hats and appropriate clothing. You will develop and keep a tan but remember this gives you only partial protection and that you are still more likely to get skin cancer than people living in cold climates.

- If you live in a temperate or cold climate but enjoy holidays in the sun think about whether you want a suntan in view of the risks involved. It may look attractive and healthy for a short while, but you will look hot and red when it is building up, especially if you are fair, and when you come home you will peel unattractively (although you can prolong your tan by putting oil in your bath water and covering yourself with moisturizer).

- If you still want a tan (!) here are some tips:

  1. Strong sunlight can seriously burn your skin within ten minutes, especially if you are fair. So start tanning cautiously and build up gradually. Remember that burning or peeling means you have lost your preciously acquired tan and that you will have to start again.
  2. Sunlight is strongest between eleven and three o'clock, so try to do any sunbathing outside these hours. It will also be stronger at altitude, or if reflected off light surfaces such as snow, white walls, water and sand.
  3. Water cools you down, giving you a false sense of security. In fact it makes you more vulnerable to sunburn, reflecting more sunlight back at you and washing off your sunscreen.
  4. Choose sunscreen preparations most suited to your skin type. They now display a sun protection factor (SPF) which ranges from 2 to 20. An SPF of 2 (low) means that skin should be able to tolerate the sun for twice as long when using this product; an SPF of 4 means four times as long and so on. Good protection is provided by an SPF over 6. Colourless sunscreens are useful for places like lips, noses and cheeks.
  5. Beware of products that claim they speed tanning. These products may contain chemicals that enhance the effect of sunlight on the skin.
  6. Use plenty of moisturizer to prevent your skin drying out.
  7. If you do burn your skin apply calamine or similar soothing cream and take painkillers. If you get no relief see your

doctor who may suggest a steroid-containing ointment to reduce inflammation.

- Too much sun damages your skin but it can also affect your whole body, making you seriously ill with heat exhaustion or sunstroke. Here are some useful tips to prevent this happening:

  1. Drink plenty of fluids but avoid alcohol.
  2. Do not exercise and sweat profusely without replacing lost fluid. It may also be advisable to take salt tablets or sprinkle your food liberally with salt to replace salt lost in sweat.
  3. Some research suggests that vitamin A tablets may help prevent sunstroke.
  4. Cool yourself down with tepid showers, air-conditioning, and a fan.
  5. Consult a doctor earlier rather than later if you cannot keep your temperature down, have a severe headache or feel faint.

- Support environmental groups who are trying to protect the ozone layer. If this layer continues to be eroded at its present rate we will experience major changes in our health (e.g. more skin cancer, as has already happened) and in our environment – the 'hothouse effect'.

SWOLLEN FEET

Feet swell when the watery part of the blood collects round the tissues of the ankle. It happens in hot weather, or to people who stand or sit a lot, especially older people when the mechanism for returning the fluid back up the legs is not working as well as it used to. People with varicose veins or a heart condition are particularly prone to swollen ankles.

Self-health

- Sit with your feet higher than your hips so gravity helps drain the fluid away.
- Wear support stockings or socks. You can buy these in the chemist or ask your doctor for advice.

- Don't sit or stand for long periods. If you cannot avoid doing so, keep the calf muscles on the move by relaxing and tensing them alternately. This will force the fluid up the legs.

- If these suggestions fail, see your doctor who may wish to investigate and treat you further.

SYPHILIS

Syphilis is a sexually transmitted disease caused by the bacterium *spirochaeta pallida*. There are three stages of the disease:

1. About four weeks after sexual contact a pimple followed by an ulcer appears on the penis, vagina, lip, or wherever contact has been made with infection. Lymph glands nearby may swell.
2. About twelve months later a rash appears all over the body, lasting a week or two. You may also have a fever and feel unwell.
3. One to thirty years later the serious symptoms of dementia, large, slow-growing abscesses, heart and artery disease and difficulty with walking and balance appear. Death will follow thereafter.

Self-health

- Stick to one sexual partner to reduce your chances of getting syphilis.

- Use a condom if your partner could be infected.

- After a sexual encounter which could infect you, check for any unexplained pimples or ulcers on your genitals, anus, lips or mouth. If you find anything suspicious see your family doctor immediately or go to a hospital special clinic. It is vital you do not ignore symptoms simply because they seem to be disappearing. The disease is still in your body and needs treatment. Women are at special risk because their symptoms are often very mild.

- You need early treatment with antibiotics to prevent the

disease passing into stages two and three. Make sure you complete your course of antibiotics so that all bacteria are killed.

- If you have syphilis do not have sex with anyone else until your doctor says it is safe to do so. If you have had sex with someone while you were unaware that you had syphilis, you must inform that person immediately, even if it is embarrassing and difficult. Syphilis is a dangerous disease if left untreated.

T

TEMPERATURE

Most people's normal body temperature is 37°C but there is great variation so it is worth taking your temperature when you are well so you know what is normal for you.

Your temperature may be taken with a mercury-filled thermometer, but the recent digital thermometers or skin temperature indicator strips, which change colour to match the temperature, are often more convenient.

The mouth is the most accurate place to take the temperature – but remember not to have a hot drink just before or you may get a shock! Under the arm is useful for children and people who are not well or are having difficulty breathing but you will need to add about 0.5°C to the reading you get. Allow two minutes when taking the temperature in the mouth and three minutes under the arm. The temperature indicator strips use the skin and are probably the least accurate thermometers.

Self-health

HIGH TEMPERATURE

- In adults the temperature rises in close relation to the severity of the illness; anything over 39°C is serious.

- In children rises and falls are more variable and it is quite possible for a child to have a temperature without being obviously ill. However, children do seem to have a critical level (39–40°C) after which they suddenly become very ill. Again, this level varies from child to child.

- A high temperature is one of the body's ways of coping with an illness. It may make the person feel shivery, unwell, nauseated, confused, even delirious, and in some children it may cause fits (see separate entry), and so it should be reduced if possible:

1. First take your child's temperature as a baseline so you know whether it is going up or down.
2. Medicines are the best way to reduce the temperature quickly. Paracetamol is best for children because it has few side effects and comes in syrup or elixir form to make it easy for young children to take.
3. Never try to 'sweat out' illnesses by heating your child's room – it could be dangerous. Instead cool the room to about 39°C.
4. Remove all the bedclothes except for a sheet.
5. Strip your child down to pants or vest – most feel uncomfortable naked.
6. Many doctors and books advise tepid sponging of your child's whole body as a useful way of reducing temperature. In theory this is true but our experience is that it is impractical and upsetting for the child. So reserve it for special occasions, such as the temperature rising fast, or any temperature over 40°C or any child who has had a febrile fit in the past. A cold fan is often an easier and more popular way of getting the temperature down.
7. Your child's temperature should drop within half an hour of taking the above measures. If it has not, you should call your family doctor.

LOW TEMPERATURE

- See **Hypothermia**.

TENNIS ELBOW

Despite its name you need never have lifted a tennis racket to get this condition. The medical name is lateral epiconylitis. The symptoms are pain on the outside of the elbow joint, which becomes tender to touch and increasingly painful on certain movements.

It is a common condition usually caused by repetitive movements such as gripping and twisting, causing soreness where the muscle joins the bone just beyond the elbow joint. It does not produce swelling and has nothing to do with arthritis.

It often causes pain and aching at night. During the daytime it is made worse by gripping or twisting (e.g. when playing tennis) or if you bang the elbow.

Self-health

- Tennis elbow will often get better simply by stopping the repetitive activity which brings it on.

- Athletes who find themselves prone to it may get some protection and relief by using a tennis elbow clamp, available at most sports shops.

- If it is slow to settle, your doctor might recommend some local treatment. This may help but do not be surprised if it takes a year or more. Eventually the condition will get better naturally.

TETANUS

Tetanus (also known as lockjaw) is a disease caused by the poison (toxin) of a bacteria called clostridia tetani which lives in soil and animal (especially horse) faeces. Worldwide there may be up to one million cases a year, mainly in unimmunized babies and children. In Britain there are fewer than thirty cases a year.

Most cases occur when the poison enters the body through wounds caused by car accidents. But other injuries like thorn or nail injuries and animal bites can also cause it, so no wound is so small that you should not be concerned about tetanus.

Symptoms begin from two days to several months after the injury. The abdominal, arm, leg and spinal muscles become rigid and suffer painful spasms. The spasms may affect the breathing muscles, too, causing death in about ten per cent of patients, despite treatment.

Self-health

- It is vital that every member of the family has an immunization course of injections. This should start within the first six months of life with a joint vaccination against tetanus, diphtheria and whooping cough, repeated once three to six months later and again before the age of five. This should be followed by five-yearly booster injections to maintain protection.

Most casualty departments will give you an automatic booster following an injury, so enquire if you do not receive one and think you may need one.

Some people have a reaction to the booster. If you are such a person tell any doctor or nurse who wishes to give you a booster so they can decide whether and how to proceed. Less reactive injections have been developed made with human rather than animal serum which may be better for you.

- All wounds should be carefully cleaned with an antiseptic, making sure all dirt is removed. Seek medical help if you cannot manage yourself, especially with deep wounds.

- If you suspect you are getting tetanus see a doctor without delay. The sooner you receive an injection to neutralize the poison, followed by antibiotics, the more likely you are to make a full recovery.

THREADWORMS

The worm *Enterobius vermicularis* may infect the intestine, causing colic (in children) and an itchy anus (very commonly) or itchy vagina in young girls. All types of homes are affected, even the cleanest.

First the worm gets into your or your child's gut when you eat contaminated food or are in close contact (especially at night) with an infected person. In the gut, it grows larger until the female worm crawls out into the anus and lays up to 10,000 eggs which cause the itching. You or your child may scratch, get the eggs under fingernails, into bedclothing or even directly into the mouth by sucking fingers, and so the cycle of reproduction continues.

Self-health

- If your child complains of an itchy anus at night have a look (at night). You may see 10–13 mm white worms wriggling round the anus. There may be quite a few so be prepared! But don't worry, they are not causing your child serious harm apart from the itch.

- If you know you have threadworms in the family every member should try to be as hygienic as possible.

1. Hands should be washed after going to the lavatory, before meals, and after handling the pet (which may also be infected).
2. Pyjamas rather than nightgowns should be worn so the chance of direct contact between hands and the anus is reduced.
3. Fingernails should be clipped to reduce the chances of carrying eggs.
4. Bed linen and underwear should be washed frequently because the eggs can survive for two or three weeks.

- All members of the family will need treatment if one member has threadworms. A medicine (repeated two weeks later) is given to kill the worms and flush them out. This is painless and, combined with good hygiene, almost always solves the problem.

THROAT, SORE

An uncomfortable, raw feeling at the back of the throat is a common symptom. It is usually caused by the viruses responsible for colds or influenza, and sometimes by bacteria such as the streptococcus. Some people are so sensitive to smoke that they will develop a sore throat if exposed to it.

Self-health

- If you have a cold or flu keep away from other people to avoid spreading germs.

- Avoid smoky atmospheres and cold, raw weather.

- Take throat lozenges or painkillers in recommended doses. Soothing drinks can also be helpful.

- If your sore throat is not getting any better after forty-eight hours or if there is no obvious reason for it, see your family doctor.

- Just occasionally a sore throat is due to a quinsy abscess on one or both tonsils. This will be seen as a white, pussy area on the tonsils. In children this abscess can grow so large and inflamed that it prevents the free flow of air in and out of their mouths, causing them to become breathless and distressed. In these emergency circumstances you should take your child immediately to casualty for urgent treatment.

THROMBOSIS

A thrombus is a blood clot which partially or completely blocks a vein. If the vein is close to the skin it may cause thrombophlebitis. If the vein is deep it is called deep vein thrombosis (DVT).

The symptoms are pain and swelling of the calf and/or thigh. Sometimes the veins stand out prominently, or the skin may look red and inflamed.

Self-health

- There are many causes of thrombosis but some people are at special risk:

    1. People over sixty-five.
    2. Anyone who is overweight.
    3. Anyone with a blood disease, e.g. leukaemia (see separate entry).
    4. Women who smoke and have been on the Pill for over five years.
    5. Anyone who lies in bed (or sits in a chair) for long hours at a time (e.g. disabled, injured or sick people).
    6. Anyone who has had an operation.

- The secrets of prevention are:

    1. Keep as mobile as possible, even if this means exercising your knee, ankle and calf muscles in bed. Lying unnecessarily long in bed after an operation or childbirth should also be avoided.

2. Try not to become overweight.
3. Do not smoke (see **Smoking**).
4. Keep your legs up on a stool or sofa when sitting.
5. Avoid standing in one place for a long time. If you cannot avoid standing, walk on the spot for a few seconds at a time every minute or so.
6. Wear support stockings if your legs have a tendency to swell.
7. If you are on the Pill consider alternative forms of contraception (see separate entry).
8. If you have any unexplained symptoms in your legs consult your family doctor. You should also tell the doctor about them if you are going for an operation.

THRUSH, MOUTH AND SKIN

Thrush (also known as candidiasis or moniliasis) is infection with the yeast *candida albicans*. It affects the mouth, nails, and the skin of breastfolds, genitals, buttocks, and underarms.

The skin becomes shiny, red, itchy and mildly inflamed with a clear border between infected and non-infected skin. Inside the mouth there is soreness and flecks of white, especially around dentures if you wear them.

Self-health

• Affected skin should be washed only with mild soap and always dried well to discourage the yeast, which flourishes in moist places.

• If you have recurrent thrush dust the area with one of the proprietary powders recommended by your chemist.

• Try not to wear synthetic materials (which can't 'breathe') close to your skin.

• Lose weight if you are overweight.

• Avoid keeping unprotected hands in water (e.g. washing up) for long periods if your nails are affected. Wear gloves, or take advantage of your skin condition to organize someone else to do this chore!

- Thrush is a common cause of nappy rash (see separate entry).

- If your mouth tends to be affected:

  1. Practise oral dental hygiene (see **Gum Disease**).
  2. Clean dentures every night.
  3. Sterilize your children's dummies to prevent the spread of infection.
  4. If you are asthmatic you may find your steroid inhaler brings on thrush. Try different forms of inhaler (e.g. the 'Volumatic') which spread the steroid medicine more evenly.
  5. People receiving radiotherapy should consult their doctor about how to prevent and treat thrush.

- Avoid steroid-containing creams because they make thrush worse.

THRUSH, VAGINAL

Vaginal thrush is known as thrush because the discharge is coloured rather like the bird's plumage. It is caused by the yeast *candida albicans* (and may be known as candidiasis or moniliasis).

The yeast lives in the vagina (and bowel) of many women without causing symptoms. But others, for reasons not fully understood, develop symptoms. These include a thick, creamy discharge with curd-like consistency, together with itching round the opening of the vagina, which may become red and swollen.

Self-health

- Thrush is not necessarily a sexually transmitted disease because it may occur in sexually non-active people. So you need feel no embarrassment about getting advice and help, or telling your partner.

- However, you can get thrush from sexual contact so the fewer partners you have the less likely you are to get it.

  If a man wears a condom it is extremely unlikely he will either catch thrush or pass it on.

- After you have opened your bowels always wipe from the vagina backwards to the anus so you do not spread the yeast from the bowels to the vagina.

- Research does not support the widely held view that nylon underwear or tights bring on thrush. However, avoiding synthetic clothing does seem common sense and is worth trying if thrush is a recurring problem for you.

- Avoid vaginal deodorants (tempting to use if you have a discharge), bubble baths, perfumed soap and talcum powder, which may make you prone to thrush.

- Taking the contraceptive pill may also make you more prone to thrush. Consider alternative forms of contraception (see separate entry), or if you continue with the Pill use anti-thrush pessaries at the times in your cycle when you usually get symptoms.

- Antibiotics change the bacteria in your vagina and make thrush more likely. If this is a problem for you, use anti-thrush pessaries while taking the antibiotics.

- Poor general health and stress make some women prone to thrush.

- If you have an attack of thrush, doctors' opinions vary about whether it is worth treating your partner to prevent the infection being passed back and forth between you. Most agree it is probably not worthwhile, although it is sensible for him to use a condom.

- Don't persist with intercourse if it is painful, because you will make the thrush worse.

- Diet probably does not affect your likelihood of getting thrush although some women find a diet low in yeasts (e.g. avoiding cheeses, some breads, alcohol, unpeeled fruits, grapes) and low in refined carbohydrates helpful.

- Complete the course of treatment your doctor prescribes to give yourself the best chance of getting rid of the yeast. If used properly, pessaries will cure over ninety per cent of cases.

- Do not expect creams applied to the outside of the vagina to either prevent or cure thrush. The infection is deep in the vagina and needs treatment there.

THYROID GLAND, OVERACTIVITY (THYROTOXICOSIS)

The thyroid gland is found on each side of the windpipe in the neck. It produces the hormone thyroxine which controls the body's metabolic rate, i.e. rate at which chemical processes take place. About one in 3,000 people suffers from a condition known as thyrotoxicosis in which the gland produces too much hormone. The effect is to make the person hyperactive but also anxious, fidgety, easily tired, and with poor concentration. He or she is prone to palpitations, loses weight despite eating an excellent diet, may suffer from diarrhoea, doesn't notice the cold and may have protuberant, red, and sore eyes. Many also have a lump in their necks due to swelling of the gland.

Self-health

- You cannot prevent thyrotoxicosis and the most important thing you can do is to recognize the symptoms early and consult your family doctor. Treatment will take the form of medicines to control the amount of thyroxine hormone produced, or radioactive iodine taken as a drink, or surgery, or a combination of all three. The outlook is generally very good for people properly treated.

- If you have high blood pressure, angina or heart disease, it is particularly important you are treated early because all these conditions are made worse by thyrotoxicosis.

THYROID GLAND, UNDERACTIVITY (MYXOEDEMA/HYPOTHYROIDISM)

The thyroid gland is found on each side of the windpipe in the neck. It provides the hormone thyroxine which controls the body's metabolic rate (the rate at which chemical processes take place). About one in 750 people cannot make enough thyroxine, which causes a condition known as myxoedema or hypothyroidism. In young babies it is known as mongolism or Down's syndrome.

Symptoms are very varied and may come on over so many

years that you do not recognize the changes. Because all the chemical processes slow down, you cannot think or act quickly. You feel lethargic and weak and put on weight despite a normal diet. Your hair may start to fall out and become thin and lifeless and your skin become dry and thickened, so your face, hands and feet look puffy and swollen. This thickening affects your vocal cords too so your voice becomes deeper than normal. Both men and women lose their sex drive. In severe cases sufferers may become very cold and confused and it is even possible to fall into a coma and die.

Self-health

- In the past, in some mountainous areas, the amount of naturally occurring iodine (needed for thyroxine) in the soil was so small that people could not get enough iodine from their food. As a result they developed swellings in the neck, or goitres, particularly women at the time of puberty or during pregnancy when the need for thyroxine is greatest. Nowadays, however, most diets contain more than enough iodine, especially as many countries add iodine to their drinking water.

- There is nothing you can do to prevent myxoedema except to recognize the symptoms early and get treatment. This consists of taking thyroxine tablets for the rest of your life. Myxoedema is a particular danger to elderly people who may live in cold homes already to save money and who can easily slip into a coma without anyone noticing.

TIC, FACIAL

A tic is a repetitive, purposeless movement of the face also known as a habit spasm. Your eye may blink repeatedly or one side of your mouth twitch or you may clear your throat constantly.

Self-health

- Try to avoid unnecessary stresses and strains or learn to cope with them better (see chapter on Stress and Mental Health) because tics are often brought on by stress, anxieties, or insecurities.

- Tics are common in children. There is nothing to gain by drawing attention to them or being cross with the child. Ignored, they usually disappear after two or three months.

- If they have not disappeared after two or three months consult your family doctor. Medicines, acupuncture or even surgery can be useful.

TONGUE, FURRED

Furring of the tongue is caused by surface cells, particles of food, smoke and other substances building up over the surface. A certain amount is normal but a thick coating is abnormal.

Self-health

- Good dental hygiene (see **Dental Care**) will keep your mouth healthy and make your tongue less likely to become furred.

- During illness your tongue may become furred because you are drinking and eating less so it does not need to be active. The food you eat may also be softer and blander than normal and so lack the necessary abrasive effect to keep the tongue clean.
    Try to counter these problems by drinking plenty. Plenty of fluids will help clean the tongue and stimulate saliva which also has a cleansing effect.

- Furred tongues can be cleaned with a toothbrush – don't be too rough to start with.

- If furring continues despite your own efforts for more than two or three weeks, consult your family doctor.

TONGUE, SORE

The tongue is a wonderfully mobile, useful organ which has great powers of healing itself. Most problems heal themselves with no or minimal treatment.

Self-health

- Ulcers are common. See **Ulcer, Mouth** for advice.

- Painful, inflamed cracks can be prevented by good dental hygiene (see **Dental Care**). Beware too of chipped teeth or badly fitting dentures, which will damage the tongue.

- Occasionally a painful, red tongue combined with anaemia (see separate entry) is caused by iron or vitamin deficiency. So if your tongue is red and sore for more than two or three weeks see your family doctor, who will probably check your blood and, if you are anaemic, advise on your diet, which should include plenty of iron- and vitamin-rich foods such as liver, bread, eggs and green, leafy vegetables.

- If you get a painful (or painless) lump on your tongue you should consult your family doctor to make sure it is not a tumour.

- Try not to smoke (see **Smoking**). Smokers have more than average problems with their tongue, including more tumours.

TONSILLITIS

Tonsillitis is inflammation of the tonsil glands of the throat caused by a virus or bacteria. It occurs most commonly in children. The symptoms are feeling unwell, a sore throat and a high temperature, followed by difficulty in swallowing, cough, stomach pain and vomiting (children only), and enlarged glands of the neck.

Self-health

- Try to keep your child away from others who have the symptoms of tonsillitis. The difficulty is that children are most infectious before symptoms appear. The incubation period for tonsillitis is three to five days.

- Once symptoms develop keep your child at home. Offer plenty of drinks and don't worry if he or she doesn't feel like eating for a few days. Cold drinks or puddings help cool an inflamed throat.

- Keep the temperature down with regular paracetamol, fans and cool sponging if necessary (see **Temperature**).

- If symptoms last longer than forty-eight hours without getting better see your family doctor.

TOXOCARIASIS

Toxocariasis is an illness caused by a roundworm which lives in dogs' and cats' intestines. The worm lays eggs which pass outside in the animals' faeces, usually contaminating soil (a recent survey of British public parks found twenty-five per cent of soil samples were contaminated). These eggs are then picked up by humans, usually children, on the hands, and swallowed. The eggs pass to all parts of the body where they hatch into larvae and then worms.

About one in ten people has been infected with toxocariasis, many without knowing it. If present, symptoms are very similar to those of flu. Very occasionally the worm gets into the eye, causing blindness.

Self-health

- Dogs and cats should be wormed regularly (e.g. three-monthly), particularly bitches with puppies. Both bitch and puppies should be wormed two, four, six and eight weeks after birth. Anyone getting a new puppy should worm it twice, just to make sure.

- Animals should be discouraged from licking children's faces.

- All animal faeces should be disposed of straightaway. Dog owners can use 'Poop Scoops' to clean up their pets' mess.

- If possible children should be discouraged from playing where soil is likely to be contaminated by animal faeces (e.g. round trees and pathways in parks).

TOXOPLASMOSIS

Toxoplasmosis can be a serious disease, caused by a parasite

Toxoplasma gondii which lives in animals' intestines, most commonly cats – and occasionally dogs. Humans become infected by eating undercooked meat containing the cysts of the parasite or by contact with infected animals' faeces that contain the parasite.

Twenty to forty per cent of people are infected by toxoplasmosis at some time, many noticing no symptoms at all. Others get symptoms similar to glandular fever, with tiredness, lethargy, a rash, aching joints and swollen glands. Occasionally the parasite gets into the brain of children, causing meningitis.

The most serious effects of toxoplasmosis occur when a newly pregnant woman is infected. The parasite may reach the fetus and cause it to be miscarried or born with serious eye and brain abnormalities.

Self-health

- Pregnant women (particularly in the first three to four months) should take special precautions, especially if they have not owned a cat before and are therefore unlikely to have built up resistance to the infection by having had it previously.

- The cat litter tray should be changed daily using gloves.

- Cats should be discouraged from licking you and you should wash your hands after stroking them.

- Wear gloves when gardening to prevent picking up the parasite from contaminated soil.

- Mention the cat to your family doctor if you feel unwell for no obvious reason during pregnancy. A simple blood test will discover whether you have the illness and your doctor can then decide whether to treat you with antibiotics. These medicines will reach the fetus and may reduce the harm the parasite is doing.

TRANQUILLIZERS

Tranquillizers (also called benzodiazepines) are mainly used as anti-anxiety medicines and sleeping pills (e.g. Mogadon). They have replaced barbiturates because they have fewer side effects and are safer.

Self-health

- Anxiety is the word doctors use to describe a condition in which irrational, anxious, confused, sometimes terrified feelings are so overwhelming that they prevent a person from living a normal life. Relaxation exercises (see chapter on Stress and Mental Health) and psychotherapy are helpful but many people also need anti-anxiety medicines to start them on the road to recovery.

- There are crisis times in everybody's life when it is difficult to sleep. Most people can cope but some people find that they need a sleeping pill. There is nothing wrong with this provided you do not allow the need to spread from weeks into months so that you become dependent upon the medicine.

- Most people get some side effects from tranquillizers. These include headache, a 'muzzy' head, poor concentration, poor memory, a dry mouth, and dizziness, clumsiness and confusion. Never combine alcohol with tranquillizers because it will make the side effects worse. Elderly people are also more likely to suffer – particularly confusion and memory loss.

- Symptoms of dependence include palpitations, headache, sweating, anxious feelings, sleeplessness, and difficulty concentrating. These are so bad when you try to stop the medicine that you quickly realize you cannot. If you notice these symptoms you should consult your doctor immediately. With expert help you will be able to break the habit.

TRAVEL, DISABLED PEOPLE

Many travel agents specialize in booking holidays and travel for disabled people but all agents should have the necessary information in print for you to be able to select a suitable holiday.

Self-health

PLANNING

1. Do not plan to travel alone unless you are confident you can cope on your own without help while you are away.
2. Find out as much as you can about the place you are visiting. Travel agents and national tourist organizations can often help. Detailed information about access can be a problem. Contact RADAR for its Holidays and Travel Abroad guide, including its Country by Country section which gives details of individual access.
3. Plan ahead and book early.

BOOKING

1. There is no purpose in hiding your disabilities from the travel agent – you will simply end up with unsuitable accommodation and have an unhappy experience.
2. You should make clear in advance what type of access you need and whether you have any special problems, such as incontinence or eating difficulties.
3. If you are going to use a wheelchair make sure the travel agent knows you are expecting to find:
   a. Ramped or level access to your accommodation.
   b. Ground-floor accommodation or rooms with a lift large enough to take your wheelchair plus companion.
   c. A bedroom large enough to move about in with a wheelchair, and to get to the bathroom if en suite.
   d. Local shops and amenities within reasonable reach of the accommodation.
4. Make sure in advance all airlines, airport authorities, shipping companies, coach companies, and railways are aware of your disabilities and able to provide help should it be needed.

• Generous holiday insurance cover is essential. Many insurance companies exclude a 'pre-existing medical condition' from their holiday insurance policies. So check with the company you are proposing to insure with before signing. If you have difficulty finding a company that does not exclude your disability contact RADAR for details of companies who specialize in disabled people.

- Your airline (occasionally shipping or coach company) may insist on a medical certificate of fitness to travel. Find out from the travel agent whether this will be needed. A note from your family doctor explaining your disabilities and medicines is also a good idea should you encounter problems while away.

- Make a checklist of any extra equipment you may need to take (e.g. commode, rubber sheets or protective underwear if you are incontinent). Assume you will not be able to buy these wherever you are going.

- Find out from your travel agent whether any special equipment you have to take will be liable to excess baggage charges or whether it will get special dispensation.

TRAVELLING ABROAD

There are some simple precautions that will help make sure your trip abroad, on holiday or business, is a success not a disaster.

Self-health

- Take a small first-aid kit with you. Include sticking plaster, antiseptic cream, water sterilization tablets and insect repellent.

- Check the safety of local drinking water. If in doubt sterilize it first, including the water you use for cleaning your teeth. Boil it for one minute or use sterilization tablets. Milk should be boiled unless it is pasteurized.

- Be careful not to eat contaminated foods. Raw vegetables, unpeeled fruit, raw shellfish, cream, ice-cream, ice cubes, underdone meat or fish, uncooked cold or reheated foods are risky. Freshly cooked foods are best.

- Wash your hands before eating, particularly when camping or caravanning.

- Avoid heatstroke and sunburn (see separate entries).

- Avoid sexually transmitted diseases, including AIDS (see separate entry). Sheaths (condoms) offer some protection. Seek medical advice early if you think you may need treatment.

- It is unwise to have your skin pierced (e.g. tattooing, ear piercing, acupuncture) unless you are certain all equipment used is sterile.

- Keep a record on your person at all times of any serious medical condition from which you may suffer.

- Consult your doctor before leaving about appropriate immunization and vaccinations. Also ask about malaria (see separate entry).

- Rabies (see separate entry) is a serious illness all over the world (including Europe) and can be fatal. Avoid dogs who are behaving unusually and see a doctor immediately if you are bitten.

- Emergency medical treatment:

  1. **European Community Countries**. In these countries you can get treatment free or at reduced cost provided you have Form E111 (available from all social security offices in the UK) with you. If you do not have an E111 form with you, contact the local health insurance offices.
  2. **Countries with reciprocal health agreements**. Some countries have arranged for UK visitors to have some treatment free or at reduced cost. Find out before treatment starts, if possible, what is free and what you will have to pay for. The following countries have this agreement: Anguilla, Australia, Austria, British Virgin Islands, Bulgaria, Channel Islands, Czechoslovakia, the Falkland Islands, Finland, the German Democratic Republic (East Germany), Hong Kong, Hungary, Iceland, Isle of Man, Malta, Montserrat, New Zealand, Norway, Poland, Romania, St Helena, Sweden, the Turks and Caicos Islands, the USSR and Yugoslavia.
  3. **Other countries**. In other countries you will need health insurance before you become ill if you are to avoid paying for treatment yourself. Always check all the small print before leaving.

- When you come home:

  1. Consult your doctor if you have been bitten by an animal,

or think you may have a sexually transmitted disease. Tell
your doctor too if you have any unusual symptoms that you
can't explain.

2. Finish taking any course of tablets (e.g. for malaria) that
   you may have been given.
3. If you donate blood, tell the staff that you have been
   abroad.
4. Claim on any health insurance (including Form E111
   holders) as soon as you get back if you have not already
   done so.

TRAVEL SICKNESS

Travel sickness is unpleasant, especially if it stops you doing
your job or ruins your holiday. There are some simple
precautions you can take to reduce your chances of getting it.

Self-health

- Choose your method of travel carefully. For example if you are
  airsick don't take a small plane to a remote spot high in the
  Andes or you may end up surprising the pilot!

- Check local conditions for the best time to travel to give
  yourself the best chance of a calm flight or sea crossing or easy
  car ride to your destination.

- **Car**
  1. If you're a passenger watch the road, not the inside of the
     car.
  2. Make sure children can see out of the window.
  3. Avoid reading, which makes most people sick, especially
     children.
  4. Keep the car well ventilated.
  5. Try fitting an electricity conductor to the back bumper
     which just touches the ground. It may stop some people
     feeling sick.

- **Boat**
  1. Sit in the middle of the boat where there is less movement.
     Keep on deck away from strong smells like diesel and
     cooking.

2. Keep your eyes fixed on the horizon, not on the heaving deck.
3. Starving yourself to keep your stomach empty will not prevent you being sick, quite the reverse. Eat a steady stream of dry, non-fatty foods like bread, ham rolls and rice.

- **Aeroplane**
  - Sit in the middle of the aeroplane where there is less movement, and avoid the kitchen area.

  - Drink plenty of fluids such as orange juice, and avoid alcohol.

  - Don't eat exotic, spicy food. Stick to dry food which will absorb your gastric juices.

- **Non-medicinal remedies**
  1. Some people find glucose – either as tablets to suck (Dextrosol) or in a drink (Emetrol) – very helpful. Start taking the glucose about thirty minutes before your journey begins. Diabetics beware, because this extra glucose may make control of the amount of sugar in your blood difficult.
  2. There is some scientific evidence, going back to the Romans and Greeks, to show that ginger may be effective – either as a piece of root ginger or as crystallized ginger.

- **Medicines**. There are many medicines available from the chemist to prevent travel sickness. Experiment to find the one that suits you best. They all have side effects (see chart), usually in proportion to how effective they are. They should all be taken well before the journey starts or they will not have a chance to work. Here is a selection:

  1. Promethazine (Avomine) is effective for long journeys and rough conditions. But it has a tendency to make some people very drowsy.
  2. Hyoscine hydrobromide (Kwells) is useful for short journeys such as crossing the Channel because its effects last only about four hours.
  3. Dimenhydrinate (Dramamine) and meclozine (Sea-Legs) are useful for moderate-length journeys in moderate conditions.
  4. Cinnarizine (Stugeron or Marzine RF) is weaker than the

Side effects of travel-sickness medicines

1. They all cause drowsiness to some extent. Drivers and pilots especially should beware.
2. They all make the effects of alcohol, tranquillizers and other medicines greater. Check with your doctor or chemist first.
3. If you are pregnant get advice from your doctor or chemist before buying a travel-sickness medicine. You may be able to manage without one.
4. If you have glaucoma take neither hyoscine nor the antihistamines (e.g. Avomine, Dramamine, Sea-Legs, Stugeron or Marzine RF) because these medicines will make the condition worse.

---

other medicines and makes you less drowsy. It is much favoured by sailors in small boats.

- Children are more prone to travel sickness than adults and usually grow out of the problem. Here are some simple tips to make trips less of a nightmare:

1. Never discuss the possibility of travel sickness in front of your children.
2. Keep them well distracted with games and fun.
3. Avoid greasy, sickly food (like hamburgers and chips) and encourage plenty of drinks of water or fruit juice. Fizzy drinks can give young children stomach ache.
4. Children aged between five and twelve can take the medicines listed above but reduced in quantity as per instructions.
5. Children under five should probably not take hyoscine hydrobromide at all.
6. If all else fails promethazine elixir (Phenergan) is a reliable standby for all ages.

TRICHOMONAS

One of the most common causes of a sore vulva or vagina often accompanied by a strongly smelling yellow or greenish discharge is a tiny organism (called a protozoan) *trichomonas vaginitis*. This lives quietly in the vagina of about ten per cent of women causing no problems, having probably got there by sexual contact. It can also live unnoticed in the penis of some men. Why it should start causing symptoms is unknown.

Self-health

- You should take the precautions and self-health measures described for thrush (see separate entry).

- Treatment from your doctor is easy and effective, primarily using medicines (tablets or vaginal suppositories such as metronidazole) which kill the organism. These medicines should not be taken if you are pregnant, especially in the first three months, so warn your doctor if there is a possibility of pregnancy. Your sexual partner should also be treated.

TUBERCULOSIS

Tuberculosis (TB) can affect many parts of the body and is caused by *mycobacterium tuberculosis.* There are two strains of the bacteria: the human kind is spread by droplets in the air and usually causes lung tuberculosis; the cattle type is spread through the milk of cows with infected udders.

The disease causes general symptoms of feeling unwell, loss of weight and appetite, tiredness, and unexplained fever and sweats (especially at night). It also causes local symptoms depending on which organs it affects, e.g. cough, bloody sputum and breathless in lung TB; back pain and deformity in spinal TB.

Self-health

- If you have a baby you should tell your doctor if there is TB in the family, so the baby can be given the BCG vaccination. This is the most certain way of preventing your children getting TB.

- In the UK children aged twelve to fourteen are routinely tested at school to see whether they have immunity against TB; if they do not they receive a BCG vaccination.

- Keep in good health and you are more likely to be able to fend off TB.

- Keep away from anyone with TB until their sputum has been tested and found to contain no bacteria.

- Public health measures such as healthy food, clean water supply and good housing are very important in the fight against TB.

- In the UK milk is tested to make sure it does not contain TB. Beware of milk in countries where it is not tested because this is a common way of catching TB.

- If you are concerned that you or a member of your family might have TB, consult your family doctor. It can be treated very successfully nowadays with antibiotics.

TYPHOID

Typhoid is a contagious disease caused by the bacterium *salmonella typhi*, which live in human faeces. It spreads by getting into food (e.g. shellfish) or water which is then eaten or drunk. Ten to fourteen days later the first symptoms of high fever (e.g. a temperature of 40°C), abdominal pain, constipation followed by diarrhoea (often bloody) and later a rash develop.

Self-health

- Anyone travelling outside northern Europe or North America should be vaccinated against typhoid. This involves two injections ten to twenty-eight days apart, which gives three years' protection. Vaccination offers the surest protection against typhoid.

- Select your food carefully in countries where there may be typhoid – particularly avoid water, or food that may have come into contact with contaminated water, e.g. shellfish and salads (see **Travelling Abroad**).

- Wash your hands after going to the lavatory and make sure you don't dry them on something (e.g. a dirty towel) that may be contaminated.

- If you think you may have developed typhoid you should see your doctor immediately. There is nothing to be gained by delaying; young and old people are particularly at risk from bleeding or rupture of the bowel. If you have diarrhoea you should drink plenty of fluids to replace lost fluid. Antibiotics may reduce the severity and length of your symptoms, which can last for one to eight weeks.

Screening

- Tests on specimens of your faeces will reveal whether you still have the infection. If you do you should not prepare food for other people and, if practical, should be the only user of one lavatory. If not practical, take special hygienic precautions. Once your faeces are clear of infection you can resume your normal life.

- After having typhoid about three per cent of people become carriers of the disease, often in their gall bladder. They have no symptoms and do not know they are infecting food. Families can be infected by each other, but typhoid occurs most dramatically when a food-handler in a restaurant infects many people. Such people should not be difficult to track down because they have always had typhoid in the past.

TYPHUS

Typhus is caused by *rickettsia*, tiny organisms half way between bacteria and viruses. There are various types, which are spread in different ways, e.g. in the faeces of lice (epidemic typhus), the faeces of fleas (endemic typhus), and the bite of ticks (Rocky Mountain spotted fever). Seven to fourteen days after infection the symptoms of high temperature, headache, limb pains and rash, usually affecting the trunk, begin to appear.

Self-health

- Louse and flea-borne typhus can be prevented by killing all lice and fleas and getting rid of their faeces.

- An insecticide powder can be puffed into the underclothing of those at risk. Protective clothing and insect repellents also help.

- Food stores should be protected from rats to prevent flea-borne typhus.

- People at risk should be immunized. Three injections are given at intervals of seven to ten days, followed by booster injections every six to twelve months.

- People at risk can also be protected by taking a very small dose of antibiotic (e.g. doxycycline 100 mg/weekly).

U

ULCER, MOUTH

Mouth ulcers are painful breaks in the lining of the mouth. They usually appear for no apparent reason. Occasionally they may be caused by a jagged or rough tooth or a denture. See also **Cold Sores**. One in ten people may have ulcers at any one time, varying from a single one to clusters.

Self-health

- Consult your dentist if you think a tooth or dentures are causing your ulcers.

- Many people notice they get ulcers if they are having a stressful time, or have anxieties and worries, or feel depressed or run down. The secret is to learn to cope better, practise relaxation techniques (see chapter on Stress and Mental Health), and eat a healthy diet, particularly plenty of vitamin C.

- Some women notice mouth ulcers at regular times during their period. There are unfortunately no known ways of preventing these.

- The pain of mouth ulcers can largely be prevented by steroid-containing tablets or mouthwashes available without prescription at your local pharmacy.

Screening

- Most ulcers should have healed within three weeks. If yours have not, see your dentist or family doctor so they can make sure you do not have a rare but serious cause, such as a tumour of the mouth.

ULCER, STOMACH

Ulcers are raw areas or breaks in the lining of the stomach and
duodenum (the section of the gut just beyond the stomach). They
are also known as peptic ulcers. In the West, about one in five
men and one in ten women have ulcers at some stage in their
lives, normally middle age. The main symptom is heartburn (see
separate entry), usually one or two hours after a meal or in the
early hours of the day, which is relieved temporarily by milk,
food and antacids. Sometimes the pain is very severe, going
through into your back. You may also lose your appetite and feel
sick. If the ulcer lies near the outlet of the stomach it slows food
passing through and makes you feel bloated and uncomfortable.
Ulcers run in families and are especially linked with blood
group O.

Self-health

- Follow the advice for heartburn (see separate entry).

- Reduce unnecessary stress in your life (see chapter on Stress
  and Mental Health) because stress can cause ulcers in some
  people.

- If you smoke try to give up (see **Smoking**).

- Drink less coffee, tea and cola, and avoid spicy foods, because
  they stimulate the production of stomach juices which irritate
  the lining of the stomach.

- Beware of aspirin and anti-arthritis medicines particularly.
  They may cause ulcers or make them worse. If these medicines
  are essential, take them with food and always tell your doctor
  what effect they are having on you.

- Reduce your alcohol intake, because alcohol stimulates
  stomach juices.

- In the past, milk or bland food was always recommended to
  people with peptic ulcers because they were thought to help
  by mopping up the gastric juices. Nowadays doctors are not so
  certain that milk is such a good thing because it may stimulate
  the stomach to produce more juices and in the long run make
  the condition worse. However, many people benefit from milk

and milky foods so the picture is by no means clear. The best approach is to experiment to see which foods help or worsen your symptoms.

- Similarly doubt has been thrown on to the value of small, frequent meals for ulcer sufferers. Again, experiment for yourself.

- Antacids bought from the chemist have a useful role, especially if you know you have overdone things. If you need antacids regularly for weeks or months at a time consult your family doctor. There may be changes to your lifestyle which your doctor can recommend, or stronger medicines which will cure the ulcer.

Screening

- One of the serious side effects of an ulcer can be bleeding from it. This can show itself by making the faeces black in colour and tarry in consistency. If you notice these features see your family doctor immediately (remember that taking iron tablets will have this effect too). More commonly, bleeding causes anaemia so if you are anaemic for no obvious reason you and your family doctor should consider an ulcer as a possible cause.

ULCER, VARICOSE

As you grow older (and especially if you have varicose veins) the circulation in your legs becomes slower and injuries take longer to heal. One common place for problems to occur is above the ankle on the inner leg, where a knock may cause a break in the skin which, instead of healing, gradually gets larger, forming an ulcer. At this stage it may be painless but if it becomes infected it may become painful. It will need special care and attention if it is to heal properly. Either or both legs may be affected. Women suffer from varicose ulcers twice as often as men.

Self-health

- See **Varicose Veins**.

- If you have varicose veins wear support stockings and be careful not to injure your lower legs.

- Do not stand in one place for long periods. If you have to, exercise the calf muscles by walking on the spot and standing on tiptoe.

- When sitting raise the affected leg to the level of your hips, or higher if possible.

- Take some moderate exercise, such as walking, every day to stimulate the circulation.

- Avoid using a whole variety of antiseptic ointments and washes. Your skin may become allergic to them, preventing the ulcer from healing.

- Most ulcers will need professional help if they are to heal successfully so consult your family doctor if you have a leg ulcer that is not healing.

V

VAGINAL INFECTIONS

It is normal for the vagina to produce a clear, or slightly milky (occasionally yellow) fluid. This secretion helps to keep it clean and healthy. During pregnancy, at certain times during your menstrual cycle, or when you are sexually excited you may notice an increase in the amount of moisture.

But some vaginal changes are not normal and may indicate that you have an infection. These changes may include a strong-smelling, or frothy, dark-coloured discharge, soreness, itching, burning, dryness, spots, or a rash round or in the genitals, an urge to pass water more often than normal and sometimes pain while doing so.

If you think you may have an infection you should see your family doctor or go to a hospital special clinic as soon as possible. Possible infections include thrush, trichomoniasis, and gonorrhoea (see separate entries).

Self-health

- Women are at risk of vaginal infections because the urethra (the tube draining the bladder) and the anus are so close together, allowing cross infections to happen easily. Understanding this fact will help you prevent infections.

- Wash your genitals with warm water every day. Do not use strongly smelling soaps, antiseptics, bath products or sprays because they may encourage infection.

- Wear fresh pants every day.

- After passing water or opening your bowels wipe yourself with soft lavatory paper from front to back, never the other way because this will bring germs from your anus forwards.

If you are prone to infections you may also wish to wash yourself with warm water after opening your bowels.

- Most people do not need to wash before sex but if you are prone to infections you may find this helps. Both partners should wash. Passing water after sex can also help. If your partner uses a condom this reduces your chances of getting (or passing on) an infection.

- If you do need medical treatment there are one or two things you can do yourself to help:

  1. Do not have sex until the infection is healed.
  2. Tell all your sexual partners that they may be infected and need treatment.
  3. Take the full course of treatment even if symptoms quickly disappear.
  4. Wear cotton pants, and avoid clothes that retain heat and moisture (like nylon underwear or tights).
  5. Try not to scratch because it may spread the infection.

VARICOSE VEINS

Varicose veins are swollen, twisted, often knotted veins which may affect a short distance of the leg or the full length. About one women in four and one man in ten suffers from them. Apart from the swollen veins themselves you may notice discoloured, 'broken' skin, aching of the leg, especially after standing, swelling of the leg and tenderness to the touch.

Varicose veins are probably caused when the valves within the veins are not working properly, so blood cannot be pumped easily back to the heart and accumulates in the legs. Anything that helps this pumping will help prevent varicose veins appearing, or slow their development.

Self-health

- Avoid standing in one place for long. If you have to, keep your calf muscles exercised by walking on the spot or standing on tiptoe every thirty seconds for a few seconds at a time.

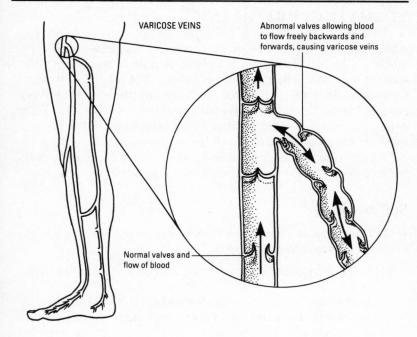

VARICOSE VEINS

Abnormal valves allowing blood to flow freely backwards and forwards, causing varicose veins

Normal valves and flow of blood

- Keep your feet up (e.g. on a stool) as much as you can. If symptoms are bad raise your feet above the level of your heart.

- Wear support stockings or tights. They are most effective if put on first thing in the morning rather than waiting until your legs have swollen. Many women find them particularly helpful during pregnancy.

- Take plenty of exercise. Walk whenever possible (e.g. use stairs rather than lifts).

- Lose weight if you are overweight.

- Constipation may make varicose veins worse so eat a high-fibre diet to make large-volume, soft faeces.

- If you ever damage a varicose vein so that it starts to bleed (often vigorously) immediately raise the leg well above your heart. This will slow the rate of bleeding so that pressing firmly over the bleeding vein will stop it.

VOMITING, PREGNANCY

About three-quarters of pregnant women suffer nausea and vomiting during the first three to four months of pregnancy. For some it may be the first sign of pregnancy. For others, however, it may start late in the pregnancy and even continue until delivery. No one knows the cause of this common problem but it is almost certainly linked to some women's over-sensitivity to the high levels of hormones in the blood during pregnancy. It is often called morning sickness because it occurs more commonly early in the day, but many women are affected at other times.

Self-health

- One simple and often effective way to prevent and cope with sickness is to adjust your diet.
  1. Avoid fatty, greasy foods; steam and grill food rather than frying it.
  2. Avoid large or spicy meals. Instead eat frequent, high-carbohydrate meals (e.g. every three hours). Toast and crackers are favourites while meat and high-protein foods are often unpopular.
  3. Some women find drinking with meals brings on the sickness. Try drinking between meals instead.
  4. Some women find getting up in the morning on an empty stomach brings on the sickness. Persuade someone (the father of your baby should be willing!) to bring you toast and tea in bed.

- If, despite your own efforts, you are finding it difficult to cope with the sickness consult your family doctor, who may be able to give you further advice or prescribe anti-sickness pills. Generally doctors are unwilling to prescribe any medicines during pregnancy, especially during the first few weeks, so you will need to be badly affected before you are given any.

- Occasionally a woman suffers so badly from vomiting that she cannot keep any food down, becomes dehydrated and puts herself and her baby at risk (known as hyperemesis gravidarum). If you find yourself in this situation you should contact your family doctor or hospital sooner rather than later so you can be treated with fluid and minerals.

WARTS

Warts (also known as verrucas) are small, solid growths on the skin caused by viruses. They are most common in adolescents aged twelve to sixteen and may affect the face, hands, feet, anus and genitals.

Self-health

- Since the virus is spread by direct contact, avoid contact with people with warts as much as possible.

- Do not go barefooted in places like swimming pools, gyms and public showers because you can pick up the virus from floors. Even shared household objects can infect you, although viruses usually survive best in damp, wet places.

- If you have warts on your hands keep them as dry as possible because water softens the wart, making it easier for the virus to spread to other people or other places on your body.

- For the same reason keep your feet dry if you have warts on them. Cork insoles and cotton socks will help.

- Try not to damage or scratch warts or the skin round warts because this will encourage them to spread. People who bite their nails often get more warts round their nails and fingers (even their lips occasionally) for this reason.

- There are many home remedies which you can try, provided they are harmless. None has been proven to work, mainly because warts often disappear without treatment for no apparent reason (and may reappear again) so it is impossible to tell whether the remedy worked or whether the wart would have disappeared anyway.

- For warts on the hands and feet you can buy paints and pastes from the chemist which will slowly burn the wart away. But you have to be careful not to burn normal surrounding skin so follow instructions carefully. If these do not work you can try forty per cent salicylic corn plasters, which are sold in packets of ten and are stronger. If your own efforts fail see your family doctor, who will consider alternative treatments.

- Never try to treat facial or genital warts yourself – they need professional care. The virus that causes them may be different and they are usually more difficult to treat.

- In many cases the simplest and least painful treatment is to ignore the warts (except genital or anal warts which should never be ignored) and wait for them to go away. However, never underestimate the psychological and social effects of warts, especially in touchy adolescents.

WHITLOW

A whitlow is an infection caused by staphylococci bacteria which occurs on the soft pad at the tip of the finger. It is different from paronychia (see separate entry).

Self-health

- Some people are more prone than others to staphylococci infections. If so, they should avoid encouraging the transfer of germs (e.g. by not using the same towels, flannels or bedclothes as others in the household).

- Wear gloves when doing housework and washing-up to prevent the hands becoming soft and infected.

- Consult a doctor immediately symptoms develop to prevent the infection becoming worse.

WHOOPING COUGH (PERTUSSIS)

Whooping cough is caused by a virus or spread by droplets from infected people (e.g. by coughing or sneezing). It tends to run in epidemics, particularly if the number of people who have been vaccinated falls. After catching the virus it takes seven to fourteen days to develop symptoms and they may last three weeks to three months, occasionally longer. The quarantine period is twenty-one days from the first 'whoop'.

The first symptoms are like those of a cold or mild flu – slight fever, feeling unwell, runny nose and cough. But instead of getting better they get worse, especially the explosive cough which ends in a 'whoop'. Quite often the bout of coughing is followed by vomiting. This nasty phase may last for two to ten weeks or may leave the child with a dry cough for another few weeks.

Whooping cough affecting unvaccinated children kills about one in every 1,000 cases. Babies under six months are most at risk, partly because they often do not 'whoop' so the diagnosis is not made. The main risks are pneumonia (see separate entry) which can cause permanent lung damage, encephalitis (see separate entry) or bursting a blood vessel in the brain during a coughing bout. Babies sometimes just stop breathing.

Self-health

- The best protection for your child is the anti-whooping cough vaccination. This is nowadays given as a course with diphtheria and tetanus vaccine. The first injection should be at the age of three months, the second six to eight weeks later, and the final one four to six months after the second.

- A few children suffer reactions to the vaccine. But the risk of such a reaction is much smaller than the risk of the disease itself; so provided there are no specific reasons why your child is at risk you should arrange the vaccination with your doctor.
  The reactions include:

  1. A small, painless lump at the injection site which disappears. This is harmless.
  2. Crying, screaming or fever occasionally occur. These settle after treatment with paracetamol.
  3. About one in 100,000 children suffers febrile fits (see **Fits**) or encephalopathy. Almost all recover without long-term problems. There is no way you can predict in advance whether your child will be affected. The problem, too, is

that both conditions can appear out of the blue so it is often impossible to know whether or not they have been caused by the vaccination.

- The following people should not have the vaccination:
  1. Any child with a fever or illness of any kind should have his or her vaccination postponed.
  2. Anyone who has had a nasty reaction to a previous whooping cough vaccination.
  3. Anyone who has had a fit (or has close relatives who have fits) should be sure to tell their doctor before vaccination.

Y

YELLOW FEVER

Yellow fever is a tropical disease caused by a virus (a togavirus). It is passed to humans by the bite of an *Aedes* mosquito. Three to six days later a headache and high temperature develop. Most people then recover but a few get liver or kidney disease or serious internal bleeding.

Self-health

- There is a safe and effective vaccine which everyone living or travelling in South America or Africa should have. You need only one injection (provided it is not within three weeks of a polio vaccination) and protection lasts at least ten years, after which a booster is needed. Infants under nine months should not be vaccinated but will inherit protection if their mothers are immune.

- Take the usual precautions against mosquitoes (see **Malaria**).

SELF-HELP GROUPS

Many self-help groups provide excellent practical advice and reassurance. Listed below are the names, addresses and telephone numbers of the major groups. In cases of difficulty locating a particular group, contact groups with similar interests. They are often able to help.

ABORTION

British Pregnancy Advisory
Service
Austy Manor
Wootton Wawen
Solihull
West Midlands, B95 6BX
Tel: 0564 793225

Brook Advisory Centre
233 Tottenham Court Road
City of Westminster
London, W1P 9AE
Tel: 071 580 2991

Pregnancy Advisory Service
11 Charlotte Street
London, W1
Tel: 071 637 8962

ABUSE OF CHILDREN

Childline
Tel: 0811 1111 (24 hours)

National Society for the
Prevention of Cruelty to
Children
67 Saffron Hill
London, EC1 8RS
Tel: 071 242 1626

Save the Children Fund
Mary Datchelor House
17 Grove Lane
London, SE5 8RD
Tel: 071 703 5400

ACUPUNCTURE

British Acupuncture Association
34 Alderney Street
London, SW1 4FU
Tel: 071 834 3353

ADOPTION

British Agencies for Adoption
and Fostering
11 Southwark Street
London, SE1 1RQ
Tel: 071 407 8800

Parents for Children
222 Camden High Street
London, NW1 8QR
Tel: 071 485 7526/7548

AGORAPHOBIA

Phobics Society
4 Cheltenham Road
Chorlton-cum-Hardy
Manchester, M21 1QN
Tel: 061 881 1937

Phobic Trust
25a The Grove
Coulsdon
Surrey, CR3 2BH
Tel: 081 660 0332

AIDS

Terrence Higgins Trust
Helpline
BM AIDS
London, WC1
Tel: 071 242 1010/
071 833 2971

ALCOHOLISM

Accept Clinic
200 Seagrave Road
London, SW6 1RQ
Tel: 071 381 3155

Al-Anon
Family Groups UK & Eire
61 Great Dover Street
London, SE1 4YF
Tel: 071 403 0888

Alcoholics Anonymous
PO Box 1
Stonebow House
Stonebow
York, YO1 2NJ
Tel: 0904 644026
London Regional Telephone
Service: 071 352 3001

ALLERGY

Action Against Allergy
43 The Downs
London, SW20 8HG
Tel: 081 947 5082

ALZHEIMER'S DISEASE

Alzheimer's Disease Society
158/160 Balham High Road
London, SW12 9BN
Tel: 081 675 6557

ANKYLOSING SPONDYLITIS

National Ankylosing
Spondylitis Society
6 Grosvenor Crescent
London, SW1X 7ER
Tel: 071 235 9585

ASBESTOSIS

SPAID
The Society for the Prevention
of Asbestosis and Industrial
Diseases
38 Drapers Road
Enfield
Middlesex, EN2 8LU
Tel: 0707 873025 (Day)
081 366 1640 (Eve)

ASTHMA

Asthma Society and Friends of
Asthma Research Council
300 Upper Street
London, N1 2XX
Tel: 071 226 2260

The British Lung Foundation
Block B
250 Kings Road
London, SW3
Tel: 071 376 5735

AUTISM

National Autistic Society
276 Willesden Lane
London, NW2 5RB
Tel: 081 451 3844

BACK PAIN

Back Pain Association
31–33 Park Road
Teddington
Middlesex, TW11 0AB
Tel: 081 977 5474/5

BEHCET'S SYNDROME

Behcet's Syndrome Society
Mrs Judith Buckle
3 Belgrave Street
Haxby Road
York, YO3 3YY
Tel: 0904 37310

BRAIN DAMAGE

Headway
National Head Injuries
Association
200 Mansfield Road
Nottingham, NG1 3HX
Tel: 0602 622382

The British Institute for Brain
Injured Children
Knowle Hall
Knowle
Bridgwater
Somerset
Tel: 0278 684060

BRITTLE BONE DISEASE

Brittle Bone Society
112 City Road
Dundee, DD2 2PW
Tel: 0382 67603

CANCER

BACUP
British Association of Cancer
United Patients
121/123 Charterhouse Street
London, EC1M 6AA
Tel: 071 608 1661

Cancer Link
46a Pentonville Road
London, N1 9HF
Tel: 071 833 2451

Cancer Prevention Society
25/27 Elmbank Street
Glasgow, G2 4PB

CEREBRAL PALSY

International Cerebral Palsy
Society
5a Netherhall Gardens
London, NW3 5RN
Tel: 071 794 9761

Spastics Society
12 Park Crescent
London W1V 4EG
Tel: 071 636 5020

CHEST DISEASES

Chest, Heart & Stroke
Association
Tavistock House North
Tavistock Square
London, WC1H 9JE
Tel: 071 387 3012/3/4

CHIROPRACTIC

British Chiropractors
Association
5 First Avenue
Chelmsford
Essex, CM1 1RX

CLEFT LIP

Cleft Lip and Palate
Association (CLAPA)
Great Ormond Street Hospital
for Sick Children
London, WC1N 2JH
Tel: 071 405 9200

COELIAC DISEASE

Coeliac Society
P.O. Box 220
High Wycombe
Bucks, HP11 2HY
Tel: 0494 37278

COLITIS

National Association for
Colitis and Crohn's Disease
(NACC)
98a London Road
St Albans
Herts, AL1 1NX
Tel: 0727 44296

COLOSTOMY

Colostomy Welfare Group
2nd Floor
38/39 Eccleston Square
London, SW1V 1PB
Tel: 071 828 5175

CONGENITAL DISPLACEMENT OF THE HIP

Congenital Displacement of the
Hip Support Group
c/o Sharon Smithard
Hope House
40 High Road
Balby
Doncaster
Tel: 0302 851117

CYSTIC FIBROSIS

Cystic Fibrosis Research Trust
Alexandra House
5 Blyth Road, Bromley
Kent, BR1 3RS
Tel: 081 464 7211

DEAFNESS

British Association of the Hard
of Hearing
7–11 Armstrong Road
London, W3 7JL
Tel: 081 743 1110

Royal National Institute for the
Deaf (RNID)
105 Gower Street
London, WC1E 6AH
Tel: 071 387 8033

DEMENTIA

Alzheimer's Disease Society
158/160 Balham High Road
London, SW12 9BN
Tel: 081 675 6557

DENTAL HEALTH

British Dental Health
Foundation
88 Gurnards Avenue
Fishermead
Milton Keynes, MK6 2BL
Tel: 0908 667063

DEPRESSION

Depressives Associated
PO Box 5
Castletown
Portland
Dorset, DT5 1BQ

Fellowship of Depressives
Anonymous
38 Chestnut Avenue
Beverley
N. Humberside, HU17 9QU

Lithium Club
24 Church End
Catworth
Huntingdon
Cambs
Tel: 08014 487

Manic Depression Fellowship
Ltd
51 Sheen Road
Richmond
Surrey, TW9 1YQ
Tel: 081 940 6235

DIABETES

British Diabetic Association
10 Queen Anne Street
London, W1M OBD
Tel: 071 323 1531

DISFIGUREMENT

Disfigurement Guidance Centre
52 Crossgate
Cupar
Fife
Scotland, KY15 5HS
Tel: 03377 281

DIVORCE

The National Federation of
Solo Clubs
Room 8
191 Corporation Street
Birmingham, B4 6RY
Tel: 021 236 2879

DOWN'S SYNDROME

Down's Syndrome Association
12–13 Clapham Common
Southside
London, SW4 7AA
Tel: 071 720 0008

DRUG ADDICTION

Accept Clinic
200 Seagrave Road
London, SW6 1RQ
Tel: 071 381 3155/2112

Drug Treatment Centre
St Stephen's Hospital
Fulham Road
London, SW10
Tel: 071 352 8161

Turning Point
CAP House
9/12 Long Lane
London, EC1A 9HA
Tel: 071 606 3947

Parents Anonymous
5 Manor Gardens
London N7
Tel: 071 263 8918

DYSLEXIA

British Dyslexia Association
Church Lane
Peppard
Oxfordshire, RG9 5JN
Tel: 04917 699

Dyslexia Institute
133 Gresham Road
Staines, TW18 2AJ
Tel: 0784 59498

DYSPHASIA

Action for Dysphasic Adults
Northcote House
37a Royal Street
London, SE1 7LL
Tel: 071 261 9572

EATING DISORDER

Anorexic Aid
The Priory Centre
11 Priory Road
High Wycombe
Bucks
Tel: 0494 21431

ECZEMA

National Eczema Society
Tavistock House North
Tavistock Square
London, WC1H 9SR
Tel: 071 388 4097

ENDOMETRIOSIS

Endometriosis Society
65 Holmdene Avenue
London, SE24 9LD
Tel: 071 737 4764

EXERCISE

Exercise Training for the
Elderly and/or Disabled
3 The Boulevard
Sheringham
Norfolk, NR26 8LJ
Tel: 0263 822479

EYE PROBLEMS

Optical Information Council
18–24 Temple Chambers
Temple Avenue
London EC4Y 0DT
Tel: 071 353 3556

Royal National Institute for the
Blind (RNIB)
224 Great Portland Street
London, W1N 6AA
Tel: 071 388 1266

FAMILY PLANNING

British Pregnancy Advisory
Service
Austy Manor
Wootton Wawen
Solihull
West Midlands, B95 6BX
Tel: 0564 793225

Brook Advisory Centres
153a East Street
London, SE17 2SD
Tel: 071 708 1234

Family Planning Association
27–35 Mortimer Street
London, W1N 7RJ
Tel: 071 636 7866

Marie Stopes House
108 Whitfield Street
London, W1P 6BE
Tel: 071 388 0662

Pregnancy Advisory Service
11–13 Charlotte Street
London, W1
Tel: 071 637 8962

FOOD ALLERGY

Food Allergy Association
c/o The Chairman
Mrs Ellen Rothera
27 Ferringham Lane
Ferring
West Sussex, BN12 5NB
Tel: 0903 41178

FRIEDREICH'S ATAXIA

Friedreich's Ataxia Group
Burleigh Lodge
Knowle Lane
Cranleigh
Surrey, GU6 8RD
Tel: 0483 272741

GAMBLING

Gamblers Anonymous
17/23 Blantyre Street
Cheyne Walk
London, SW10
Tel: 071 353 3060

GILLES DE LA TOURETTE SYNDROME

Tourette Syndrome (UK)
Association
734 High Road
Goodmayes
Ilford
Essex, IG3 8SX
Tel: 081 599 1826

GLAUCOMA

International Glaucoma
Association
Department of Ophthalmology
King's College Hospital
London, SE5 9RS
Tel: 071 274 6222 Ext. 2466/
2453

GLYCOGEN STORAGE DISEASE

Association for Glycogen
Storage Disease (UK)
9 Lindop Road
Hale
Altrincham
Cheshire, WA15 9DZ
Tel: 061 980 7303

GROWTH PROBLEMS

Association for Research into
Restricted Growth
24 Pinchfield
Maple Cross
Rickmansworth
Herts, WD3 2TP
Tel: 0923 770759

Child Growth Foundations
2 Mayfield Avenue
London, W4
Tel: 081 995 0257

HAEMOPHILIA

The Haemophilia Society
PO Box 9
16 Trinity Street
London, SE1 1DE
Tel: 071 928 2020

HANDICAPPED

The Across Trust
Crown House
Morden
Surrey, SM4 5EW
Tel: 081 540 3897

Disabled Living Foundations
380–384 Harrow Road
London, W9 2HU
Tel: 071 289 6111

Physically Handicapped and
Able-Bodied (PHAB)
Tavistock House North
Tavistock Square
London, WC1H 9HX
Tel: 071 388 1963

Royal Society for Mentally
Handicapped Children and
Adults (MENCAP)
123 Golden Lane
London EC1
Tel: 071 253 9433

The Salvation Army
Association for the
Handicapped
101 Queen Victoria Street
London, EC4P 4EP
Tel: 071 236 5222

HEAD INJURY

Headway
National Head Injuries
Association
200 Mansfield Road
Nottingham, NG1 3HX
Tel: 0602 622382

HEART DISEASE

British Heart Foundation
102 Gloucester Place
London, W1H 4DH
Tel: 071 935 0185

Chest, Heart & Stroke
Association
Tavistock House North
Tavistock Square
London, WC1H 9JE
Tel: 071 387 3012/3/4

Coronary Prevention Group
60 Great Ormond Street
London, WC1N 3HR
Tel: 071 833 3687

Heart to Heart
Box 7
High Street
Pershore
Worcs WR10 1AA

Heartline
12 East Road
Langford
Beds, SG18 9QF
Tel: 0462 700233

HODGKIN'S DISEASE

Hodgkin's Disease Association
PO Box 275
Haddenham
Aylesbury
Bucks HP17 8JJ

HOMEOPATHY

The British Homeopathic
Association (BHA)
27a Devonshire Street
London, W1N 1RJ
Tel: 071 935 2163

HOSPITAL PATIENTS

The Talking Books Library
12 Lant Street
London, SE1 1QH
Tel: 071 407 9417

The National Association of
League of Hospital Friends
38 Ebury Street
London, SW1W 0LU
Tel: 071 730 0103

National Association for the
Welfare of Children in
Hospital
Argyle House
29/31 Euston Road
London, NW1 2SD
Tel: 071 833 2041

HUNTINGTON'S CHOREA

Association to Combat
Huntington's Chorea
34a Station Road
Hinckley
Leics, LE10 1AP
Tel: 0455 615558

HYDROCEPHALUS

Association for Spina Bifida
and Hydrocephalus
22 Upper Woburn Place
London, WC1H OEP
Tel: 071 388 1382/8 lines

HYPERACTIVITY

Hyperactive Children's
Support Group
71 Whyke Lane
Chichester
West Sussex
Tel: 0903 725182

HYSTERECTOMY

Hysterectomy Support Group
11 Henryson Road
London, SE4 1HL
Tel: 081 690 5987

ILEOSTOMY

Ileostomy Association of Great
Britain and Ireland
Amblehurst House
Black Scotch Lane
Mansfield
Notts NG18 4PF
Tel: 0623 28099

INDUSTRIAL DISEASE

SPAID
The Society for the Prevention
of Asbestosis and Industrial
Diseases
38 Drapers Road
Enfield
Middlesex, EN2 8LU
Tel: 0707 873025 (Day)
081 366 1640 (Eve)

INFANTILE HYPERCALCAEMIA

Infantile Hypercalcaemia
Foundation (Williams
Syndrome)
37 Mulberry Green
Old Harlow
Essex, CM17 0EY
Tel: 02792 7214

INFERTILITY

National Association for the
Childless
Birmingham Settlement
318 Summer Lane
Birmingham, B19 3RL
Tel: 021 359 4887/2113

KIDNEY DISEASE

The British Kidney Patient
Association
Bordon
Hants, GU35 9JP
Tel: 04203 2021/2

National Federation of Kidney
Patients' Associations
c/o Mrs Margaret Jackson
Acorn Lodge
Woodsetts
Worksop
Notts, S81 8AT
Tel: 0909 562703

The Renal Society
64 South Hill Park
London, NW3 2SJ
Tel: 071 794 9479

LANGUAGE DISORDERS

Association for all Speech
Impaired Children
347 Central Markets
London, EC1A 9NH
Tel: 071 236 3632/6487

Invalid Children's Aid
Association
126 Buckingham Palace Road
London, SW1W 9SB
Tel: 071 730 9891

National Centre for Cued
Speech
29/30 Watling Street
Canterbury
Kent, CT1 2UD
Tel: 0227 450757

LARYNGECTOMY

The National Association of
Laryngectomy Clubs
Fourth Floor
39 Eccleston Square
London, SW1V 1PB
Tel: 071 834 2857

LEFTHANDEDNESS

Anything Lefthanded
65 Beak Street
London, W1R 3LF
Tel: 071 437 3910

LEG AND FOOT DEFORMITIES

STEPS
c/o Sue Banton
8 Princess Road
Urmston
Manchester, M31 3SS
Tel: 061 747 7014

LEUKAEMIA

Leukaemia Research Fund
43 Great Ormond Street
London, WC1N 3JJ
Tel: 071 405 0101

Leukaemia Care Society
PO Box 82
Exeter, EX2 5DP
Tel: 0392 218514

LIVER DISEASE

Michael McGough Foundation
Against Liver Disease in
Children
PO Box 494
Western Avenue
London, W3 0SH
Tel: 081 992 3400 ext. 6131

LUPUS ERYTHEMATOSIS

Lupus Group
6 Grosvenor Crescent
London, SW1X 7ER
Tel: 071 235 0902/5

MARITAL GUIDANCE

The Catholic Marriage
Advisory Council
151 Lansdowne Road
London, W11 3AJ
Tel: 071 727 0141

Clinic of Psychotherapy
26 Belsize Square
London, NW3 4HU
Tel: 081 903 6455

The Isis Centre
Little Clarendon Street
Oxford, OX1 2HU
Tel: 0865 56648

Relate (The National Marriage
Guidance Council)
Herbert Gray College
Little Church Street
Rugby, CV21 3AP
Tel: 0788 73241

Scottish Marriage Guidance
Council
26 Frederick Street
Edinburgh, EH2 2JR
Tel: 031 225 5006

MASTECTOMY

The Mastectomy Association
26 Harrison Street
(off Grays Inn Road)
London, WC1H 8JG
Tel: 071 837 0908

MEDICAL ACCIDENTS

Action for the Victims of
Medical Accidents (AVMA)
24 Southwark Street
London, SE1 1TY
Tel: 071 403 4744

MENTAL HEALTH

British Institute of Mental
Handicap
Wolverhampton Road
Kidderminster
Worcestershire, DY10 3PP
Tel: 0562 850251

British Society for Music
Therapy
69 Avondale Avenue
East Barnet
Herts, EN4 8NB
Tel: 081 368 8879

Campaign for People with
Mental Handicap
12a Maddox Street
London, W1R 9PL
Tel: 071 491 0727

Centre for Educating
Handicapped Children at
Home
636 Wilmslow Road
Didsbury
Manchester, M20 0AH
Tel: 061 445 2411

MIGRAINE

British Migraine Association
178a High Road
Byfleet
Weybridge
Surrey, KT14 7ED
Tel: 09323 52468

The Migraine Trust
45 Great Ormond Street
London, WCIN 3HD
Tel: 071 278 2676

MILK ALLERGY

Milk Allergy Self-Help Group
(MASH)
34 Crown Lane
London, N14 5ES
Tel: 081 368 3132

MINIMAL BRAIN DYSFUNCTION

In Touch
10 Norman Road
Sale
Cheshire, M33 3DF
Tel: 061 962 4441

MISCARRIAGE

Miscarriage Association
18 Stoneybrook Close
West Bretton
Wakefield
W. Yorkshire, WF4 4TP
Tel: 092 485 515

National Childbirth Trust
(NCT)
Alexandra House
Oldham Terrace
London, W3 6NH
Tel: 081 992 8637

MOBILITY

Disability Alliance
25 Denmark Street
London, WC2H 8NJ
Tel: 071 240 0806

Disabled Drivers' Association
Drake House
18 Creekside
London, SE8 3DZ
Tel: 081 692 7141

Disabled Drivers' Motor Club
Ltd
1a Dudley Gardens
London, W13 9LU
Tel: 081 840 1515

Disabled Living Foundation
380–384 Harrow Road
London, W9 2HU
Tel: 071 289 6111

Equipment for the Disabled
Mary Marlborough Lodge
Nuffield Orthopaedic Centre
Headington
Oxford, OX3 7LD
Tel: 0865 750103

London Regional Transport
Unit for Disabled Passengers
Tel: 071 222 5600 ext. 3299

Mobility Aid and Guide Dog
Association (MAGDA)
1 Palmer Road
Carlisle, CA2 7NE

Motability
Gate House
West Gate
Harlow
Essex, CM20 1HR
Tel: 0279 635666

Royal Association for
Disability and Rehabilitation
(RADAR)
25 Mortimer Street
London, W1N 8AB
Tel: 071 637 5400

MOTOR NEURONE DISEASE

Motor Neurone Disease
Association
61 Derngate
Northampton, NN1 1EU
Tel: 0604 22269/250505

MUCOPOLYSACCHARIDE DISEASES

Society for
Mucopolysaccharide Diseases
30 Westwood Drive
Little Chalfont
Bucks
Tel: 02404 2789

MULTIPLE BIRTHS

Twins and Multiple Births
Association
41 Fortuna Way
Aylesby Park
Grimsby
South Humberside, DN37 9SJ

MULTIPLE SCLEROSIS

Action Research into Multiple
Sclerosis (ARMS)
4a Chapel Hill
Stansted
Essex, CM24 8AG
Tel: 0279 81553
(administration)
071 222 3123 (counselling
service)

Multiple Sclerosis Society of
Great Britain and Northern
Ireland
25 Effie Road
Fulham
London, SW6 1EE
Tel: 071 736 6267

MUSCULAR DYSTROPHY

Muscular Dystrophy Group of
Great Britain and Northern
Ireland
Nattrass House
35 Macauley Road
London, SW4 0QP
Tel: 071 720 8055

MUSIC THERAPY

British Society for Music
Therapy
69 Avondale Avenue
East Barnet
Herts, EN4 8NB
Tel: 081 368 8879

MYALGIC ENCEPHALOMYELITIS

Myalgic Encephalomyelitis
Association
PO Box 8
Stanford-le-Hope
Essex, SS17 8EX
Tel: 03756 42466
(Mon–Thurs mornings only)

MYASTHENIA GRAVIS

British Association of
Myasthenics
9 Potters Drive
Mariners Park
Hopton-on-Sea
Norfolk, NR31 9RW
Tel: 0502 731904

NERVOUS DISEASES

Amandus Club
Atkinson Morley Hospital
Wimbledon
London, SW20 0NE
Tel: 081 946 7711 ext. 133

NEUROFIBROMATOSIS

Link: The Neurofibromatosis
Association
London House
26–40 Kensington High Street
London, W8 4PF
Tel: 071 938 2222 ext 2226

NEUROMUSCULAR DISEASES

Motor Neurone Disease
Association
61 Derngate
Northampton, NN1 1UE
Tel: 0604 22269/250505

NIEMANN-PICK DISEASE

Research Trust for Metabolic
Diseases in Children
9 Arnold Street
Nantwich
Cheshire, CW5 5QB
Tel: 0270 626834
(24-hour service) 0270 629782

NOONAN SYNDROME

Noonan Syndrome Support
Group
Sheila Brown
27 Pinfold Lane
Cheslyn Hay
Walsall
Staffordshire, WS0 7HP
Tel: 0922 418419

NUTRITION

British Holistic Medical
Association
179 Gloucester Place
London, NW1 6DX
Tel: 071 262 5299

British Nutrition Foundation
15 Belgrave Square
London, SW1X 8PS
Tel: 071 235 4904

Community Health Foundation
East West Centre
188 Old Street
London, EC1 9EG
Tel: 071 251 4076

Coronary Prevention Group
60 Great Ormond Street
London, WC1N 3HR
Tel: 071 833 3687

Ketogenic Kids
Mrs Irene Cullen
32 Chepstow Avenue
Sale
Cheshire, M33 4QP
Tel: 061 969 2005

London Food Commission
PO Box 291
London, N5 1DU
Tel: 071 633 5782

Vegan Society
33–35 George Street
Oxford, OX1 2AY
Tel: 0865 722166

Vegetarian Society of the
United Kingdom Ltd
Parkdale
Dunham Road
Altrincham
Cheshire, WA14 4QG
Tel: 061 928 0793

Vegetarian Centre and
Bookshop in London
53 Marloes Road
London, W8 6LA
Tel: 071 937 7739

ONE-PARENT FAMILIES

Exploring Parenthood
Omnibus Workspace
39–41 North Road
London, N7 9DP
Tel: 071 607 9647

Gingerbread
35 Wellington Street
London, WC2E 7BN
Tel: 071 240 0953

National Council for One-
Parent Families
255 Kentish Town Road
London, NW5 2LX
Tel: 071 267 1361

SPLASH
(Single Parent Links and
Special Holidays)
Empire House
Clarence Street
Swindon
Wiltshire, SN1 2JF
Tel: 0793 613220

Families Need Fathers
BM Families
London, WC1N 3XX

MATCH
(Mothers Apart from Their
Children)
BM Problems
London, WC1N 1XX

Meet-a-Mum Association
(MAMA)
c/o Kate Goodyer
3 Woodside Avenue
South Norwood
London, SE25 5DW
Tel: 081 654 3137

Mothers' Union
Mary Sumner House
24 Tufton Street
London, SW1P 3RB
Tel: 071 222 5533

OPREN

Opren Action Group
Miss Kathleen Gresham
13 Carlton Close
Debenham
Norfolk
Tel: 0362 67483

OSTEOGENESIS IMPERFECTA

Brittle Bone Society
112 City Road
Dundee, DD2 2PW
Tel: 0382 67603

OSTEOPATHY

British College of Naturopathy
and Osteopathy
Frazer House
6 Netherall Gardens
London, NW3 5RR
Tel: 071 435 8728

British Osteopathic
Association
8/10 Boston Place
London, NW1 6QH
Tel: 071 262 5250/1128

General Council and Register
of Osteopaths
1–4 Suffolk Street
London, SW1Y 4HG
Tel: 071 839 2060

OSTEOPETROSIS

Research Trust for Metabolic
Diseases in Children
9 Arnold Street
Nantwich
Cheshire, CW5 5QB
Tel: 0270 626834
(24-hour service) 0270 629782

OSTEOPOROSIS

National Osteoporosis Society
PO Box 10
Barton Meade House
Radstock
Bath BA3 3YB
Tel: 0761 32472

OSTOMY CARE

Colostomy Welfare Group
38/39 Ecclestone Square
London, SW1V 1PB
Tel: 071 828 5175

Ileostomy Association of Great
Britain and Ireland
Amblehurst House
Black Scotch Lane
Mansfield
Notts NG18 4PF
Tel: 0623 28099

The Kingston Trust
The Drove
Fuzzy Drove
Basingstoke
Hants, RG22 5LU
Tel: 0256 52320

PAGET'S DISEASE

National Association for the
Relief of Paget's Disease
413 Middleton Road
Manchester, M24 4QZ
Tel: 061 643 1998

PAIN

Intractable Pain Society of
Great Britain and Ireland
Pain Relief Clinic
Basingstoke District Hospital
Aldermaston Road
Basingstoke
Hants, RG24 9NA
Tel: 0256 473202

PARENTHOOD

Association for Breastfeeding
Mothers
131 Mayow Road
London, SE26 4HZ
Tel: 081 778 4769

British Organisation of Non-
Parents (BON)
BM Box 5866
London, WC1N 3XX
Tel: 0372 52467

Cope (UK)
19–29 Woburn Place
London, WC1H OLY
Tel: 071 278 7048

Crysis
BCM Crysis
London, WC1N 3XX
Tel: 071 404 5011

Earlybirth Association
16 Warnham Rise
Hollingbury
Brighton
East Sussex, BN1 8DF
Tel: 0273 559634

FAIR (Family Action
Information and Rescue)
BCM Box 3535
PO Box 12
London, WC1N 3XX

National Childbirth Trust
Alexandra House
Oldham Terrace
London, W3 6NH
Tel: 081 992 8637

PARKINSON'S DISEASE

Parkinson's Disease Society
36 Portland Place
London, W1N 3DG
Tel: 071 323 1174

PATIENTS

Patients Association
18 Victoria Square
London, E2
Tel: 081 981 5676

PELVIC INFLAMMATION

Pelvic Inflammatory Disease
Group
Jessica Pickard
61 Jenner Road
London, N16 7RB

PENSIONERS

National Federation of
Retirement Pensions
Associations
Melling Road
91 Preston New Road
Blackburn
Lancs, BB2 6BD
Tel: 0254 52606

Pensioners Link
17 Balfe Street
London, N1 9EB
Tel: 071 278 5501/4

PERTHES DISEASE

Perthes Association
49 Great Stone Road
Northfield
Birmingham
Tel: 021 477 4415

PHOBIAS

Phobic Action
Greater London House
547/551 High Road
Leytonstone
London, E11 4PR
Tel: 081 558 6012

Phobics Society
4 Cheltenham Road
Chorlton-cum-Hardy
Manchester, M21 1QN
Tel: 061 881 1937

Phobic Trust
25a The Grove
Coulsdon
Surrey, CR3 2BH
Tel: 081 660 0332

PHYSICALLY HANDICAPPED

Physically Handicapped and
Able Bodied
Tavistock House North
Tavistock Square
London, WC1H 9HX
Tel: 071 388 1963

POLIO

British Polio Fellowship
Bell Close
West End Road
Ruislip
Middlesex, HA4 6LP

PORT WINE STAINS

Disfigurement Guidance Centre
52 Crossgate
Cupar
Fife
Scotland, KY15 5HS
Tel: 03377 281 (8 a.m.–8.30 p.m.
daily)

POSTNATAL DEPRESSION

Association for Postnatal
Depression
7 Gowan Avenue
Fulham
London, SW6 6HR
Tel: 071 731 4867

PRADER-WILLI SYNDROME

Prader-Willi Syndrome
Association (UK)
Mrs J. Williams
30 Follett Drive
Abbots Langley
Herts, WD5 0LP
Tel: 0923 674543

PRECONCEPTUAL CARE

Foresight (The Association for
the Promotion of
Preconceptual Care)
Mrs Peter Barnes
The Old Vicarage
Church Lane
Witley
Godalming
Surrey, GU8 5PN
Tel: 042879 4500

PRE-ECLAMPTIC TOXAEMIA

Pre-eclamptic Toxaemia
Society (PETS)
Dawn James
33 Keswick Avenue
Hullbridge
Essex, 3SS 6JL
Tel: 0702 231689

PREMATURE BABIES

Nippers – National
Information for Parents of
Prematures:
Education, Resources and
Support
c/o The Sam Segal Perinatal
Unit
St Mary's Hospital
Praed Street
London, W2
Tel: 071 725 6666

PREMENSTRUAL SYNDROME

National Association for
Premenstrual Syndrome
Mrs Debbie Frith
2nd Floor
25a Market Street
Guildford
Surrey, GU1 4LB
Tel: 09592 4371 (evenings)

PRE-RETIREMENT

Pre-Retirement Association of
Great Britain and Northern
Ireland
19 Undine Street
London, SW17 8PP
Tel: 081 767 3225/6

PSORIASIS

Psoriasis Association
7 Milton Street
Northampton, NN2 7JG
Tel: 0604 711129

PSYCHIATRIC REHABILITATION

Psychiatric Rehabilitation
Association
The Groupwork Centre
21a Kingsland High Street
London, E8 2JS
Tel: 071 254 9753 (24-hour
answering service)

PSYCHOTHERAPY

Clinic of Psychotherapy
26 Belsize Square
London, NW3 4HU
Tel: 081 903 6455

The Psychotherapy Centre
1 Wythburn Place
London, W1H 5WL
Tel: 071 723 6173

RADIOS AND TV FOR THE BEDRIDDEN

Wireless for the Bedridden
81b Corbets Tey Road
Upminster
Essex, RM14 2AJ
Tel: 04022 50051

RAPE

Rape Crisis Centre
PO Box 69
London, WC1X 9NJ
Tel: 071 278 3956 (office
hours)
071 837 1600 (24-hour service)

RAYNAUD'S DISEASE

Raynaud's Association Trust
40 Bladon Crescent
Alsager
Cheshire, ST7 2BG
Tel: 09363 5167

RESTRICTED GROWTH

Association for Research into
Restricted Growth
Pam Rutt   Chairman
24 Pinchfield
Maple Cross
Rickmansworth
Herts, WD3 2TP
Tel: 0923 770759

RETINITIS PIGMENTOSA

British Retinitis Pigmentosa
Society
Greens Norton Court
Greens Norton
Towcester
Northants, NN12 8BS
Tel: 0327 53276

RETIREMENT

National Confederation of
Retirement Pensions
Associations
Melling House
91 Preston New Road
Blackburn
Lancs, BB2 6BD
Tel: 0254 52606

Retired Executives Action
Clearing House (REACH)
89 Southwark Street
London, SE1 0HD
Tel: 071 928 0452

REYE'S SYNDROME

National Reye's Syndrome
Foundation
Mrs Gillian Denney
15 Nicholas Gardens
Pyrford
Woking
Surrey, GU22 8SD
Tel: 09323 46843

SAFETY

Consumer Safety Unit
Department of Trade and
Industry
10–18 Victoria Street
London SW1H 0NN
Tel: 071 215 3215

Royal Society for the
Prevention of Accidents
(RoSPA)
Cannon House
The Priory
Queensway
Birmingham B4 6BS
Tel: 021 233 2461

Child Accident Prevention
Trust
28 Portland Place
London W1N 3AL
Tel: 071 636 2545

Disabled Living Foundation
380–384 Harrow Road
London W9 2HU
Tel: 071 289 6111

SALVATION ARMY

Salvation Army
280 Mare Street
London, E8 1HE
Tel: 081 985 1181

SAMARITANS

Samaritans
17 Uxbridge Road
Slough
Berkshire, SL1 1SN
Tel: 0753 32713/4

SARCOIDOSIS

Sarcoidosis Association UK
Mrs Anita Cook
19 Ashurst Close
Blackbrook, St Helens
Merseyside, WA11 9DN
Tel: 0744 28020

SCHIZOPHRENIA

National Schizophrenia
Fellowship
78/79 Victoria Road
Surbiton
Surrey, KT6 4NS
Tel: 081 390 3651 (3 lines)

Schizophrenia Association of
Great Britain
International Schizophrenia
Centre
Bryn Hyfred
The Crescent
Bangor
Gwynedd, LL57 2AG
Tel: 0248 354048

SCLERODERMA

Maria Scleroderma Therapy
Trust
47 Freame Way
Gillingham
Dorset, SP8 4RA
Tel: 07476 4448 or 0494
783741

SCOLIOSIS

The Scoliosis Association (UK)
380–384 Harrow Road
London, W9 2HU
Tel: 071 289 5652

SEXUAL PROBLEMS

Albany Trust
24 Chester House
London, SW1W 9HS
Tel: 071 730 5871

SPOD
(Association to Aid the Sexual
and Personal Relationships of
People with a Disability)
286 Camden Road
London, N7 OBJ
Tel: 071 607 8851/2

SHELTER

Shelter
88 Old Street
London, EC1V 9AX
Tel: 071 253 0202

SHOPLIFTERS

Crisis Counselling for Alleged
Shoplifters
c/o National Consumer
Protection Council
London, NW4 4NY
Tel: 081 202 5787
081 958 8859 after 7 p.m.

SICKLE CELL ANAEMIA

Sickle Cell Information Centre
St Leonard's Hospital
Nuttall Street
London, N1 5LZ
Tel: 071 739 8484 ext. 369

Sickle Cell Society
Green Lodge
Barrets Green Road
London, NW10 7AP
Tel: 081 961 7795

SKIN CAMOUFLAGE

Disfigurement Guidance Centre
52 Crossgate
Cupar
Fife
Scotland, KY15 5HS
Tel: 03377 281 (8 a.m.–
8 p.m. daily)

SLEEP PROBLEMS

Narcolepsy Association UK
c/o Central Community Health
Council
1 St Ann's Churchyard
Manchester, M2 7LN

National Association for
Parents of Sleepless Children
PO Box 38
Prestwood
Great Missenden
Buckinghamshire, HP16 OSZ

SMOKING

Action on Smoking and Health
(ASH)
5–11 Mortimer Street
London, W1N 7RH
Tel: 071 637 9843

SOLVENT ABUSE

Re-Solv
St Mary's Chambers
19 Station Road
Stone, Morden
Surrey, SM4 5DX

SPASTICS

Association of the Parents and
Friends of Spastics
Rotary Centre for Spastics
7 Queen's Crescent
St George's Cross
Glasgow, G4 9BW
Tel: 041 332 4616

Scottish Council for Spastics
22 Corstorphine Road
Edinburgh, EH12 6PH
Tel: 031 337 9876

The Spastics Society
12 Park Crescent
London, W1N 4EQ
Tel: 071 636 5020

SPEECH IMPAIRMENT

Association for all Speech
Impaired Children
347 Central Markets
London, EC1A 9NH
Tel: 071 236 3632/6487

National Centre for Cued
Speech
29/30 Watling Street
Canterbury
Kent, CT1 2UD
Tel: 0227 450757

SPORTS

Sports Council
16 Upper Woburn Place
London, WC1H 0QP
Tel: 071 388 1277

British Sports Association for
the Disabled
Hayward House
Barnard Crescent
Aylesbury
Bucks, HP21 8PP
Tel: 0296 27889

Scottish Sports Association for
the Disabled
Glenrothes
Tel: 0592 771 700

SPINA BIFIDA

Association for Spina Bifida
and Hydrocephalus
22 Upper Woburn Place
London, WC1H 0EP
Tel: 071 388 1382 (8 lines)

Scottish Spina Bifida
Association
190 Queensferry Road
Edinburgh, EH4 2BW
Tel: 031 332 0743

SPINAL INJURIES

Scottish Spinal Cord Injury
Association
Princes House
5 Shandwick Place
Edinburgh, EH2 4RG
Tel: 031 228 3827

Spinal Injuries Association
Yeoman House
76 St James's Lane
London, N10 3DF
Tel: 081 444 2121

STEP FAMILY

Stepfamily
Ross Street Community Centre
Ross Street
Cambridge, CB1 3BS
Tel: 0223 215370

STILLBIRTHS

Stillbirth and Neonatal Death
Society (SANDS)
Argyle House
29–31 Euston Road
London, NW1 2SD
Tel: 071 833 2851

STRESS

Organisation for Parents Under
Stress
106 Godstone Road
Whyteleafe, Surrey, CR3 0EB
Tel: 081 645 0469

STROKE

Amandus Club
Atkinson Morley Hospital
Wimbledon
London, SW20 0NE
Tel: 081 946 7711 ext. 133

Chest, Heart & Stroke
Association
Tavistock House North
Tavistock Square
London, WC1H 9JE
Tel: 071 387 3012/3/4

SUDDEN INFANT DEATH SYNDROME

Foundation for the Study of
Infant Deaths
15 Belgrave Square
London, SW1X 8PS
Tel: 071 235 1721/071 235 0965

SUICIDE

The Samaritans
17 Uxbridge Road
Slough
Bucks, SL1 1SN
Tel: (0753) 32713

SYRINGOMYELIA

ANTS (Ann's Neurological
Trust Society)
Miss Ann Conroy
Jocelyn Lodge
Keythrope
Rugby
Leicester, LE7 9XJ
Tel: 053 756244

SYSTEMIC LUPUS ERYTHEMATOSIS

Lupus Group Arthritis Care
6 Grosvenor Crescent
London, SW1X 7ER
Tel: 071 235 0902/3/4/5

TAY SACHS DISEASE

Tay Sachs and Allied Diseases
Association
17 Sydney Road
Barkingside
Ilford
Essex, IG6 2ED
Tel: 081 550 8989

TEETH

British Dental Health
Foundation
88 Gurnards Avenue
Fishermead
Milton Keynes, MK6 2BL
Tel: 0908 667063

THALASSAEMIA

United Kingdom Thalassaemia
Society
107 Nightingale Lane
London, N8 7QY
Tel: 081 348 0437

TINNITUS

British Tinnitus Association
c/o 105 Gower Street
London, WC1E 6AH
Tel: 071 387 8033

TOURETTE SYNDROME

Tourette Syndrome (UK)
Association
734 High Road
Goodmayes
Ilford
Essex, IG3 8SX
Tel: 081 599 1826

TRACHEO-OESOPHAGEAL

TOFS (Tracheo-Oesophageal
Fistula Society)
Mrs Morris
124 Park Road
Chesterfield, S40 2LG
Tel: 0246 37996

TRANQUILLIZER ADDICTION

Accept Clinic
200 Seagrave Road
London, SW6 1RQ
Tel: 071 381 3155 and 2112

TRANSSEXUALS AND TRANSVESTITES

Beaumont Trust
BM Charity
London, WC1N 3XX
Tel: 071 730 7453 (7–11 p.m.)
Wives and Partners:
061 256 2521 (7–10 p.m.)

TUBERCULOSIS

Chest, Heart & Stroke
Association
Tavistock House North
Tavistock Square
London, WC1H 9JE
Tel: 071 387 3012/3/4

TUBEROUS SCLEROSIS

Tuberous Sclerosis Association
of Great Britain
Mrs Janet Medcalf
Little Barnsley Farm
Milton Road
Catshill
Bromsgrove
Worcs, B61 0NQ
Tel: 0527 71898

TURNER'S SYNDROME

Turner's Syndrome Society
Mrs Susan Bennett
c/o Child Growth Foundation
2 Mayfield Avenue
London, W4 1PW
Tel: 081 751 2555

TWINS AND MULTIPLE BIRTHS

Twins and Multiple Births
Association
41 Fortuna Way
Aylesby Park
Grimsby
South Humberside DN37 9SJ

ULCERATIVE COLITIS

National Association for
Colitis and Crohn's Disease
98a London Road
St Albans
Herts, AL1 1NX
Tel: 0727 44296

UROSTOMY

Urostomy Association
'Buckland'
Beaumont Park
Danbury
Essex, CM3 4DE
Tel: 024541 4294

VACCINE DAMAGED CHILDREN

Association of Parents of
Vaccine Damaged Children
2 Church Street
Shipston-on-Stour
Warwickshire, CV36 4AP
Tel: 0608 61595

VEGETARIANISM

Vegan Society
33–35 George Street
Oxford, OX1 2AY
Tel: 0865 722166

VICTIMS

Criminal Injuries
Compensation Board
Whittington House
19 Aldred Place
London, WC1E 7EA
Tel: 071 636 9501

WEIGHT PROBLEMS

Weight Watchers (UK) Ltd
11 Fairacres
Dedworth Road
Windsor
Berkshire, SL4 4UY
Tel: 07538 56751

WOMEN'S HEALTH

Women's Health Information
Centre
52 Featherstone Street
London, EC1Y 8RT
Tel: 071 251 6580

Women's National Cancer
Control Campaign
1 South Audley Street
London, W1Y 5DQ
Tel: 071 499 7532/4

Index

(Headings and page references in bold denote A–Z)